Sustainable Agriculture Reviews

Volume 55

Series Editor
Eric Lichtfouse
Aix-Marseille University
CNRS, IRD, INRAE, Coll France, CEREGE
Aix-en-Provence, France

Other Publications by Dr. Eric Lichtfouse

Books
Scientific Writing for Impact Factor Journals
https://www.novapublishers.com/catalog/product_info.php?products_id=42242

Environmental Chemistry
http://www.springer.com/978-3-540-22860-8

Sustainable Agriculture
Volume 1: http://www.springer.com/978-90-481-2665-1
Volume 2: http://www.springer.com/978-94-007-0393-3

Book series
Environmental Chemistry for a Sustainable World
http://www.springer.com/series/11480

Sustainable Agriculture Reviews
http://www.springer.com/series/8380

Journal
Environmental Chemistry Letters
http://www.springer.com/10311

Sustainable agriculture is a rapidly growing field aiming at producing food and energy in a sustainable way for humans and their children. Sustainable agriculture is a discipline that addresses current issues such as climate change, increasing food and fuel prices, poor-nation starvation, rich-nation obesity, water pollution, soil erosion, fertility loss, pest control, and biodiversity depletion.

Novel, environmentally-friendly solutions are proposed based on integrated knowledge from sciences as diverse as agronomy, soil science, molecular biology, chemistry, toxicology, ecology, economy, and social sciences. Indeed, sustainable agriculture decipher mechanisms of processes that occur from the molecular level to the farming system to the global level at time scales ranging from seconds to centuries. For that, scientists use the system approach that involves studying components and interactions of a whole system to address scientific, economic and social issues. In that respect, sustainable agriculture is not a classical, narrow science. Instead of solving problems using the classical painkiller approach that treats only negative impacts, sustainable agriculture treats problem sources.

Because most actual society issues are now intertwined, global, and fast-developing, sustainable agriculture will bring solutions to build a safer world. This book series gathers review articles that analyze current agricultural issues and knowledge, then propose alternative solutions. It will therefore help all scientists, decision-makers, professors, farmers and politicians who wish to build a safe agriculture, energy and food system for future generations.

More information about this series at http://www.springer.com/series/8380

Vaibhav Kumar Maurya
K. M. Gothandam • Shivendu Ranjan
Nandita Dasgupta • Eric Lichtfouse
Editors

Sustainable Agriculture Reviews 55

Micro and Nano Engineering in Food Science Vol 1

Springer

Editors
Vaibhav Kumar Maurya
Centre for Food Research and Analysis
National Institute of Food Technology
Entrepreneurship and Management
(NIFTEM)
Sonipat, Haryana, India

Shivendu Ranjan
Faculty of Engineering and the Built
Environment
University of Johannesburg
Johannesburg, South Africa

Eric Lichtfouse
Aix-Marseille University
CNRS, IRD, INRAE, Coll
France, CEREGE
Aix-en-Provence, France

K. M. Gothandam
School of Bio Sciences and Technology
Vellore Institute of Technology
Vellore, Tamil Nadu, India

Nandita Dasgupta
Department of Biotechnology
Institute of Engineering and Technology
Lucknow, Uttar Pradesh, India

ISSN 2210-4410 ISSN 2210-4429 (electronic)
Sustainable Agriculture Reviews
ISBN 978-3-030-76812-6 ISBN 978-3-030-76813-3 (eBook)
https://doi.org/10.1007/978-3-030-76813-3

This Springer imprint is published by the registered company Springer Nature Switzerland AG
The registered company address is: Gewerbestrasse 11, 6330 Cham, Switzerland

"Dedicated to the food technologists trying to enrich the food with notorious nanodelivery system"

Vaibhav, Gothandam, Shivendu,
Nandita, and Eric

Preface

Think Circular

This book is the first of several volumes on micro- and nanoengineering in food science published in the series Sustainable Agriculture Review. Food quality is crucial for health and survival of humans and other living organisms. Nanotechnology has been a time-tested tool in revolutionizing different sectors such as pharmacy, healthcare, textiles, pulp and paper, energy, transport, agriculture, and information technology. Currently, the application of nanotechnology in the food sector is in its burgeoning state across the globe. "Let food be thy medicine and medicine be thy food," although this was quoted 2500 years ago, it can be achieved in true sense, as the properties of micro-/nanoparticles can be exploited to design and develop quality food with desired functionalities such as extended shelf life; smart packaging; enhanced bioavailability of bioactive compounds; improved taste, texture, and appearance; and smart sensing of contaminants and foodborne pathogens. In particular, this book features the application of nanotechnology in food science with a significant and up-to-date review focusing on fundamental concepts, current trends, limitations, and future directions. Distinguished engineers, researchers, and technologists from renowned institutions have contributed chapters that deliver a comprehensive depiction of their particular subjects.

In its premise, the book states essential concepts of micro- and nanoengineering approaches and effective integration of other disciplines to design micro-/nanomaterials which are compatible for food application. Due to the contribution of unique chapters from leading researchers, this book has become a reference source for research scholars, teachers, scientists, and postgraduate and graduate university students, who are attracted to the field.

The first chapter, by **Sahani** et al., excellently highlights the different forms of nano- and microengineered structures that are currently being deployed in the food sector. The application of engineered nanomaterials in the food sector, their health hazards, and safety regulations for their safe use in food industries have been comprehensively addressed in Chap. 2 by **Lugani** et al. In Chap. 3, **Huerta-Jimenez**

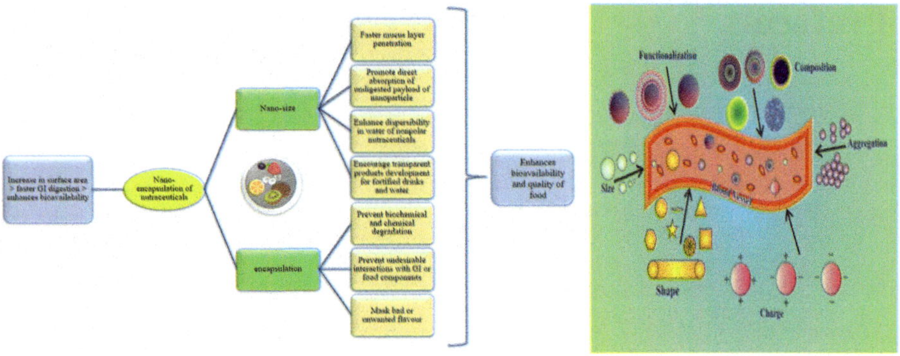

Fig. 1 Effect of nano-encapsulation of nutraceuticals on their bioavailability (Verma and Pandey from Chap. 1 and Mala et. al from Chap. 10)

et al. have discussed the application of ultrasound in micro-/nanomaterial fabrication. In Chap. 4, **Calamak** emphasizes the current know-how and approaches for the production of micro-/nanoparticles for active food compounds and application in new-generation foods along with their future progress, and **Mishra** et al. have comprehensively reviewed the encapsulation techniques adopted for herbal extract in Chap. 5. Improving bioavailability of nutrients through nanotechnology has been discussed by **Verma** and **Pandey** in Chap. 6. The application of cyclodextrins as an encapsulating wall material for bioactive food compounds has been addressed by **Kumar** and **Singhal** in Chap. 7. Bacteriophage in the food industry has been comprehensively reviewed by **Sain** and **Jayaprakash** in Chap. 8. In Chap. 9, **Tyagi** and **Bhattacharya** discuss the potential of biosensors in the food industry, while **Mala** et al. have comprehensively reviewed the pros and cons of nanomaterials as mineral supplements in poultry feed in Chap. 10 (Fig. 1).

Thanks for reading

Sonipat, Haryana, India — Vaibhav Kumar Maurya
Vellore, Tamil Nadu, India — K. M. Gothandam
Johannesburg, South Africa — Shivendu Ranjan
Lucknow, Uttar Pradesh, India — Nandita Dasgupta
Aix-en-Provence, France — Eric Lichtfouse

Contents

About the Editors

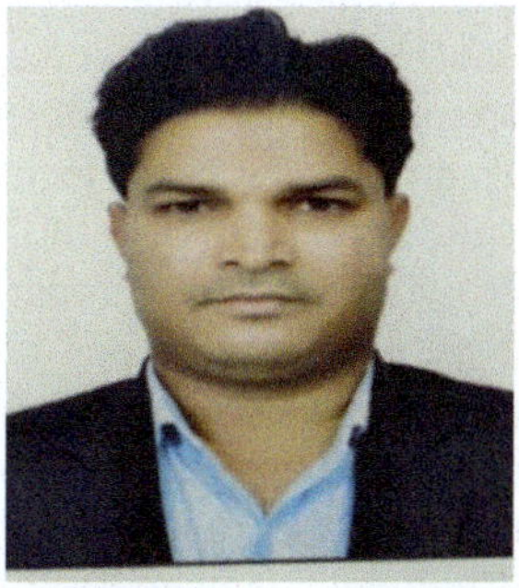

Vaibhav Kumar Maurya is currently is working as a quality analyst in the Center for Food Research & Analysis, National Institute of Food Technology Entrepreneurship and Management (Institute of National Importance under the Ministry of Food Processing Industries, Govt. of India), in Sonepat, Haryana, India. His area of research is multidisciplinary: nano-food technology; nano-agritechnology; nanobiotechnology; nano-toxicology; microencapsulation and nanodelivery system for food bioactives (vitamins, phytochemicals, and other food bioactives); analytical method development and validation for detection and quantification of pesticide, aflatoxins, plant growth regulators, veterinary drug, phytochemicals, metals, and other food bioactives using LC-MS/MS, HPLC, AAS, ICP-OES, and FTIR; thermal methods of analysis (TGA, DTA, DSC); atomic and molecular spectroscopy (UV-VIS, IR, AAS, ICP-OES); elemental analysis (flame photometry, CHNS); rheological methods (rheometry); and sound theoretical knowledge and interpretation of most analysis techniques (FTIR, TGA, DSC, Rheometer, CHNS). He has published many scientific articles in international peer-reviewed journals.

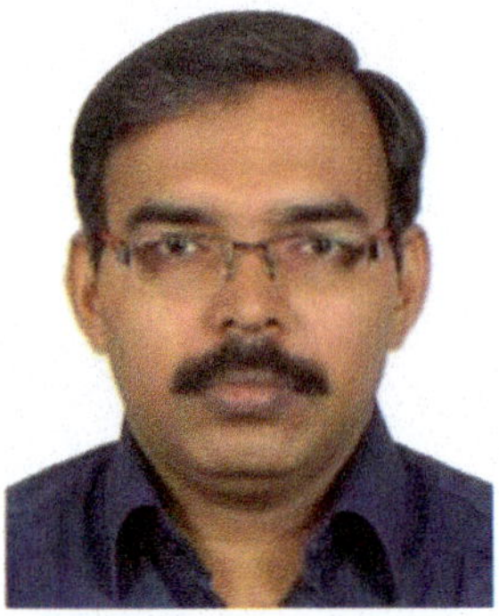

K. M. Gothandam is currently working as a professor in the School of Bio Sciences and Technology at VIT University, Vellore, Tamil Nadu, India. His main area of research is plant biotechnology and environmental biotechnology. He has published many scientific research and review articles in international peer-review journals, and also refereed for many journals with high-impact factor.

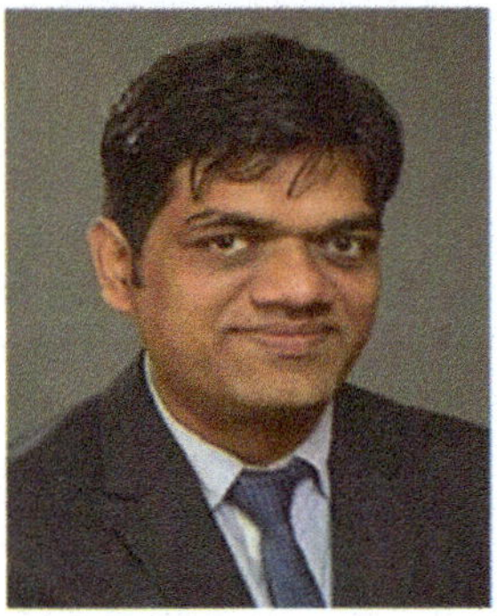

Shivendu Ranjan has completed his B.Tech. and Ph.D. in biotechnology from VIT University, Vellore, India, and has expertise in nano(bio)technology and is an elected fellow of Bose Scientific Society (FBSS). He is currently working as head of research and technology development at E-Spin Nanotech Pvt. Ltd., SIDBI Center, Indian Institute of Technology, Kanpur, India. After joining E-Spin Nanotech, IIT Kanpur, he has successfully developed prototypes for many products and three patents. He is also serving as a senior research associate (adjunct) in the Faculty of Engineering & Built Environment, University of Johannesburg, Johannesburg, South Africa. Shivendu is also guiding the Atal Innovation Centre, Bhubaneswar, Odisha, giving his technical inputs to the center. Atal Innovation Centre is part of the Atal Innovation Mission of the NITI Aayog, Govt. of India. He is also reviewer at Iran National Science Foundation (INSF), Tehran, Iran, and jury at Venture Cup, Denmark. Shivendu had founded and drafted the concept for the first edition of the "VIT Bio Summit" in 2012, and the same has been continued till date by the university. He has worked at CSIR-CFTRI, Mysuru, India, as well as Uttar Pradesh Drugs and Pharmaceutical Co. Ltd., India, and IIFPT, Thanjavur, MoFPI, Govt. of India. At IIFPT, Thanjavur, he was involved in a project funded by a leading pharmaceutical company, Dr. Reddy's Laboratories, and has successfully engineered microvehicles for model drug molecules. His research interests are multidisciplinary and include micro-/nanobiotechnology, nanotoxicology, environmental nanotechnology, nanomedicine, and nanoemulsions. He is an associate editor of *Environmental Chemistry Letters* – a Springer journal. Shivendu has published six edited books and one authored book with Springer, Switzerland. He has published many scientific articles in international peer-reviewed journals and has authored many book chapters as well as review articles. He has received several awards and recognitions from different national and international organizations.

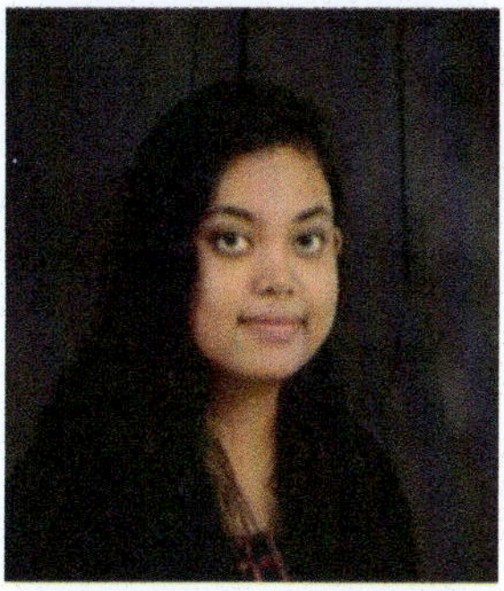

Nandita Dasgupta has completed her B.Tech. and Ph.D. from VIT University, Vellore, India, and is an Elected Fellow (FBSS) of Bose Science Society. She has major working experience in micro-/nanoscience and is currently working as assistant professor in the Department of Biotechnology, Institute of Engineering and Technology, Lucknow, India. Earlier, at LV Prasad Eye Institute, Bhubaneswar, India, she worked on mesenchymal stem cell-derived exosomes for the treatment of uveitis. She has exposure of working at university, research institutes, and industries including VIT University, Vellore, Tamil Nadu, India; CSIR-Central Food Technological Research Institute, Mysore, India; Uttar Pradesh Drugs and Pharmaceutical Co. Ltd., Lucknow, India; Indian Institute of Food Processing Technology (IIFPT), Thanjavur; and the Ministry of Food Processing Industries, Govt. of India. At IIFPT, Thanjavur, she was involved in a project funded by a leading pharmaceutical company, Dr. Reddy's Laboratories, and has successfully engineered microvehicles for model drug molecules. Her areas of interest include micro-/nanomaterial fabrication and its applications in various fields – medicine, food, environment, and biomedical agriculture. She has published 13 edited books and 1 authored book with Springer, Switzerland. Nandita is an associate editor of *Environmental Chemistry Letters* – a Springer journal with an impact factor of 4.867.

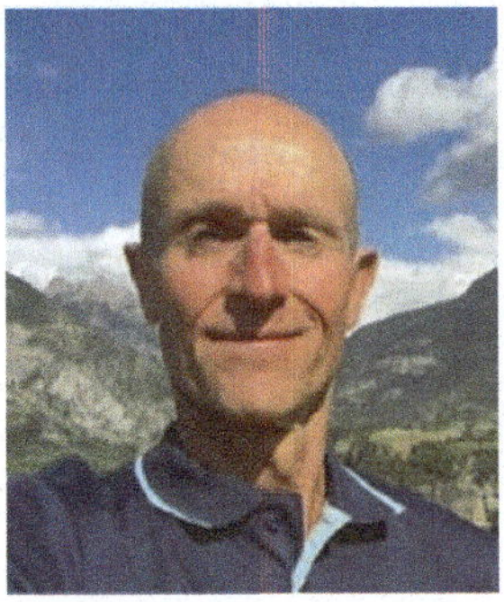

Eric Lichtfouse Ph.D., born in 1960, is an environmental chemist working at the University of Aix-Marseille, France. He has invented carbon-13 dating, a method allowing to measure the relative age and turnover of molecular organic compounds occurring in different temporal pools of any complex media. He is teaching scientific writing and communication, and has published the book *Scientific Writing for Impact Factors*, which includes a new tool – the micro-article – to identify the novelty of research results. He is founder and chief editor of scientific journals and series in environmental chemistry and agriculture. He founded the European Association of Chemistry and the Environment. Eric received the Analytical Chemistry Prize by the French Chemical Society, the Grand Prize of the Universities of Nancy and Metz, and a Journal Citation Award by the Essential Indicators. This text book describes in particular the micro-article, a new tool to identify the novelty of experimental results.

Contributors

Alma Delia Alarcon-Rojo Faculty of Animal Science and Ecology, Autonomous University of Chihuahua, Chihuahua, Chih, Mexico

Arvind Department of Dairy Science and Food Technology, Institute of Agricultural Sciences, Banaras Hindu University, Varanasi, India

Bhaswati Bhattacharya Department of Basic and Applied Sciences, National Institute of Food Technology Entrepreneurship and Management (NIFTEM), Sonipat, Haryana, India

Semih Calamak Department of Basic Pharmaceutical Sciences, Faculty of Pharmacy, Hacettepe University, Ankara, Turkey

Luis Manuel Carrillo-Lopez National Council of Science and Technology, Mexico City, Mexico
Faculty of Animal Science and Ecology, Autonomous University of Chihuahua, Chihuahua, Chih, Mexico

Ivan Adrian Garcia-Galicia Faculty of Animal Science and Ecology, Autonomous University of Chihuahua, Chihuahua, Chih, Mexico

Mariana Huerta-Jimenez National Council of Science and Technology, Mexico City, Mexico
Faculty of Animal Science and Ecology, Autonomous University of Chihuahua, Chihuahua, Chih, Mexico

N. S. Jayaprakash Centre for Bioseparation Technology, Vellore Institute of Technology, Vellore, Tamil Nadu, India

Ravichandran Keerthana Department of Biotechnology, Mepco Schlenk Engineering College, Sivakasi, Tamil Nadu, India

Yogesh Kumar Department of Food Science and Technology, National Institute of Food Technology Entrepreneurship and Management, Sonipat, Haryana, India

Yogita Lugani Department of Biotechnology, Punjabi University, Patiala, Punjab, India

Rajendran Mala Department of Biotechnology, Mepco Schlenk Engineering College, Sivakasi, Tamil Nadu, India

Sadhna Mishra Centre of Food Science and Technology, Institute of Agriculture Science (Banaras Hindu University), Varanasi, India

Preetha Mohan Department of Biotechnology, Mepco Schlenk Engineering College, Sivakasi, Tamil Nadu, India

Simmi Oberoi Department of Community Medicine, Government Medical College, Patiala, India

Vijayeta Pal School of Materials Science and Technology, Indian Institute of Technology, Banaras Hindu University, Varanasi, Uttar Pradesh, India

Anand Kumar Pandey Department of Biotechnology Engineering, Institute of Engineering and Technology, Bundelkhand University, Jhansi, India

Gurdeep Rattu Basic and Applied Science, National Institute of Food Technology Entrepreneurship and Management (NIFTEM), Kundli, Haryana, India

Shalini Sahani Department of Material Science and Engineering, Gachon University, Seongnam, South Korea

Avtar Sain Centre for Bioseparation Technology, Vellore Institute of Technology, Vellore, Tamil Nadu, India

Yogesh Chandra Sharma Department of Chemistry, Indian Institute of Technology (Banaras Hindu University), Varanasi, India

Somya Singhal Department of Food Engineering and Technology, Tezpur University, Tezpur, Assam, India

Varee Tyagi Department of Basic and Applied Sciences, National Institute of Food Technology Entrepreneurship and Management (NIFTEM), Sonipat, Haryana, India

Shalja Verma Department of Biochemical Engineering and Biotechnology, Indian Institute of Technology, New Delhi, India

Chapter 1
Micro and Nanoengineered Structures in Food Sector

Shalini Sahani, Sadhna Mishra, and Yogesh Chandra Sharma

Abstract The drastic population explosion has enhanced the demand of food supply in large quantity. This has pressurized the manufacturing units involved in agriculture sector to accelerate its working efficiency for maximum food production using minimum raw materials so that mass across the globe can be served in economical way. In this direction, Nanotechnology has given a new perspective to food sector to provide good quality and healthy food to people out there at reasonable cost. Currently, the application of nanotechnology in the food sector is in its burgeoning state across the globe. Nanotechnology in food engineering has stressed on the characterization, fabrication, and manipulation of nanostructures or nanomaterials synthesized from naturally occurring precursors. Microengineering develops micro-level food processes which are used in nanotechnology for analytical analyses. This offers less sample volume along with more sensitive detection capacity and reduced process cost by decreasing the quantity of required reagents. Nanotechnology finds several applications in food industry such as nanodevices or nanosensors, nanoencapsulation, anticaking agent, nanoadditives, neutraceuticals, nano-packaging, edible nanocoatings, and gelating agents used in food processing and food packaging. The nanostructures utilized in food science have improved the taste, texture and persistence or durability of food ingredients. Recently many nanostructures are explored in food industry such as biopolymeric particles, liposomes, emulsions, composites, inorganic particles, and hydrogels. These nano and micro structures improve the solubility of food ingredients in vivo, along with enhance-

S. Sahani (✉)
Department of Material Science and Engineering, Gachon University, Seongnam, South Korea

S. Mishra
Centre of Food Science and Technology, Institute of Agriculture Science (Banaras Hindu University), Varanasi, India

Y. C. Sharma
Department of Chemistry, Indian Institute of Technology (Banaras Hindu University), Varanasi, India
e-mail: ysharma.apc@iitbhu.ac.in

V. K. Maurya et al. (eds.), *Sustainable Agriculture Reviews 55*, Sustainable Agriculture Reviews 55, https://doi.org/10.1007/978-3-030-76813-3_1

ment in bioavailability and controlled release. This chapter highlights the different forms of nano and micro engineered structures which are currently being deployed in food nanotechnology to tune the characteristics of conventional food and their applications. Additionally, a critical overview on recent shortcomings associated to nanotechnology in food science along with detailed future perspective is also highlighted later. Since very few reports are found which provide the sound knowledge regarding nanostructures used in food sector, so this study is especially a very detailed description about recent advancements in the application of different nanomaterials as food additives and packaging stuffs.

Keywords Nanotechnology · Microengineering · Nanoencapsulation · Nanocoatings · Anticaking agent

1.1 Introduction

In the era of population explosion, Food and Agricultural Organization (FAO), a branch of the United Nations has estimated that global population would be achieving the par of 9 billion by 2050 which certainly will cause the shocking 70% increment in food demand till then. The increasing demand for good quality and healthy food are compelling the research fraternity to explore the pathways to improve the food quality with least alteration of the nutritional content of the food product. But these changes might be also having a negative impact on the actual nature of biological samples by deteriorating it (Fu et al. 2014; Dasgupta et al. 2015). However, nanotechnology in food chemistry has improved food processes that use enzymes which are used to hydrolyze to anti-nutritive ingredients and increase the bioavailability of essential food nutrients, minerals and vitamins. Nanotechnology results in the excellent encapsulation and faster delivery rate of the bioactive food ingredients compared to the conventional encapsulating agents. Additionally, nanotechnology has developed many novel and innovative techniques in the food industry and also in the biomedical and pharmaceutical industry. The inception of nanotechnology amazed the whole universe with several new possible adventures in food science and technology (Singh et al. 2017a, b). Gradually this became the boon to food industry with some astonishing applications to mock of improved taste, flavor, color, texture, durability of foodstuffs, excellent absorption of bioactive materials, abundant availability of nutraceuticals, supplements for vital bioelements, food antimicrobials, long-lasting food packaging materials with improved mechanical strength and antimicrobial properties, nano-sensors for traceability of health hazards, bionano-sensors to check food quality during transport and storage along with encapsulation or coating of food components or additives (Jafari and McClements 2017; Sharma et al. 2020; Bajpai et al. 2019; Shukla et al. 2019; Srivastava et al. 2018). The word "nano" is sourced from the Greek language and it means 'dwarf'. The ideology regarding nanotechnology was laid down by Richard

Feynman in the year of 1959; however, later Norio Taniguchi coined 'nanotechnology' in 1974 (Hulla et al. 2015). A nanostructure object finds an intermediate size between nano and micro range that can be processed into various other forms. There is no wonder that very soon nanotechnology would change the entire concept of conventional ways of research and development in food science by engineering biological molecules for several applications in the food sector. Interestingly, day by day new set of changes is getting incorporated into food items giving us novel characteristics in food materials (Gupta et al. 2016). Nanotechnology in food engineering has given a lot of attention on the fabrication and characterization of nanostructures synthesized from naturally occurring precursors. Nanotechnology has evolved many methodologies to fabricate these nano-materials. A nanomaterial finds its intermediate size between 1-1000 nm that can be processed into other forms (Singh et al. 2017a, b). Further, it is "structured" to microlevel by using soft/hard templates. Nanostructured materials have at least one dimension in nanometer in form of nanoparticles, nanorods, nanowires, thin films with nanoscale thickness, and bulk materials with nanoscale building blocks (Pathakoti et al. 2017). According to the dimensional features, nanoengineering materials are categorized into zero-dimensional as nanoparticles, nanoclusters, quantum dots, and fullerenes; one-dimensional as nanowires, nanorods or nanotubes; two-dimensional as nano-thin films or membranes; three-dimensional as nanocomposites and dendrimers (Pathakoti et al. 2017; Das et al. 2019). As the unique properties of nanostructures such as physical, chemical, and biological properties are significantly different than their macro-material counterparts, they have changed the entire chemistry and comprehension of biological and physicochemical properties of food. The significance of nanotechnology in food science apprehends its role in the quality improvement of food materials as it alters the texture, appearance, taste, nutritional value, life in a positive way so that it could fulfill the requirement as food supplements providing them novel qualities. Nanotechnology has also tremendous benefits for food packaging using biodegradable biopolymers, which show multiple merits i.e. mechanical strength and heat-resistant properties. Since nanotechnology has excellent potential to produce innovative and novel products in the food sector, it can overcome so many challenges in food science and technology such as the production of edible nano-carriers developed by economically viable methods for mass consumption.

This study presents the various kinds of nanostructures used in the current food sector and their manufacturing techniques along with their impact on food quality in food science and later their negative influences are also thoroughly discussed.

1.2 Nano- and Microstructured Materials in Food

Nanotechnology used in food chemistry has been influencing the vital aspects of food industry right from the synthesis of new edible food products and food-sensors to their storage (Singh et al. 2017a, b). Recently many nanostructures are explored in food industry such as biopolymeric particles, liposomes, emulsions, composites, inorganic particles, and hydrogels. These nanostructures improve solubility, bioavailability, selective and controlled release along with protection of bioactive components during food processing (Jafari and McClements 2017; Maurya and Aggarwal 2017).

1.3 Biopolymeric Particles

Inceptively, biopolymer nanoparticles were made up of albumin and non-biodegradable polyacrylamide and poly (methylacrylate) (Kumar et al. 2018). But very soon risk of chronic toxicity as a result of overloading of non-degradable polymers e.g. polyacrylamide and poly methylacrylate) nanoparticles was realized and limitation on their use was imposed (Verma et al. 2020). Consequently, synthetic biodegradable polymers received tremendous attention in food processing. There are some synthetic biodegradable polymers such as polyalkylcyanoacrylate, poly (lactic-co-glycolic acid) and polyanhydride are used in food processing and food sensing (Verma et al. 2020). There were some shortcomings reported with above-mentioned biopolymer compounds due to their hydrophobicity which led to the inappropriate encapsulation of therapeutic bioactives such as nucleic acid, peptides, and proteins with hydrophilic nature (Rostamabadi et al. 2019). Additionally, the toxicity level of synthetic biopolymer is also found very much considerable for their application in the food sector. Therefore hydrophilic biopolymer compounds have been explored at large scale.

Polysaccharide-based nanoparticles improve the biocompatibility of cell toxic materials which together with new immobilization technique can be easily ejected out of the body. Currently, the development in novel bionanoparticle-derived pharmaceutical formulations has designed nanoparticles from naturally occurring polysaccharides for the in vivo administration of vital components such as nucleic acids (Khalid et al. 2020).

The following schematic diagram in Fig. 1.1 depicts the varieties of edible biopolymers used in food industry currently.

1.3.1 Preparation Methodologies

Protein and polysaccharide-based nanoparticles can be prepared by several methods; emulsification, desolvation and electrospray drying technique (Shishir et al. 2018; Maurya et al. 2020a, b).

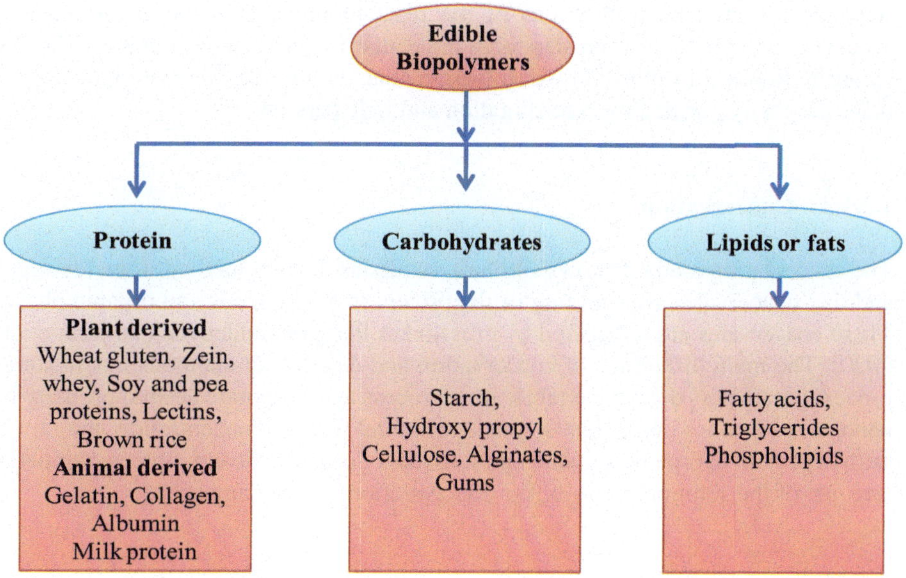

Fig. 1.1 A schematic representation of various edible biopolymers which are applied in food chemistry as novel nano and micro-structures

1.3.1.1 Emulsification

Nano-emulsion formation is processed by spontaneous emulsification on mixing an aqueous and organic phase. The organic phase consists of oil, lipophilic surfactant and water-miscible solvent whereas aqueous phase consists of hydrophilic surfactant and water (Kale and Deore 2017). This technique involves the emulsification of an organic solvent with an aqueous solution at high agitation resulting in the formation of nanoparticles in 50–100 nm followed by the dissolution of hydrophobic material. Afterwards, the organic solvent is evaporated resulting in stable dispersion of nano-particles. A major shortcoming of this method is the requirement of organic solvent because residues of organic solvent might be toxic for its biological application (Maurya et al. 2020b).

1.3.1.2 Desolvation

Desolvation is basically for the fabrication of nanoparticles which involves sluggish addition of natural salts or alcohol as a desolvation factor, to the biopolymeric solution (Turasan et al. 2020). The desolvation factor affects the physical structure of the protein. There is the formation of protein clump after the critical level of desolvation, later it reacts with a chemical substance (glutaraldehyde) via cross-linking resulting in the formation of nanoparticles. The two-step desolvation process was initially developed for the synthesis of gelatin nanoparticles. In the first desolvation step, the low molecular fractions of the reaction mixture in the supernatant is decanted, while in the second step, high molecular fractions present in the sediment are again dissolved followed by desolvation at acidic pH. Later, resulting nanoparticles are easily purified by centrifugation and redispersion.

1.3.1.3 Coacervation

The coacervation method shows similarity with desolvation method. It yields small and tiny coacervates after mixing of the protein in the aqueous and organic phase. These coacervates are connected by crosslinker like glutaraldehyde (Turasan et al. 2020). The main difference of coacervation and desolvation methods lies in some process parameters during the fabrication process to incorporate desired property in nanoparticles. These parameters consist of initial protein concentration, the molar ratio of protein to organic solvent, addition rate of organic solvent, process temperature, pH of the solution, cross-linker concentration, and stirring speed.

1.3.1.4 Electrospray Drying

This method generates relatively mono-disperse and bioactive protein nanoparticles. Electrospray drying method starts with the preparation of protein solution by dissolving the dry powder in an electro-sprayable solution (Maurya et al. 2020a). Later the dispersion of the solution followed by solvent evaporation produces dry residues of particles in desired structure and size spread on substrates. Insulin nanoparticles sized in 88–110 nm were synthesized using this method (Turasan et al. 2020). Here biological activity of the electrosprayed protein-based NPs is not disturbed by the process conditions.

1.4 Liposomes

Complete nutrition provides bioactive compounds with several benefits to health in a positive way. Nanoliposome has shown exciting opportunities for the food sector in encapsulation and controlled release of food materials, bioavailability, stability, higher durability. Nanoliposomes provide the controlled and specific delivery of nutraceuticals, nutrients, enzymes, vitamins, antimicrobials, and additives (Liu et al. 2015; Maurya et al. 2020b). Liposomes have been a suitable carrier for a wide variety of substances to biological, biochemical, pharmacological, and agricultural targets. The proteoliposomes are known as liposomes incorporating one or more proteins. Typically, liposomes are known as spherulites due to their basic spherical shape. It consists of either a single layer or multiple layers of amphiphilic shells. Liposomes with single bilayer shell are called as small unilamellar vesicles (less than 30 nm) or large unilamellar vesicles (30–100 nm), respectively (Khorasani et al. 2018; Maurya et al. 2020a). Nanoliposome application in food industry has offered thrilling and exotic characteristics for the protection of fragile and delicate food components. Furthermore, improved efficacy of nanoliposomes has also fastened the manufacturing of some foodstuffs, like cheese and other secondary food products. Ghorbanzade et al. (2017) reported liposome-encapsulated fish oil to fortify yogurt effectively and found the combination was more efficacious than fish oil alone. Khosravi-Darani et al. (2016) noticed a considerable increment in antimicrobial activity of Zataria multiflora essential oil encapsulated in liposomes. These few very important examples suggest the potential application of nanoliposome in food and pharmaceutical sector.

1.4.1 Preparation Methods

The selection of preparatory methods relies on the physicochemical properties of entrapping solutes and liposomes, the nature of the dispersion medium, the concentration of the entrapped solutes, potential toxicity, and efficient delivery of the vesicles (Khorasani et al. 2018). The conventional method involves evaporation of solvent from the phospholipid solution of stabilizing agent and material to be encapsulated. After adding hydrophilic material and supplying of threshold energy, the formation of multilamellar vesicles (MLVs) takes place. The conventional methods such as extrusion, sonification, and microfluidizer have been employed in nanoliposome production at large scales. In extrusion methodology, the pore-size of the filters applied in system regulates the structural modification to large unilamellar vesicles (LUV) of nanoliposomes using very high pressure (Wang et al. 2016). Sonification method is commonly used protocol for nanoliposome synthesis. Both probe sonification and bath sonification are used in nanoliposome synthesis (Veneti et al. 2016). This technique consists some flaws i.e. very low internal volume/encapsulation efficiency, entrapment of large molecule, and metal leaching from probe material. In sonification method, there are several process parameters such as temperature, sonication time, sample volume, sonicator tuning, and lipid composition (or concentration) which actually govern the mean pore size of vesicle and polydispersity index of vesicles. Next, microfluidizer being an energy intensive method employs a microfluidizer with no use of toxic solvents (diethyl ether and chloroform) but utilizes the high pressures (up to 12,000 psi) to direct the flow stream through microchannels resulting in cavitation with shear which impacts inside the interaction chamber and reduces particles size forming nanoliposomes at the end.

There are some other techniques to prepare nanoliposomes such as the reverse-phase evaporation technique, ether injection technique, freeze-thaw method, and rapid solvent-exchange method. In the food sector, liposomes and nanoliposomes are needed to be prepared on a large scale (Khorasani et al. 2018). But it is equally important for them to meet health standards. This owes to the fact that all conventional methods for liposome production incorporate the application of various nonfood-grade toxic chemicals and making the use of liposome troublesome in the food industry for in vivo application (Panahi et al. 2017; Maurya et al. 2020b). Furthermore, higher sheer forces or high pressure can potentially alter the physicochemical properties of nanoliposomes which is not desirable at all for its in vivo application. Hence alternative methodologies should have been explored such as Mozafari method, a thermal treatment-based technique where nanoliposomes can be synthesized using a single apparatus without using any toxic chemical and high shear forces (Panahi et al. 2017).

1.5 Emulsions

Nano-emulsions are a colloidal suspension of 50 nm to 1000 nm. They are utilized for varieties of purposes such as flavour additives to food ingredients and beverages as taste enhancers, food décor and fortification (Vala et al. 2017; Maurya and Aggarwal 2019a, b). Emulsions furnish various positive characteristic as it does not compromise with physicochemical nature and flavour of food ingredient. These self-assembled nano-emulsions execute the delivery of essential vitamins, steroids, minerals, antioxidants and other functional components in vivo. Nano-emulsions are uniformly distributed colloidal phase comprising of an oil phase distributed in an aqueous phase. Here, each drop of oil is circled by emulsifying molecules forming an interface layer with a particle size of 50–500 nm (Ingale and Chaudhari 2018). There are two types of nano-emulsions depending on kind of phases taken: oil/water or water/oil. Nonetheless, oil/water-based nano-emulsions are given more priority as they can be used to prepare edible coatings by incorporating various lipophilic materials bound in a hydrophilic polymeric matrix (Pramanik and Pramanik 2016). Various lipophilic substances are reported for the preparation of nano-emulsions such as essential oils derived from plants, fatty acids, carotenoids, antioxidants, phytosterols, and quinines (Pisoschi et al. 2018). There are varieties of plant-derived lipophilic materials used in the formation of nanoemulsions including antioxidants, fatty acids, phytosterols, essential oils and quinones (Salvia-Trujillo et al. 2017). Since nano-emulsions are found to be thermodynamically unstable owing to aggregation, coalescence, flocculation, Oswald's maturation, and gravitational forces over the period (de Oca-Ávalos et al. 2017), these nano-emulsions are stabilized by the addition of natural biopolymers for their application as a potential delivery system (Maurya and Aggarwal 2017).

1.5.1 Preparation of Nano-Emulsions

Nano-emulsion generally comprises an aqueous phase, an oil phase and an emulsifying agent (Gupta et al. 2016). An emulsifier decreases the interfacial tension between the oil and aqueous phases facilitating emulsions. Moreover, emulsifiers also stabilize of nano-emulsions. The physicochemical properties of nano-emulsions depend upon the nature of all three above mentioned components. Usually, O/W based nano-emulsion has got more application as it has a core-shell-type structure where the shell is made up of amphiphilic material or surfactant surrounds the core of lipophilic material.

1.5.1.1 Oil Phase

The oil phase in food-grade nano-emulsions is usually derived from nonpolar molecules, such as an ester of fatty acids or triglycerides (TG), waxes, mineral oils and other lipophilic bioactive compounds. The triglycerides are mainly extracted from either vegetable oil or animal fats. The physicochemical characteristics of the oil phase govern the properties of prepared nano-emulsion accordingly.

1.5.1.2 Aqueous Phase

Similarly, the aqueous phase in food-grade nano-emulsions is derived from polar molecules such as carbohydrates, proteins, acids, minerals or alcohols with water. Like the oil phase, the choice of the aqueous phase strongly affects the physicochemical properties of the produced nano-emulsion.

1.5.1.3 Stabilizers

Stabilizers are used to stabilize the NPs in emulsion and it regulates the nano-emulsion formation to a great extent (Gupta et al. 2016). Various amphiphilic compounds are used as emulsifier such as proteins, phospholipids, surfactants, and polysaccharides. There are varieties of stabilizers compounds categorized as emulsifiers, ripening retarders, texture modifiers and weighting agents in nano-emulsion formation. However, emulsifiers are highly applicable stabilizers for the production of nano-emulsions (Gupta et al. 2016).

1.5.2 Production of Nano-emulsions

Nano-emulsion is a high energy or non-equilibrium system which is formed by supplying external energy driving forces as its formation disturbs the equilibrium from a stable energy state (Pisoschi et al. 2018). Nano-emulsions can be formulated by two broad energy required methodologies including high and low energy supplements. The operating conditions used in above mentioned both techniques impact the size and composition of emulsion particles. In high energy technique for nano-emulsion formation, energy supplying devices apply the highly energized disruptive forces and allow the extensive mixing with simultaneous addition of surfactant

(5–10%). This leads to the formation of tiny droplets with a specific size of nano-emulsions. While in low energy approaches, the formation of tiny oil droplets in triphasic systems depends on environmental temperature and composition affecting the size of the formed drops in nano-emulsions (Pisoschi et al. 2018).

1.5.2.1 High-Energy Emulsification Methods

Several mechanical devices are employed in the high-energy approach for the production of tiny droplets of emulsion. These mechanical devices are high-pressure valve homogenizers, microfluidizers, ultrasound homogenizer, and other high-speed devices (Charcosset 2016). The major concerns related to nanoemulsion production through high energy approach lie in its toxic additives such as synthetic surfactants, polymers, oils and harmful organic solvents assimilated during synthesis. This problem can be tackled out by using food grade agents e.g. flavoured oil, triglyceride oil, proteins, lipids, and polysaccharides which are ethically acceptable for food application and economically viable for further lab to land scaling. Moreover, synthesis routes with low energy approach are not still widely in vogue for nano-emulsion production while high energy synthesis routes are widely implemented for nano-emulsion production at commercial level which is not desirable from economic point of view (Maurya and Aggarwal 2019b). Therefore, low energy approach must be investigated for their viability for nano-emulsion production at industrial scale. Additionally, the fate of a very small emulsion droplet having nano size in vivo is not properly studied so there may be some scope of potential toxicity because properties of emulsion differ at the nanoscale from the bulk state. That's why the application of nano-emulsion in food industry should be verified for its extent of toxicity in vivo.

1.5.2.2 Low-Energy Emulsification Methods

The low-energy methods utilize the internal chemical energy constituting the system. The formation of nano-emulsions takes place via phase transitions owing to the fluctuation either in the temperature or compositions of constituents. The composition of the system, water/stabilizer/oil ratio, nature of aqueous phase, an oil phase, and stabilizer with their ionic strength, temperature, time, and agitation rate decide the size of a droplet in emulsion (Dasgupta et al. 2016). There are several low energy methods such as membrane emulsification method, spontaneous emulsification method, solvent displacement, phase inversion temperature method, phase inversion composition method, and emulsion inversion point method. Remarkably, low-energy intensive methods are known to generate smaller droplets than high-energy approaches but low-energy approaches are limited to only specific oils and emulsifiers. Here, in low energy methods, proteins or polysaccharides cannot be used as stabilizing agents and high surfactant dose is also needed to form nano-emulsions. Such limitations make the use of low energy methods least applicable in food chemistry (Karthik et al. 2017). There are several applications of nanoemulsions in very important aspects of the food sector. These nanoemulsions are employed for encapsulation of lipophilic components, to improve drug bioavailability and pharmacological effects, to improve digestibility characters of food ingredients (Maurya and Aggarwal 2019a. b).

1.6 Composites

Nanocomposites materials have proved themselves as potential alternatives in food packaging because of their functionality and low cost (Sharma et al. 2017). Nanocomposites are polymer matrices incorporated by inorganic or organic nanofillers with particular geometries (fibres, flakes, spheres, whiskers, sheets, and fibres) having any of their three dimensions in nano range (Sharma et al. 2017; Bratovcic et al. 2015). There are several nanofillers explored so far i.e. clays, metal oxides, carbon nanotubes, and cellulose fibrils of nano dimension (Sharma et al. 2017). Several synthetic polymers along with natural polymers have been used in food packaging for decades. However, being concerned about environmental impacts, biodegradable and natural biopolymers are focused at large scale. Several biodegradable synthetic polymers such as polyvinyl alcohol, polylactide, and polyglycolic acid are now in vogue for nanocomposites formation. The aspect ratio of filler materials is defined as the ratio of the largest to the smallest dimension of filler material. This plays a crucial role in the formation of the composite. The filler material with the highest aspect ratio acquires higher surface area which further corresponds to higher values of reinforcing properties. Infact, nanobiocomposite consisting biopolyesters exhibits enhanced gas, vapour and UV barrier which further manifest controlled release of bioactives and efficiency of food preservatives derived from natural plant extract having antimicrobial and antioxidant properties for food bio-packaging applications. Especially, bio-nanocomposite made up of either matrix or reinforcement or both derived from natural resources which are biodegradable, can be tempting candidate for nanocomposites in food sector. Infact, various bio-hybrid nanocomposites have been found with desirable functional and structural properties alongwith higher extent of biodegradability and bioavailability.

1.6.1 Types of Nanofillers

1.6.1.1 Clay and Silicate Nano-platelets

Clay and silicates, as nano-fillers have gained tremendous attention attributing to their wide availability. The clay and silicate nano-platelets with thickness in nanorange are found the best candidate as nano-fillers. So, silicates combined with polymers execute magnificent barrier properties. This provides the diffusive path for an infiltrate resulting in intercalated or exfoliated nanocomposites. Montmorillonite clay is extensively used nano component along with various types of polymer matrices (polyethene, nylon, polyvinyl chloride, etc.) in nanocomposites formation (Sharma et al. 2017). Nonetheless, the application of synthetic polymers matrix causes in vivo application of nanocomposites troublesome but bio-nanocomposite solves the aforementioned issue of potential toxicity. Natural clay reinforced in biopolymers matrices resolves the problem of potential toxicity in vivo and other environmental issues (Sharma et al. 2017).

1.6.1.2 Cellulose

Cellulose is a highly strong natural polymer. Cellulosic materials are abundantly available in nature and environment friendly. Cellulose nanofibers provide higher surface area and enhance the nanoparticle activity. These additional characteristics enable the cellulose derived nanocomponents more attractive materials for nano-composites assembly (Benítez and Walther 2017). Generally, there are two general types of reinforcements derived from cellulose i.e. microfibrils and whiskers. The microfibrils (or nanofibers) chains of cellulose are intercalated with hydrogen bonds where each microfibril is composed of crystalline and amorphous elementary fibril. Furthermore, the extracted crystalline part of fibrils separated by acid hydrolysis is coined as whiskers or nanocrystals. Recently, cellulose nanofibers-banana starch based nanocomposite has been found an efficient value-added food packaging system from waste raw materials (Tibolla et al. 2019). Duan et al. (2018) explored Ag nanoparticles anchored on cellulose nanofibrils composite with superior antibacterial activity in food packaging.

1.6.1.3 Carbon Nanotubes

Carbon nanotubes are subdivided into two major classes; single-wall nanotube or multiwalled nanotubes (Yola and Atar 2019). The single-walled nanotube has a cylindrical shape with a thickness of one carbon atom and multiwalled nanotube is identified as a flock of concentric tubes. These carbon tubes with very high aspect ratios and elastic modulus exhibit excellent tensile strength. Carbon nanotubes are also known to exhibit antimicrobial property. The carbon nanotubes have been extensively incorporated into packaging system due to their enormous strength. Moreover, carbon nanotube also acts as detector for micro-organisms, toxic proteins and food spoilage system. A nanocomposite material consisting allyl isothiocyanate and carbon nanotubes manifested an excellent preservation of shredded cooked chicken meat for 40 days with least alteration in physicochemical characteristics of shredded cooked chicken meat (King et al. 2018).

1.6.1.4 Starch

Starch based nanocomposites have also been extensively exploited over decades in food packaging applications owing to their abundance, biocompatibility, non-toxicity, low cost, biodegradability, and stability in air (El Achaby et al. 2017). In fact, starch is the most abundant biomass-derived material. This also ensures the biocompatibility of starch based nanocomposites. Starch nanocrystals or nanoparticles are successfully tested and found very much suitable for their food applications as potential stabilizers in nanoemulsions and delivery system for bioactive compounds (Campelo et al. 2020). Starch nanoparticles are also observed to improve the mechanical and barrier properties of biopolymer films extracted from plants.

1.6.1.5 Chitosan

Chitosan, a popular heteropolysaccharide is known for its biocompatibility and metal complexation tendency (Divya and Jisha 2018). The polycationic nature of chitosan is responsible for its antimicrobial activity (Ahmed and Aljaeid 2016). The following schematic diagram in Fig. 1.2 depicts the different methodologies to prepare nanocomposites incorporating different structural and functional properties.

Several nanocomposites materials have been observed to exhibit excellent antimicrobial properties, oxygen scavenging ability, enzyme immobilization, and sensing for temperature or oxygen level which make them ideal nano-packaging system but obstacles still remain unsolved regarding perfect compatibility between matrix and filler to provide complete dispersion of nanoparticles. The compatibility issue between the duos must be thoroughly explored before in vivo application.

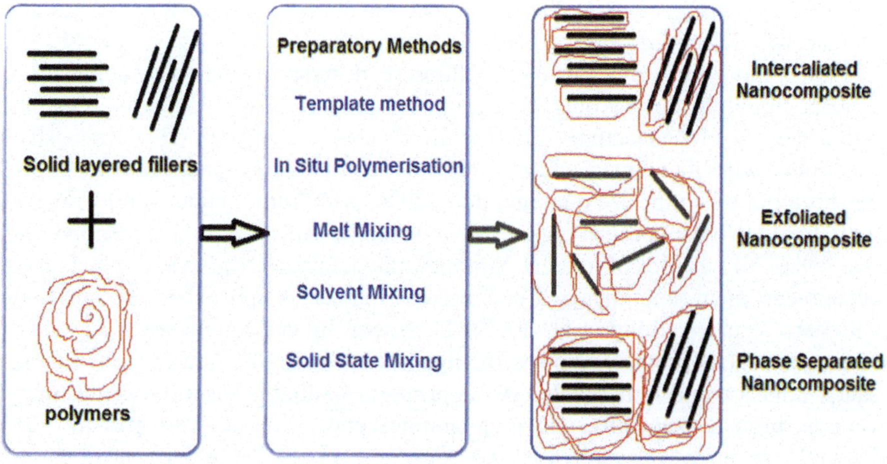

Fig. 1.2 A schematic representation of nanocomposites formation through various synthetic routes

1.7 Inorganic Particles

Various metals and metal oxide-based nanoparticles have been utilized either in coating or packaging of food materials (dos Santos et al. 2020; Kalpana and Rajeswari 2017). The active metal either directly reacts with food components or performs an individual task of antimicrobial activity. The possible phenomenon happening in antimicrobial action might be the direct contact with the microbial cell body and further rupturing cell envelope and electron transfer; oxidizing cell components; formation of secondary reaction species which ultimately destroy the microbial cell. Amongst the all-metal nano-particles, silver nano-particles are the most phenomenal nano-particles due to their effective antimicrobial activity against several pathogens for examples virus, bacteria, and fungi. Silver nanoparticles disrupt the cell functions through direct binding with vital components of cell. Secondly, different structural forms of TiO_2 have been considered for its antibacterial properties (Periasamy et al. 2015). Its well-known antibacterial capacity is confined with UV irradiation. Moreover, the biocidal activity of TiO_2 is regarded to its initial oxidative attack on the cell membrane by hydroxyl radicals modifying the Coenzyme A-dependent enzyme activity and DNA damage. Gold nanoparticles are probably the most investigated and reported ones in the literature with few examples currently in clinical trials for rheumatoid arthritis and cancer therapy. Additionally, varieties of metal oxides like SiO_2, ZnO, MgO, and others are used in the formation of nanocomposites. Inorganic nanoparticles such as MgO, ZnO and CaO have also reflected anti-microorganism activity towards pathogen control (Oun and Rhim 2017). Recently, the biocompatibility of calcium phosphate or hydroxyapatite has also been leveraged in the food sector as nano-fillers. As calcium phosphate is soluble in an acidic medium as it can be utilized for transportation of therapeutics in the body without any sort of accumulation. Bimetallic iron and copper nanoparticles are detected to exhibit synergistically enhanced activity for the inactivation of *E. coli* and MS2 coliphage, compared to single-metal nanoparticles i.e. Fe-nanoparticles or Cu- nanoparticles (Kim et al. 2019).

Now a day's quantum dots (QDs), fluorescent nano-crystals have achieved significant limelight due to outstanding optical properties with superior sensitivity, photostability, high selectivity and resolution (Song et al. 2015). They can easily be functionalized with anticancer drugs and other compounds of interest. A lot of effort has been put to synthesize quantum dots (QDs) with higher photoactivity and least toxicity in UV-NIR spectral region so that it can be utilized for the faster and selective release of analytes of interest. Similarly, lanthanides are also found to deal with such issues when functionalized with organic ligands as they exhibit excellent optical characteristics (Song et al. 2015). The metal-ligand complexes are a class of rare-earth metals protected by organic ligands exhibiting luminescence with a very sharp emission and remarkable optical properties suitable for bioimaging (upconversion, high Stokes-shift, and long luminescence lifetime) (Song et al. 2015). Recently, extensive research is driven onto chemical modification of metal core with ligands to improve the quantum yield.

1.7.1 Preparation Methods

There are two preferential methods for the production of inorganic nanoparticles i.e. top-down and bottom-up approaches (Pathakoti et al. 2017). The top-down synthesis route breaks macro-sized bulk materials to nano-scale using various means of degradation. There are varieties of nanostructure's preparation techniques in the top-down method such as ball milling, high-pressure homogenization, microfluidization, and ultrasound emulsification (Robles-García et al. 2016). Ball milling is the most widely used technique followed by thermal pretreatment to reduce the size of bulk material called 'solid-state route'. Sometime it may be via mechanical grinding of macro materials and subsequent stabilization of the synthesized nanomaterial by adding the specific protecting agents. But the serious drawback with the top-down approach has been its sluggish rate of production that is why it is disabled for mass-scale production (Robles-García et al. 2016). Apart from this, there are several other drawbacks which include surface imperfection, contaminations, and stress and strain in nano-particle along with wastage of material. The bottom-up approach is just the reverse case of the former one. The fundament difference from the top-down approach involves the generation of nano-particles from individual atoms via their self-assembly in a natural and self-regulating manner. The bottom-up methods such as co-precipitation, sol-gel, auto-combustion route, etc., for the production nano-materials have better luck to produce the nanostructures with least defects, more homogenous texture, and uniform with tunable size throughout the crystal network.

1.8 Hydrogels

Hydrogels are as hydrophilic gels with three dimensional cross-linked networks of polymer chains. Hydrogels are derived from colloidal gels having water as the dispersion medium. Hydrogels are smart structural and functional entities which respond over the varieties of stimuli such as pH, temperature, pressure, ionic strength, and presence of catalyst or enzyme. Hydrogels mock the living tissue of organisms owing to their softness, flexibility, and biocompatibility in vivo. Therefore, they are extensively applied in the food and pharmaceutical industries (Ahmad et al. 2019; Batista et al. 2019). Hydrogels manifest many important features i.e. softness, flexibility, swelling, absorbent capacity and water storage properties (Truong et al. 2015). Hydrogels are manufactured via the addition of cross-linking edible polymers to water or water-like solvent followed by allowing the heterogeneous system to swell. Hydrogels might be synthesized using natural or synthetic edible polymers having hydrophilic functionalities such as -OH, -COOH, $-NH_2$, $-CONH_2$ etc. attached to their backbone. Several physical forms of hydrogels are in use nowadays in food and biochemical industries (Ali and Ahmed 2018). The hydrogel can be derived either from natural or synthetic polymers. Alginate, xanthan, and dextran are few natural polymers and are capable of forming hydrogels (Gyles et al. 2017). Poly (vinyl alcohol), polymethacrylic acid (PMAA), polyacrylic Acid (PAA) poly N-vinylpyrrolidone (PVP), polyethylene glycol diacrylate/dimethacrylate (PEGDA/PEGDMA), polyethylene glycol acrylate/methacrylate (PEGA/PEGMA), and polystyrene (PS) are commonly used as synthetic polymers (Sithole et al. 2017). Edible polymers derived plant and animal are the basic component of hydrogel schematically shown in following Fig. 1.1. There are different forms of hydrogels used in food technology so far and has been illustrated in Fig. 1.3.

1.8.1 Methods for Preparation of Hydrogel

Usually, formation of hydrogel depends upon the nature of cross-linking in above mentioned edible polymers. Two major techniques are physical and chemical cross-linking involved in hydrogel production (Ali and Ahmed 2018; Qu and Luo 2020) summarized in Fig. 1.4.

1.8.2 Applications of Edible Polymer-Based Hydrogels

Due to three-dimensional structure, hydrophilic networks, and polymeric chains linked through physical or chemical bonds, hydrogels can be a very suitable carrier system for bioactive compounds. Their exclusive physico-chemical properties have been manifested in Fig. 1.5.

Nonetheless, the physicochemical properties of hydrogel of nano-dimension and its interaction with biological system must be checked before its administration

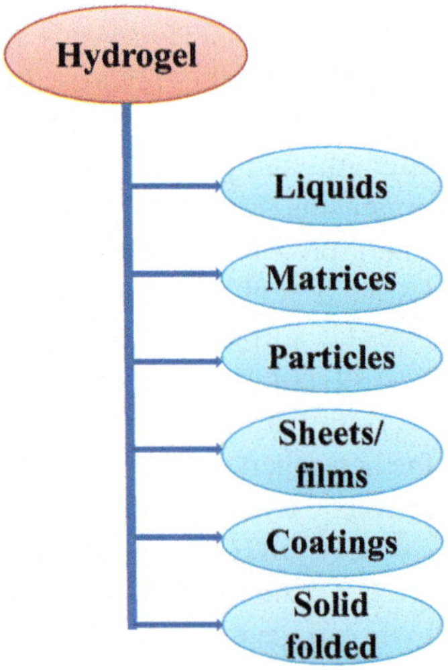

Fig. 1.3 Schematic depiction of various forms of hydrogels employed in food science

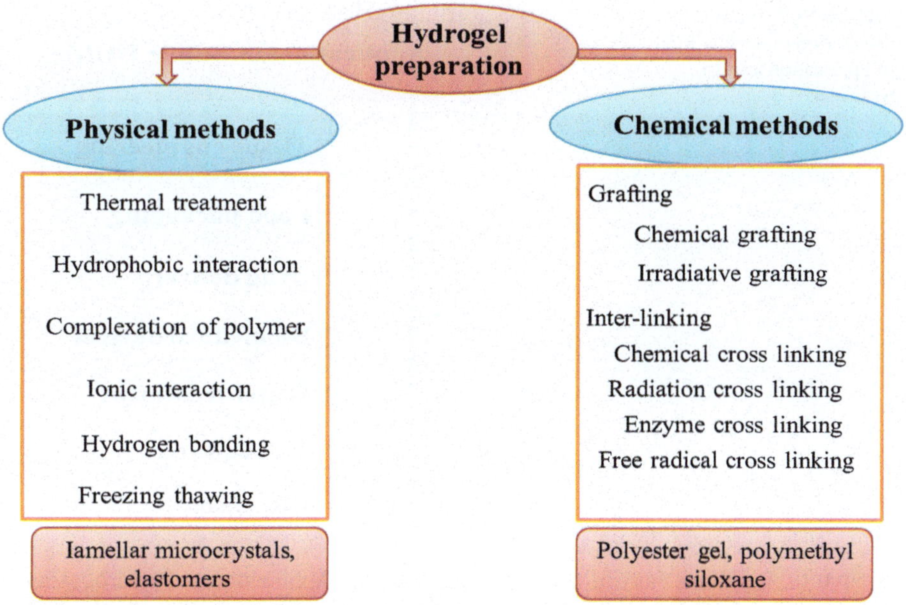

Fig. 1.4 Summary of preparation methods for hydrogel to be used in food sector

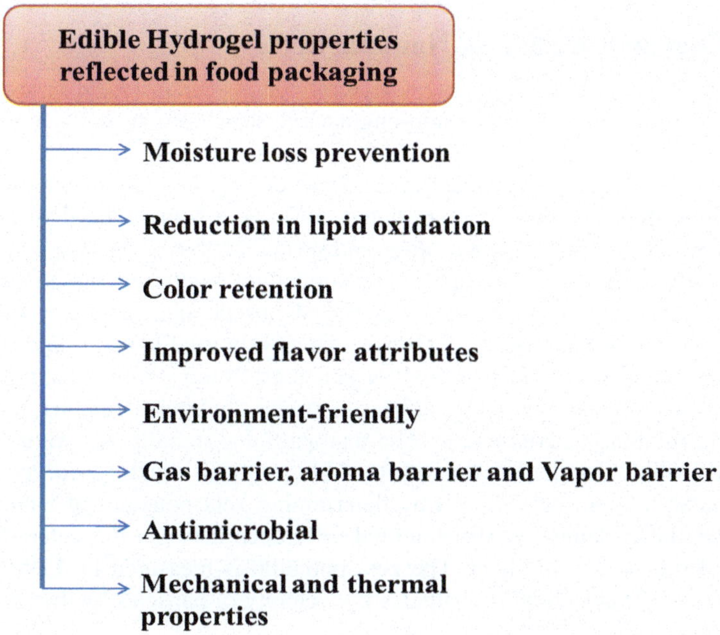

Fig. 1.5 Schematic illustration of physicochemical properties of nanostructured hydrogel

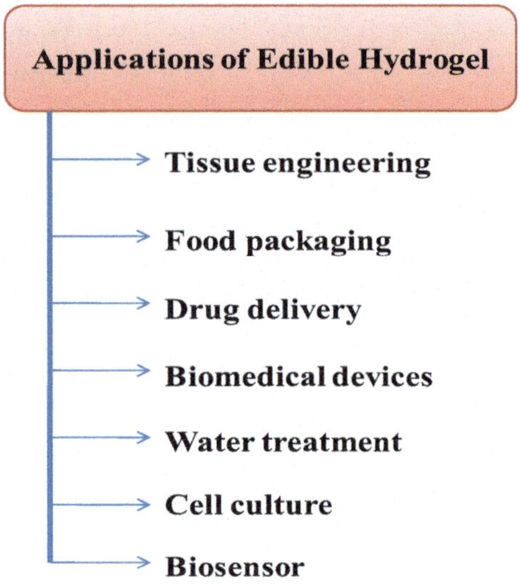

Fig. 1.6 Schematic illustration of several kinds of application area of hydrogel

in vivo to avoid any sort of toxicity. The potential applications of hydrogel mentioned in Fig. 1.6, have been investigated in wide spectrum of food packaging, pharmaceutical and other industries depending upon their exclusive physico-chemical properties elaborated in Fig. 1.5 (Kołodyńska et al. 2016).

1.9 Characterization of Nanoparticles

There are different forms of nano-engineered structures such as biopolymeric nanoparticles, liposomes, nanoemulsions, nanocomposites, inorganic nanoparticles, and hydrogels which are involved in food chemistry to tune the characteristics of conventional food ingredients represented in Fig. 1.7. Nanoparticles are generally characterized by their size, morphology and surface charge using several instrumental methods (Chirayil et al. 2017). Dynamic light scattering (DLS) or photon-correlation spectroscopy (PCS) is the fastest and most popular method of determining the particle size of nanoparticles. DLS is extensively used to determine the size of Brownian nanoparticles in colloidal suspensions. Nanoparticle tracking analysis (NTA) is a methodology that analyzes particles in liquids relating the rate of Brownian motion to particle size. The nanoparticles stability is a very important parameter which decides the durability of bio-polymer affecting storage capacity. Particle stability can be assessed by determining zeta potential of nanoparticles. Zeta potential is defined as the potential difference between the outer Helmholtz layer and the surface of shear. The zeta potential is measured by Laser Doppler Anemometry. This technique evaluates the velocity of particles by the shift caused

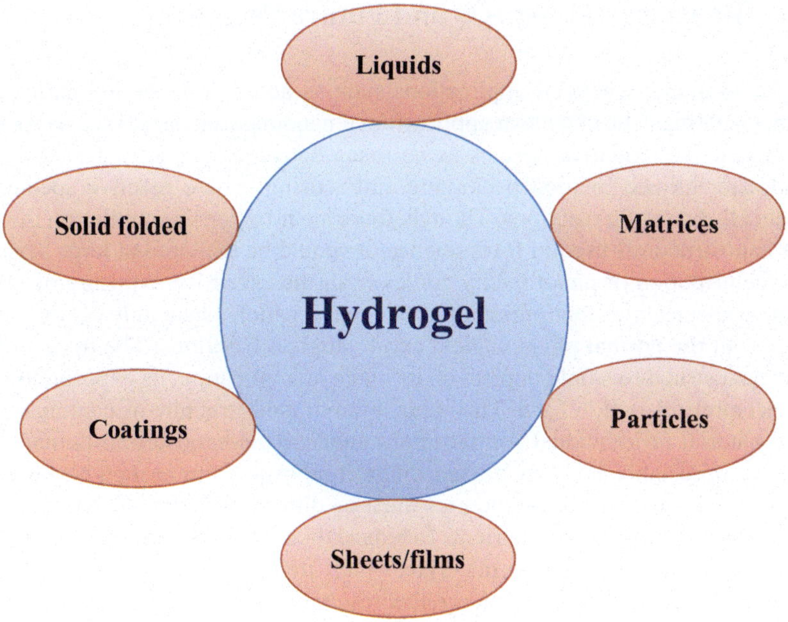

Fig. 1.7 An illustration of several micro and nano structured materials seeking very important application in food sector

in the interference fringe produced by the intersection of two laser beams. The surface morphology of nanoparticles exerts a profound impact on the physicochemical properties that affect their interaction with the chemical reagents. There are several analytical tools to monitor the morphology of nanoparticles. Microscopic characterizations such as scanning electron microscopy (SEM), tunneling electron microscopy (TEM) and atomic force microscopy (AFM) determine morphology or surface roughness of the nanoparticles. X-ray diffraction (XRD) is the primary tool for investigating the phase and crystal structure of particles. Fourier transform infrared spectroscopy (FTIR) is a supplementary technique of XRD. This gives information about functional moieties present in protein and polysaccharides. This also suggests their structural changes during food processing. In addition to above discussed structural, particle size and surface area characterizations, optical characterizations are also crucially important to realize the deep insight mechanism of nanostructures executing any mean of photo-interactions during their application in food sector. The optical properties of nanostructures can easily be investigated using ultraviolet–visible (UV–Vis), photoluminescence (PL) and null ellipsometer. Additionally, the ultraviolet–visible diffuse reflectance spectrometer (DRS) is an advanced equipment to measure the optical absorption, transmittance and reflectance just by using only one assembly (Khan et al. 2019).

1.10 Toxicological Aspects and Future Perspective

Besides so many beneficial applications such as antimicrobials and antioxidants, and nanocoatings, the extensive application of nanomaterial causes the overproduction of reactive oxidative species as so many active inorganic and organic compounds are utilized in food packaging and sensing. These reactive species may trigger cell-damaging reactions. Though, there are no extensive studies on the toxicity of nanostructures used in food science, it should be explored at large scale. The major contribution of nanotoxicity comes from the excessive exposure of reacting oxidative species dysfunctioning the cells in vivo which adequately become unable to carry out the normal physiological and biological functions. The toxicity extent of any nanostructure would depend on its mode of application, its exposure time and its concentration used in food. The application of nanostructure as coating or packaging material in individual format might enhance the exposure to human beings but gets appreciably low when used multi composite form alongwith other food ingredients. Moreover, nanostructures must be diluted for their application in food as carriers of bioactives and nutrients to reduce their concentration in vivo. The dilution should be performed with materials which are native to food such as proteins, polysaccharides, and lipids making the resultant entity with negligible toxicity (Singh et al. 2017a, b). Recently, nanolaminates as surface coatings are prepared of polysaccharides, proteins, and lipids showing zero hazard potential whereas nanostructures as encapsulating agents are composed of polylactic acid, an edible polymer. These diluting agents are known to be non toxic and biodegradable in nature. Next, the spraying of iron-carbon nanoparticles did not cause their migration form application sites while it occurred when they were injected in pumpkins (Corredor et al. 2009). Injection of nanostructures might be the reason for the insertion of nanoparticles and their further accumulation in biological systems. In another observation, Au nanoparticles were observed to migrate from the water column to the marine food web in laboratory-constructed estuarine mesocosms containing sea water, sediment, sea grass, microbes, biofilms, snails, clams, shrimp and fish (Ferry et al. 2009). Ag nanoparticles were noticed to be migrated from a commercial baby feeding bottle and a food box containing Ag nanoparticles assured by surface morphological and elemental analysis (Ramos et al. 2016). Ag nanoparticles release was checked in the temperature range of 20–70 °C over contact time up to 10 days. Ag nanoparticles released from the food box was found with 2 to 3 times higher magnitude than that noticed in case of the baby bottle, however, the total silver content in the food box material was half of that in the baby bottle (Ramos et al. 2016). Therefore, severe nanotoxicity may cause DNA mutation, uncontrolled cell signalling, allergic pulmonary inflammation, modified cell motility, cytotoxicity, apoptosis, and incurable disease like cancer (Pathakoti et al. 2017). Athinarayanan et al. (2014) noticed the nano-silica contamination in the body where E551 has been adulterated in food ingredients. Similarly, silver and zinc oxide NPs are found to leach into food material from their packaging stuff whereas silver NPs significantly leach into the meat exudates (Pathakoti et al. 2017). Chen et al. (2013) reported the release of nano titania from chewing gum and gotten accumulated in the human body causing severe toxicity. In a study executed by Bettini et al. (2017), food-grade nano titanium dioxide (TiO_2), a white pigment used in common foodstuffs as E171, including confectionary causes an increased risk of chronic intestinal inflammation and carcinogenesis on daily oral TiO_2-NP intake. In fact after monitoring its regular exposure in rats orally for 1 week at human relevant levels, titanium was detected in the immune cells of Peyer's patches (PP). This observation must be carefully taken into consideration for the risk assessments because human beings may be susceptible to Th17-driven autoimmune diseases and to colorectal cancer due to regular TiO_2 uptake from dietary sources. Brandelli (2019) reported in vivo toxicity of several metal oxides nanoparticles and metal species nanoparticles with antimicrobial properties such as Ag, ZnO, TiO_2 causing serious health hazards over long-term oral exposure. However, the development of nanotechnology in the food industry should not be objected rather must be embraced consciously keeping all the above-mentioned facts into consideration. The effect of nanotoxicity can be assuaged through a proper risk assessment of physicochemical properties of nanomaterials along with their absorption, biodistribution, metabolism, and excretion in vivo with utmost seriousness before their application in the food sector (Prociak et al. 2015). Various above mentioned nanostructures are successfully employed in food sector so far also summarized in Table 1.1.

1.11 Conclusions

This book chapter briefs the potential and beneficial innovations made by nanotechnology which further influence the food quality and ultimately the public health. There are different forms of nano-engineered structures such as biopolymeric nanoparticles, liposomes, nanoemulsions, nanocomposites, inorganic nanoparticles, and hydrogels which are involved in food chemistry to tune the characteristics of conventional food ingredients. They tune the taste, flavour, colour, texture, and durability of foodstuffs. They exhibit excellent absorption of bioactive materials. They enhance the availability of nutraceuticals in vivo and also act as supplements for vital bioelements. Owing to aforementioned virtues, these nanostructures find their tremendous applications in the food industry such as nanodevices or nanosensors, nanoencapsulation agents, anticaking agent, nano-additives, neutraceuticals, nano-packaging systems, edible nanocoatings, gelating agents. The demand of non-toxic food products with nano-particle which comprises essential and vital elements, is continuously increasing day by day. But these changes might be having a negative impact on the actual nature of biological samples by deteriorating it. Above all, the exclusive properties of nanostructures which are quite different than their bulk form may occasionally cause hazardous side effects in flora and fauna of our ecosystem. Hence, there should be some stringent and explicit guidelines to comprehend the crucial information regarding nanostructures about their size, dose, surface reaction and other interactions with food ingredients for the assessment of their

Table 1.1 An illustration of the summary of various nano and micro structures employed in food stuff along with their application mode

Nanostructures	Preparation techniques	Application	Remarks	References
Biopolymeric compound				
Rice bran albumin nanoparticles	Ultra homogenizer	Bioactive loading	Increased in vitro bioactivity and in vivo bioavailability	Liu et al. (2018)
Nisin-loaded pectin nanoparticles	Complexation method	Antimicrobial properties as food preservative	Wide spectrum antimicrobial activity against gram-positive bacteria	Krivorotova et al. (2016)
Methylcellulose	Anti-solvent precipitation	Stabilizing agent	Rheological properties of the obtained emulsions can be tuned by altering their compositions	Zeng et al. (2017)
Beeswax, propolis wax	Glyceryl behenate	Carrier for bioactives	Development of highly functional nanostructured lipid carriers	Soleimanian et al. (2018)
Saturated canola oil	Polyethylene glycol (PEG) and Sodium lauryl sulfate (SLS)	Nano-scale solid lipid particles with a high content of a hydrophilic bioactive;	Carrier for bioactives	Couto et al. (2017)
Zein core surrounded by a caseinate or caseinate–dextran shell	Caseinate–dextran conjugates were formed using the Maillard reaction	Encapsulation of bioactives such as resveratrol	Carrier for bioactives, development of effective delivery systems for incorporating lipophilic nutraceuticals into functional foods and beverages	Davidov-Pardo et al. (2015)
Liposomes				
Layer-by-layer assembly of lactoferrin and BSA on liposomes (Hybrid nanoparticles)	Electrostatic deposition	Functional molecular delivery systems in food and nutrition areas	Control physical–chemical and digestion stability	Liu et al. (2017)
Folated pluronic F127 (FA-F127) modified liposomes	–	Delivery system of curcumin	Significantly higher cytotoxicity towards KB cells, folic acid modified liposomes provide a novel strategy to improve chemotherapeutic efficacy of hydrophobic bioactive compounds	Li et al. (2020a, b)

(continued)

Table 1.1 (continued)

Nanostructures	Preparation techniques	Application	Remarks	References
Phospholipid and pluronic F127 (F127-Lps) liposomes	Film evaporation method	Carrier for bioactives i.e. curcumin	Enhanced entrapment efficiency and stability	Li et al. (2020a, b)
Phosphatidyl choline	–	As potent preservative and conservation agents	Increased antimicrobial activity against *E. Coli* O157:H7	Khosravi-Darani et al. (2016)
Phosphatidyl choline	–	To encapsulate flavoring and nutritive agents, antimicrobial activity in food	Improving the flavor of ripened cheese, targeted delivery of functional food ingredients, synergistic delivery of ascorbic acid and tocopherols for promoting antioxidant activity in foods, the stabilization of minerals (such as iron) in milk	Khanniri et al. (2016)
Nanometric bilayer phospholipids vesicle	–	As promising encapsulation technology for the nutraceutical industry	Protection of sensitive bioactive molecules, storage stability, high loading capacity, enhanced bioavailability, and sustained-release mechanism	Khorasani et al. (2018)
Emulsions				
Food grade vitamin E acetate nanoemulsion	Fabricated using the edible mustard oil and surfactant Tween-80 by low energy approach	Bioactivity, antioxidant, and antimicrobial activity	Increase the shelf life of fruit juice	Dasgupta et al. (2016)
Essential oil (EO) nanoemulsions	Low energy approach	Natural antimicrobials and preservatives in the food industry	Delivery system both in vitro and in vivo product	Donsì and Ferrari (2016)
Long chain omega-3 polyunsaturated fatty acids (LCω3PUFA)	Quillaja saponin as emulsifier	Increase lcω3pufa bioavailability	Use in functional food	Bush et al. (2019)

(continued)

Table 1.1 (continued)

Nanostructures	Preparation techniques	Application	Remarks	References
Composites				
Nano-ZnO_2 over	Carboxymethyl cellulose (CMC)	Edible coatings	Extension of shelf life	Saba and Amini (2017)
Sulfur nanoparticles (SNP)/chitosan	Solution casting method	Antimicrobial films	High potential to be used as antimicrobial food packaging films	Lin et al. (2019)
(Eudragit EPO, Eudragit S100 or ethyl cellulose) polymer-blended quinine nanocomposite particles	Spray-drying technique	As test masker	Masking bitter tastes in the field of food and pharmaceutical industry	Taki et al. (2017)
Inorganic particles				
Gold and silver nanoparticles	Environmental-friendly green synthesis method using quercetin as reducing agent	Sensor for bioactives	Lactose biosensor with high sensitivity and stability	Bollella et al. (2017)
Gracilaria vermiculophylla extract films containing zinc oxide	Film formation using glycerol and sorbitol were added as plasticizers	Food packaging material	Smoked salmon packaging	Baek and Song (2018)
Zinc oxide nanoparticles	–	Food packaging material	Excellent antimicrobial activity against foodborne pathogens *salmonella typhimurium* and *staphylococcus aureus*	Akbar et al. (2019)
Hydrogels				
Poly(gelatin-*co*-dmaam)/CA–BE	Redox polymerization technique	Food packaging material	Mechanical and water resistance properties, antimicrobial activity against *Escherichia coli*, *Bacillus subtilis* and *Staphylococcus aureus*, antioxidant and anthocyanin properties	Alpaslan (2019)
Whey and soy protein-based hydrogels	–	Site-specific delivery systems	Protein-based hydrogels systems for delivery of bioactive compound	Abaee et al. (2017)

(continued)

Table 1.1 (continued)

Nanostructures	Preparation techniques	Application	Remarks	References
Hydrogel composed of xanthan, gellan and pullulan	–	Bioactive carrier system	Good viscoelastic nature and flow behaviour index	Kalia and Choudhury (2019)
Gelling matrices valorized artichoke industrial wastes from natural and blanched processed samples	Microwave hydrodiffusion and gravity (MHG)	Food preservative and storage	Preservation capacity of the bioactive properties of the samples for at least 3 years.	López-Hortas et al. (2019)

optimum use in the food sector. Moreover, there should be a proper study applying in vitro and in vivo models for toxicity assessment before their application in food or related industries. Since this has been observed that sometimes *in vitro* models do not function appropriately for estimation of pulmonary toxicity involved in mechanism followed by nanostructures, there should be a thorough understanding of their action in vivo.

Acknowledgement Authors would also show their great sense of gratitude towards UGC (Delhi) for financial assistantship as SRF to SS and SM.

References

Abaee A, Mohammadian M, Jafari SM (2017) Whey and soy protein-based hydrogels and nano-hydrogels as bioactive delivery systems. Trends Food Sci Technol 70:69–81. https://doi.org/10.1016/j.tifs.2017.10.011

Ahmad S, Ahmad M, Manzoor K, Purwar R, Ikram S (2019) A review on latest innovations in natural gums based hydrogels: preparations & applications. Int J Biol Macromol 136:870–890. https://doi.org/10.1016/j.ijbiomac.2019.06.113

Ahmed TA, Aljaeid BM (2016) Preparation, characterization, and potential application of chitosan, chitosan derivatives, and chitosan metal nanoparticles in pharmaceutical drug delivery. Drug Des Dev Ther 10:483–507. https://doi.org/10.2147/DDDT.S99651

Akbar A, Sadiq MB, Ali I, Muhammad N, Rehman Z, Khan MN, Muhammad J, Khan SA, UrRehman F, Anal AK (2019) Synthesis and antimicrobial activity of zinc oxide nanoparticles against foodborne pathogens Salmonella typhimurium and Staphylococcus aureus. Biocatal Agric Biotechnol 17:36–42. https://doi.org/10.1016/j.bcab.2018.11.005

Ali A, Ahmed S (2018) Recent advances in edible polymer based hydrogels as a sustainable alternative to conventional polymers. J Agric Food Chem 66(27):6940–6967. https://doi.org/10.1021/acs.jafc.8b01052

Alpaslan D (2019) Use of colorimetric hydrogel as an indicator for food packaging applications. Bull Mater Sci 42(5):247. https://doi.org/10.1007/s12034-019-1908-z

Athinarayanan J, Periasamy VS, Alsaif MA, Al-Warthan AA, Alshatwi AA (2014) Presence of nanosilica (E551) in commercial food products: TNF-mediated oxidative stress and altered cell cycle progression in human lung fibroblast cells. Cell Biol Toxicol 30(2):89–100. https://doi.org/10.1007/s10565-014-9271-8

Baek SK, Song KB (2018) Development of Gracilaria vermiculophylla extract films containing zinc oxide nanoparticles and their application in smoked salmon packaging. LWT Food Sci Technol 89:269–275. https://doi.org/10.1016/j.lwt.2017.10.064

Bajpai VK, Shukla S, Khan I, Kang SM, Haldorai Y, Tripathi KM, Jung SH, Chen L, Kim TY, Huh YS, Han YK (2019) A sustainable graphene aerogel capable of the adsorptive elimination of biogenic amines and Bacteria from soy sauce and highly efficient cell proliferation. ACS Appl Mater Interfaces 11(47):43949–43963. https://doi.org/10.1021/acsami.9b16989

Batista RA, Espitia PJP, Quintans JDSS, Freitas MM, Cerqueira MÂ, Teixeira JA, Cardoso JC (2019) Hydrogel as an alternative structure for food packaging systems. Carbohydr Polym 205:106–116. https://doi.org/10.1016/j.carbpol.2018.10.006

Benítez AJ, Walther A (2017) Cellulose nanofibril nanopapers and bioinspired nanocomposites: a review to understand the mechanical property space. J Mater Chem A 5(31):16003–16024. https://doi.org/10.1039/C7TA02006F

Bettini S, Boutet-Robinet E, Cartier C, Coméra C, Gaultier E, Dupuy J, Naud N, Tache S, Grysan P, Reguer S, Thieriet N, Refregiers N, Thiaudiere D, Cravedi JP, Carriere M, Audinot JN, Pierre FH, Piriou LG, Houdeau E (2017) Food-grade TiO_2 impairs intestinal and systemic immune homeostasis, initiates preneoplastic lesions and promotes aberrant crypt development in the rat colon. Sci Rep 7:40373. https://doi.org/10.1038/srep40373

Bollella P, Schulz C, Favero G, Mazzei F, Ludwig R, Gorton L, Antiochia R (2017) Green synthesis and characterization of gold and silver nanoparticles and their application for development of a third generation lactose biosensor. Electroanalysis 29(1):77–86. https://doi.org/10.1002/elan.201600476

Brandelli A (2019) The interaction of nanostructured antimicrobials with biological systems: cellular uptake, trafficking and potential toxicity. Food Sci Hum Wellness 9:8–20. https://doi.org/10.1016/j.fshw.2019.12.003

Bratovcic A, Odobasic A, Catic S, Sestan I (2015) Application of polymer nanocomposite materials in food packaging. Croatian J Food Sci Technol 7(2):86–94. https://doi.org/10.17508/CJFST.2015.7.2.06

Bush L, Stevenson L, Lane KE (2019) The oxidative stability of omega-3 oil-in-water nanoemulsion systems suitable for functional food enrichment: a systematic review of the literature. Crit Rev Food Sci Nutr 59(7):1154–1168. https://doi.org/10.1080/10408398.2017.1394268

Campelo PH, Sant'Ana AS, Clerici MTPS (2020) Starch nanoparticles: production methods, structure, and properties for food applications. Curr Opin Food Sci (In press). https://doi.org/10.1016/j.cofs.2020.04.007

Charcosset C (2016) Preparation of nanomaterials for food applications using membrane emulsification and membrane mixing. Nanotechnol Agri-Food Indust Emul Grumezescu AM Academic Press 3:37–69. https://doi.org/10.1016/B978-0-12-804306-6.00002-7

Chen XX, Cheng B, Yang YX, Cao A, Liu JH, Du LJ, Liu Y, Zhao Y, Wang H (2013) Characterization and preliminary toxicity assay of nano-titanium dioxide additive in sugar-coated chewing gum. Small 9(9-10):1765–1774. https://doi.org/10.1002/smll.201201506

Chirayil CJ, Abraham J, Mishra RK, George SC, Thomas S (2017) Instrumental techniques for the characterization of nanoparticles. Thermal and rheological measurement techniques for nanomaterials characterization, pp 1–36. Elsevier. https://doi.org/10.1016/B978-0-323-46139-9.00001-3

Corredor E, Testillano PS, Coronado MJ, González-Melendi P, Fernández-Pacheco R, Marquina C, Ibarra MR, de la Fuente JM, Rubiales D, Pérez-de-Luque A, Risueño MC (2009) Nanoparticle penetration and transport in living pumpkin plants: in situ subcellular identification. BMC Plant Biol 9(1):45. https://doi.org/10.1186/1471-2229-9-45

Couto R, Alvarez V, Temelli F (2017) Encapsulation of vitamin B_2 in solid lipid nanoparticles using supercritical CO_2. J Supercrit Fluids 120:432–442. https://doi.org/10.1016/j.supflu.2016.05.036

Das GS, Shim JP, Bhatnagar A, Tripathi KM, Kim T (2019) Biomass-derived carbon quantum dots for visible-light-induced photocatalysis and label-free detection of Fe (iii) and ascorbic acid. Sci Reports 9(1):1–9. https://doi.org/10.1038/s41598-019-49266-y

Dasgupta N, Ranjan S, Mundekkad D, Ramalingam C, Shanker R, Kumar A (2015) Nanotechnology in agro-food: from field to plate. Food Res Int 69:381–400. https://doi.org/10.1016/j.foodres.2015.01.005

Dasgupta N, Ranjan S, Mundra S, Ramalingam C, Kumar A (2016) Fabrication of food grade vitamin E nanoemulsion by low energy approach, characterization and its application. Int J Food Prop 19(3):700–708. https://doi.org/10.1080/10942912.2015.1042587

Davidov-Pardo G, Pérez-Ciordia S, Marin-Arroyo MR, McClements DJ (2015) Improving resveratrol bioaccessibility using biopolymer nanoparticles and complexes: impact of protein–carbohydrate maillard conjugation. J Agri Food Chem 63(15):3915–3923. https://doi.org/10.1021/acs.jafc.5b00777

de Oca-Ávalos JMM, Candal RJ, Herrera ML (2017) Nanoemulsions: stability and physical properties. Curr Opin Food Sci 16:1–6. https://doi.org/10.1016/j.cofs.2017.06.003

Divya K, Jisha MS (2018) Chitosan nanoparticles preparation and applications. Environ Chem Lett 16(1):101–112. https://doi.org/10.1007/s10311-017-0670-y

Donsì F, Ferrari G (2016) Essential oil nanoemulsions as antimicrobial agents in food. J Biotechnol 233:106–120. https://doi.org/10.1016/j.jbiotec.2016.07.005

dos Santos CA, Ingle AP, Rai M (2020) The emerging role of metallic nanoparticles in food. Appl Microbiol Biotechnol 104(6):2373–2383. https://doi.org/10.1007/s00253-020-10372-x

Duan C, Meng J, Wang X, Meng X, Sun X, Xu Y, Zhao W, Ni Y (2018) Synthesis of novel cellulose-based antibacterial composites of ag nanoparticles@ metal-organic frameworks@ carboxymethylated fibres. Carbohydr Polym 193:82–88. https://doi.org/10.1016/j.carbpol.2018.03.089

El Achaby M, El Miri N, Aboulkas A, Zahouily M, Bilal E, Barakat A, Solhy A (2017) Processing and properties of eco-friendly bio-nanocomposite films filled with cellulose nanocrystals from sugarcane bagasse. Int J Biol Macromol 96:340–352. https://doi.org/10.1016/j.ijbiomac.2016.12.040

Ferry JL, Craig P, Hexel C, Sisco P, Frey R, Pennington PL, Fulton MH, Scott IG, Decho AW, Kashiwada S, Murphy CJ, Shaw TJ (2009) Transfer of gold nanoparticles from the water column to the estuarine food web. Nature Nanotechnol 4(7):441–444. https://doi.org/10.1038/nnano.2009.157

Fu JY, Che HL, Tan DM, Teng KT (2014) Bioavailability of tocotrienols: evidence in human studies. Nutr Metab 11(1):1–10. https://doi.org/10.1186/1743-7075-11-5

Ghorbanzade T, Jafari SM, Akhavan S, Hadavi R (2017) Nano-encapsulation of fish oil in nano-liposomes and its application in fortification of yogurt. Food Chem 216:146–152. https://doi.org/10.1016/j.foodchem.2016.08.022

Gupta A, Eral HB, Hatton TA, Doyle PS (2016) Nanoemulsions: formation, properties and applications. Soft Matter 12(11):2826–2841. https://doi.org/10.1039/c5sm02958a

Gyles DA, Castro LD, Silva JOC Jr, Ribeiro-Costa RM (2017) A review of the designs and prominent biomedical advances of natural and synthetic hydrogel formulations. Euro Polymer J 88:373–392. https://doi.org/10.1016/j.eurpolymj.2017.01.027

Hulla JE, Sahu SC, Hayes AW (2015) Nanotechnology: history and future. Hum Exp Toxicol 34(12):1318–1321. https://doi.org/10.1177/0960327115603588

Ingale AG, Chaudhari AN (2018) Nanotechnology in the food industry. Nanotechnol Food Security Water Treatment, Springer Chem, pp 87–128. https://doi.org/10.1007/978-3-319-70166-0_3

Jafari SM, McClements DJ (2017) Nanotechnology approaches for increasing nutrient bioavailability. In: Advances in food and nutrition research, vol 81. Academic, pp 1–30. https://doi.org/10.1016/bs.afnr.2016.12.0008

Kale SN, Deore SL (2017) Emulsion micro emulsion and nano emulsion: a review. Syst Rev Pharm 8(1):39. https://doi.org/10.5530/srp.2017.1.8

Kalia S, Choudhury AR (2019) Synthesis and rheological studies of a novel composite hydrogel of xanthan, gellan and pullulan. Int J Biol Macromol 137:475–482. https://doi.org/10.1016/j.ijbiomac.2019.06.212

Kalpana VN, Rajeswari VD (2017) Biosynthesis of metal and metal oxide nanoparticles for food packaging and preservation: a green expertise. In: Food Biosynthesis. Academic, New York, pp 293–316. https://doi.org/10.1016/B978-0-12-811372-1.00010-5

Karthik P, Ezhilarasi PN, Anandharamakrishnan C (2017) Challenges associated in stability of food grade nanoemulsions. Crit Rev Food Sci Nutr 57(7):1435–1450. https://doi.org/10.1080/10408398.2015.1006767

Khalid K, Tan X, Mohd Zaid HF, Tao Y, Lye Chew C, Chu DT, Lam MK, Ho YC, Lim JW, Wei LC (2020) Advanced in developmental organic and inorganic nanomaterial: a review. Bioengineering 11(1):328–355. https://doi.org/10.1080/21655979.2020.1736240

Khan I, Saeed K, Khan I (2019) Nanoparticles: properties, applications and toxicities. Arab J Chem 12(7):908–931. https://doi.org/10.1016/j.arabjc.2017.05.011

Khanniri E, Bagheripoor-Fallah N, Sohrabvandi S, Mortazavian AM, Khosravi-Darani K, Mohammad R (2016) Application of liposomes in some dairy products. Crit Rev Food Sci Nutr 56(3):484–493. https://doi.org/10.1080/10408398.2013.779571

Khorasani S, Danaei M, Mozafari MR (2018) Nanoliposome technology for the food and nutraceutical industries. Trends Food Sci Technol 79:106–115. https://doi.org/10.1016/j.tifs.2018.07.009

Khosravi-Darani K, Khoosfi EM, Hossenini H (2016) Encapsulation of Zataria multiflora Boiss. Essential oil in liposome: antibacterial activity against E. coli O157:H7 in broth media and minced beef. J Food Safety 36:515–523. https://doi.org/10.1111/jfs.12271

Kim HE, Lee HJ, Kim MS, Kim T, Lee H, Kim HH, Cho M, Hong SW, Lee C (2019) Differential microbicidal effects of bimetallic iron–copper nanoparticles on Escherichia coli and MS2 Coliphage. Environ Sci Technol 53(5):2679–2687. https://doi.org/10.1021/acs.est.8b06077

King T, Osmond-McLeod MJ, Duffy LL (2018) Nanotechnology in the food sector and potential applications for the poultry industry. Trends Food Sci Technol 72:62–73. https://doi.org/10.1016/j.tifs.2017.11.015

Kołodyńska D, Skiba A, Górecka B, Hubicki Z (2016) Hydrogels from fundaments to application. Emerging Concept Anal Appl Hydrogels:69–100. https://doi.org/10.5772/63466

Krivorotova T, Cirkovas A, Maciulyte S, Staneviciene R, Budriene S, Serviene E, Sereikaite J (2016) Nisin-loaded pectin nanoparticles for food preservation. Food Hydrocoll 54:49–56. https://doi.org/10.1016/j.foodhyd.2015.09.015

Kumar R, Sharma RK, Singh AP (2018) Grafted cellulose: a bio-based polymer for durable applications. Poly Bull 75(5):2213–2242. https://doi.org/10.1007/s00289-017-2136-6

Li Z, Huang Y, Peng S, Chen X, Zou L, Liu W, Liu C (2020a) Liposomes consisting of pluronic F127 and phospholipid: effect of matrix on morphology, stability and curcumin delivery. J Dispers Sci Technol 41(2):207–213. https://doi.org/10.1080/01932691.2018.1562353

Li Z, Xiong X, Peng S, Chen X, Liu W, Liu C (2020b) Novel folated pluronic F127 modified liposomes for delivery of curcumin: preparation, release, and cytotoxicity. J Microencapsul 37(3):220–229. https://doi.org/10.1080/02652048.2020.1720030

Lin L, Gu Y, Cui H (2019) Moringa oil/chitosan nanoparticles embedded gelatin nanofibers for food packaging against listeria monocytogenes and Staphylococcus aureus on cheese. Food Packag Shelf Life 19:86–93. https://doi.org/10.1016/j.fpsl.2018.12.005

Liu W, Ye A, Singh H (2015) Progress in applications of liposomes in food systems. In: Microencapsulation and microspheres for food applications. Academic, London, pp 151–170. https://doi.org/10.1016/B978-0-12-800350-3.00025-X

Liu W, Kong Y, Tu P, Lu J, Liu C, Liu W, Han J, Liu J (2017) Physical–chemical stability and in vitro digestibility of hybrid nanoparticles based on the layer-by-layer assembly of lactoferrin and BSA on liposomes. Food Funct 8(4):1688–1697. https://doi.org/10.1039/C7FO00308K

Liu C, Yang X, Wu W, Long Z, Xiao H, Luo F, Shen Y, Lin Q (2018) Elaboration of curcumin-loaded rice bran albumin nanoparticles formulation with increased in vitro bioactivity and in vivo bioavailability. Food Hydrocoll 77:834–842. https://doi.org/10.1016/j.foodhyd.2017.11.027

López-Hortas L, Conde E, Falqué E, Domínguez H, Torres MD (2019) Preparation of hydrogels composed of bioactive compounds from aqueous phase of artichoke obtained by MHG technique. Food Bioprocess Technol 12(8):1304–1315. https://doi.org/10.1007/s11947-019-02301-2

Maurya VK, Aggarwal M (2017) Enhancing bio-availability of vitamin D by nano-engineered based delivery systems – an overview. Int J Curr Microbiol App Sci 6(7):340–353. https://doi.org/10.20546/ijcmas

Maurya VK, Aggarwal M (2019a) A phase inversion based nanoemulsion fabrication process to encapsulate vitamin D3 for food applications. J Steroid Biochem Mol Biol 190:88–98. https://doi.org/10.1016/j.jsbmb.2019.03.021

Maurya VK, Aggarwal M (2019b) Fabrication of nano-structured lipid carrier for encapsulation of vitamin D3 for fortification of 'Lassi'; a milk based beverage. J Steroid Biochem Mol Biol 193:105429. https://doi.org/10.1016/j.jsbmb.2019.105429

Maurya VK, Aggarwal M, Ranjan V, Gothandam KM (2020a) Improving bioavailability of Vitamin A in food by encapsulation: an update. Nanosci Med 1:117–145. Springer, Cham. https://doi.org/10.1007/978-3-030-29207-2_4

Maurya VK, Bashir K, Aggarwal M (2020b) Vitamin D microencapsulation and fortification: trends and technologies. J Steroid Biochem Mol Biol 196:105489. https://doi.org/10.1016/j.jsbmb.2019.105489

Oun AA, Rhim JW (2017) Carrageenan-based hydrogels and films: effect of ZnO and CuO nanoparticles on the physical, mechanical, and antimicrobial properties. Food Hydrocoll 67:45–53. https://doi.org/10.1016/j.foodhyd.2016.12.040

Panahi Y, Farshbaf M, Mohammadhosseini M, Mirahadi M, Khalilov R, Saghfi S, Akbarzadeh A (2017) Recent advances on liposomal nanoparticles: synthesis, characterization and biomedical applications. Artif Cells Nanomed Biotechnol 45(4):788–799. https://doi.org/10.1080/21691401.2017.1282496

Pathakoti K, Manubolu M, Hwang HM (2017) Nanostructures: current uses and future applications in food science. J Food Drug Anal 25(2):245–253. https://doi.org/10.1016/j.jfda.2017.02.004

Periasamy VS, Athinarayanan J, Al-Hadi AM, Al Juhaimi F, Mahmoud MH, Alshatwi AA (2015) Identification of titanium dioxide nanoparticles in food products: induce intracellular oxidative stress mediated by TNF and CYP1A genes in human lung fibroblast cells. Environ Toxicol Pharm 39(1):176–186. https://doi.org/10.1016/j.etap.2014.11.021

Pisoschi AM, Pop A, Cimpeanu C, Turcuş V, Predoi G, Iordache F (2018) Nanoencapsulation techniques for compounds and products with antioxidant and antimicrobial activity – a critical view. Euro J Medicinal Chem 157:1326–1345. https://doi.org/10.1016/j.ejmech.2018.08.076

Pramanik S, Pramanik G (2016) Nanotechnology for sustainable agriculture in India. In: Nanoscience in food and agriculture 3. Sustainable Agriculture Reviews, Springer Chem, pp 243–280. https://doi.org/10.1007/978-3-319-48009-1_10

Prociak JP, Stokłosa K, Banach M (2015) Nanosilver products and toxicity. Environ Chem Lett 13(1):59–68. https://doi.org/10.1007/s10311-014-0490-2

Qu B, Luo Y (2020) Chitosan-based hydrogel beads: preparations, modifications and applications in food and agriculture sectors – a review. Int J Biol Macromol 452:437–448. https://doi.org/10.1016/j.ijbiomac.2020.02.240

Ramos K, Gómez-Gómez MM, Cámara C, Ramos L (2016) Silver speciation and characterization of nanoparticles released from plastic food containers by single particle ICPMS. Talanta 151:83–90. https://doi.org/10.1016/j.talanta.2015.12.071

Robles-García MA, Rodríguez-Félix F, Márquez-Ríos E, Aguilar JA, Barrera-Rodríguez A, Aguilar J, Ruiz-Cruz S, Del-Toro-Sánchez CL (2016) Applications of nanotechnology in the agriculture, food, and pharmaceuticals. J Nanosci Nanotechnol 16(8):8188–8207. https://doi.org/10.1166/jnn.2016.12925

Rostamabadi H, Falsafi SR, Jafari SM (2019) Nanoencapsulation of carotenoids within lipid-based nanocarriers. J Control Release 298:38–67. https://doi.org/10.1016/j.jconrel.2019.02.005

Saba MK, Amini R (2017) Nano-ZnO/carboxymethyl cellulose-based active coating impact on ready-to-use pomegranate during cold storage. Food Chem 232:721–726. https://doi.org/10.1016/j.foodchem.2017.04.076

Salvia-Trujillo L, Soliva-Fortuny R, Rojas-Graü MA, McClements DJ, Martin-Belloso O (2017) Edible nanoemulsions as carriers of active ingredients: a review. Annual Rev Food Sci Technol 8:439–466. https://doi.org/10.1146/annurev-food-030216-025908

Sharma C, Dhiman R, Rokana N, Panwar H (2017) Nanotechnology: an untapped resource for food packaging. Frontiers Microbiology 8:1735. https://doi.org/10.3389/fmicb.2017.01735

Sharma A, Sharma N, Kumari A, Lee HJ, Kim T, Tripathi KM (2020) Nano-carbon based sensors for bacterial detection and discrimination in clinical diagnosis: a junction between material science and biology. Appl Mater Today 18:100467. https://doi.org/10.1016/j.apmt.2019.100467

Shishir MRI, Xie L, Sun C, Zheng X, Chen W (2018) Advances in micro and nano-encapsulation of bioactive compounds using biopolymer and lipid-based transporters. Trends Food Sci Technol 78:34–60. https://doi.org/10.1016/j.tifs.2018.05.018

Shukla S, Khan I, Bajpai VK, Lee H, Kim T, Upadhyay A, Huh YS, Han YK, Tripathi KM (2019) Sustainable graphene aerogel as an ecofriendly cell growth promoter and highly efficient adsorbent for histamine from red wine. ACS Appl Mater Interfaces 11:18165–18177. https://doi.org/10.1021/acsami.9b02857

Singh T, Shukla S, Kumar P, Wahla V, Bajpai VK, Rather IA (2017a) Application of nanotechnology in food science: perception and overview. Front Microbiol 8:1501. https://doi.org/10.1016/j.ijbiomac.2020.03.105

Singh T, Shukla S, Kumar P, Wahla V, Bajpai VK, Rather IA (2017b) Application of nanotechnology in food science: perception and overview. Front Microbiol 8:1501. https://doi.org/10.3389/fmicb.2017.01501

Sithole MN, Choonara YE, du Toit LC, Kumar P, Pillay V (2017) A review of semi-synthetic biopolymer complexes: modified polysaccharide nano-carriers for enhancement of oral drug bioavailability. Pharm Dev Technol 22(2):283–295. https://doi.org/10.1080/10837450.2016.1212882

Soleimanian Y, Goli SAH, Varshosaz J, Sahafi SM (2018) Formulation and characterization of novel nanostructured lipid carriers made from beeswax, propolis wax and pomegranate seed oil. Food Chem 244:83–92. https://doi.org/10.1016/j.foodchem.2017.10.010

Song J, Li J, Li X, Xu L, Dong Y, Zeng H (2015) Quantum dot light-emitting diodes based on inorganic perovskite cesium lead halides ($CsPbX_3$). Adv Mater 27:7162–7167. https://doi.org/10.1002/adma.201502567

Srivastava AK, Dev A, Karmakar S (2018) Nanosensors and nanobiosensors in food and agriculture. Environ Chem Lett 16(1):161–182. https://doi.org/10.1007/s10311-017-0674-7

Taki M, Tagami T, Ozeki T (2017) Preparation of polymer-blended quinine nanocomposite particles by spray drying and assessment of their instrumental bitterness-masking effect using a taste sensor. Drug Dev Ind Pharm 43(5):715–722. https://doi.org/10.1080/03639045.2016.1200070

Tibolla H, Pelissari FM, Martins JT, Lanzoni EM, Vicente AA, Menegalli FC, Cunha RL (2019) Banana starch nanocomposite with cellulose nanofibers isolated from banana peel by enzymatic treatment: in vitro cytotoxicity assessment. Carbohydr Polym 207:169–179. https://doi.org/10.1016/j.carbpol.2018.11.079

Truong VX, Tsang KM, Simon GP, Boyd RL, Evans RA, Thissen H, Forsythe JS (2015) Photodegradable gelatin-based hydrogels prepared by bioorthogonal click chemistry for cell encapsulation and release. Biomacromolecules 16(7):2246–2253. https://doi.org/10.1021/acs.biomac.5b00706

Turasan H, Bonilla J, Bozkurt F, Maldonado L, Li X, Yilmaz T, Sadeghi R, Kokini J (2020) Comparison of the fabrication methods, formation dynamics, structure, and delivery performance of solid nanoparticles and hollow layer by layer edible/biodegradable nanodelivery systems. J Food Process Eng 43:13413. https://doi.org/10.1111/jfpe.13413

Vala MH, Rafati H, Aliahmadi A, Ardalan A (2017) Nanoemulsions: a novel antimicrobial delivery system. Nano Microscale Drug Deliv Syst Elsevier 13:245–266. https://doi.org/10.1016/B978-0-323-52727-9.00013-3

Veneti E, Tu RS, Auguste DT (2016) RGD-targeted liposome binding and uptake on breast cancer cells is dependent on elastin linker secondary structure. Bioconjug Chem 27:1813–1821. https://doi.org/10.1021/acs.bioconjchem.6b00205

Verma ML, Dhanya BS, Rani V, Thakur M, Jeslin J, Kushwaha R (2020) Carbohydrate and protein based biopolymeric nanoparticles: current status and biotechnological applications. Int J Biol Macromol 154:390–412. https://doi.org/10.1016/j.ijbiomac.2020.03.105

Wang SX, Michiels J, Arien KK, New R, Vanham G, Roitt I (2016) Inhibition of HIV virus by neutralizing Vhh attached to dual functional liposomes encapsulating dapivirine. Nanoscale Res Lett 11:350. https://doi.org/10.1186/s11671-016-1558-7

Yola ML, Atar N (2019) Simultaneous determination of β-agonists on hexagonal boron nitride nanosheets/multi-walled carbon nanotubes nanocomposite modified glassy carbon electrode. Mater Sci Eng C 96:669–676. https://doi.org/10.1016/j.msec.2018.12.004

Zeng T, Wu ZL, Zhu JY, Yin SW, Tang CH, Wu LY, Yang XQ (2017) Development of antioxidant Pickering high internal phase emulsions (HIPEs) stabilized by protein/polysaccharide hybrid particles as potential alternative for PHOs. Food Chem 231:122–130. https://doi.org/10.1016/j.foodchem.2017.03.116

Chapter 2
Ultrasonication and Food-Grade Nano-Materials

Mariana Huerta-Jimenez, Luis Manuel Carrillo-Lopez, Ivan Adrian Garcia-Galicia, and Alma Delia Alarcon-Rojo

Abstract In this chapter some potential uses and benefits of nano-technology and ultrasound in food industry are presented. Nano-technology provides new agro-chemicals and new supply mechanisms to improve crop productivity and promises to reduce the use of pesticides. Nano-scale micronutrients used in nano-fertilizers report an improvement in nutrient absorption efficiency and avoiding losses. In the food sector, nano-technology is applied in intelligent packaging based on nano-sensors and polymer films that help to improve the safety and quality of food. The applications of nano-technology in animals include administration of medicines and other substances; diagnosis and treatment of diseases; traceability of an animal and its products; and management of reproduction. High-intensity ultrasound applied in food science has been used to cause mechanical, physical or chemical changes in the exposed food through cavitation. Ultrasound can modify structurally and functionally animal proteins. Some recent findings include the ability of ultrasound to enhance the diffusion of micro-encapsulated fatty acids into the meat. High intensity ultrasound has been considered as an important alternative for reducing nano-size of animal proteins and to improve nano-emulsion properties. Many potential combinations of ultrasound and nano-technology may result on improvement of quality in beef. Ultrasound also induces changes in the properties of milk and its components, while the application of nano-materials improves the quality and shelf life of milk. The convergence of both technologies, ultrasound and nano-materials, is well recognized, where the synthesis of nano-materials is carried out through the use of ultrasound as assisted technology, known as sonochemistry. Nano-materials

M. Huerta-Jimenez · L. M. Carrillo-Lopez (✉)
National Council of Science and Technology, Mexico City, Mexico

Faculty of Animal Science and Ecology, Autonomous University of Chihuahua, Chihuahua, Chih, Mexico
e-mail: mhuertaj@uach.mx; lmcarrillo@uach.mx

I. A. Garcia-Galicia · A. D. Alarcon-Rojo (✉)
Faculty of Animal Science and Ecology, Autonomous University of Chihuahua, Chihuahua, Chih, Mexico
e-mail: igarciag@uach.mx; aalarcon@uach.mx

V. K. Maurya et al. (eds.), *Sustainable Agriculture Reviews 55*, Sustainable Agriculture Reviews 55, https://doi.org/10.1007/978-3-030-76813-3_2

applications in dairy are the emulsification and homogenization of milk beverages, nano-particulated delivery systems, ingredients and additives that improve sensory and functional properties, and antibacterial and intelligent packaging. Finally, concerns have arisen regarding the safety of nano-materials and more information is needed about the risks and an optimal regulation that guarantees food security and environmental protection.

Keywords Nano-materials · Food production · Ultrasound · Packaging · Processing · Meat · Dairy

2.1 Introduction

Ultrasound offers a great potential to control, improve, and accelerate processes without damaging the quality of food and other products. It has been successfully used in processes such as; emulsification, crystallization, extraction, homogenization, increasing water diffusion, reducing drying time, activation or inhibition of enzymes, cell damage, antimicrobial activity and meat tenderizing (Alarcon-Rojo et al. 2015). High intensity ultrasound applied in an aqueous medium may cause cellular disruption by cavitation. The formation and implosion of microbubbles release energy to the medium causing structural damage in a nano- micro- or macro-scale (Kehinde et al. 2020). The potential of power ultrasound involves physical and chemical processes. Physical processes are mainly ascribed to mechanical effects of the high-intensity waves in any medium while chemical processes refer to chemical effects induced by ultrasonic cavitation in liquids also called sonochemistry. The general term for the whole area is sonoprocessing or ultrasonic processing (Gallego-Juarez 2010). The basis of the applications of high intensity ultrasound is acoustic cavitation, which occurs in regions under rapidly alternating high-amplitude pressure waves and consists of the growth and collapse of gas bubbles within a liquid medium resulting in physical modifications of food matrices.

Nano-technology provides new agrochemicals and new supply mechanisms to improve crop productivity, and promises to reduce the use of pesticides and improve the food quality by providing improved nutrient delivery, food preservation and food packaging. Precision cultivation techniques are being carried out to improve crop yields, reducing soil and water damage, reducing nitrogen loss due to leaching and emissions, as well as improving long-term nutrient uptake by the soil microorganisms.

It believed that these two technologies i.e. nanotechnology and ultrasonication can enrich agriculture and food sector with their positive effects. In the food industry the combination of nano-materials and ultrasound represents a very useful and promising processing technique, involving sound waves, their properties, and their effects on chemical, physical, and biological systems. Both technologies have the potential to transform the food industry by changing the way food is produced, processed, packaged, transported, and consumed. Hence, the current chapter focuses on the applications of ultrasonication and nanotechnology in improving the agriculture and food production along with it positive and negative impact of agriculture and food sectors.

2.2 Ultrasonication in Agriculture and Food Production

When ultrasound is applied to foods the ultrasonic agitation by sound waves with more than 20 kHz frequency breaks coarse droplets into nano-emulsions. Acoustic waves applied by sonotrode produce mechanical vibration and acoustic cavitation, and with the collapse of cavitations, strong shock waves generated break the coarse droplets (Behrend et al. 2000). An outstanding application of high intensity ultrasound is in the formation of nano-emulsions. High intensity ultrasound has been used to prepare nano-emulsions of essential oils. The bioactivity of the essential oil was increased by nano-emulsion. Further, increase in the antibacterial activity could be observed by decreasing the nano-emulsion droplet size.

Aggregates contained in food molecules are broken into smaller structures by the ultrasonic radiation. In this way, ultrasound treatment reduces particle size of myofibrillar proteins which consequently enhanced solubility of muscle proteins (Amiri et al. 2018). Since solubility is a prerequisite for other functional properties, water holding capacity, emulsifying and foaming properties as well as gel strength improved considerably after sonication. Sonication techniques are user-friendly and induce the ultra-high surface area to form disperse particles of nanometer size.

Ultrasound is currently extensively used in different areas of nano-chemistry and related fields of nano-technology, as a principal or assisting technique. Its main advantages in comparison to conventional mixing are faster processes, higher yields, and the possibility of fabrication of novel compounds, substances or materials, which are impossible or difficult to obtain via classic interactions (Kharissova et al. 2011). Kehinde et al. (2020) published an excellent review on the recent nano-, micro- and macro-technological applications of ultrasonication in food-based systems. In their review, they made an analytic exploration of recent researches and designs regarding ultrasound methodology and equipment on diverse food systems. The relative effects of ultrasonication on food formulations, components and attributes such as nano-emulsions, nano-capsules, proteins, micronutrients, sensory and mechanical characteristics are evaluatively delineated (Table 2.1).

Agri-food issues are focused on the sustainability and protection of food produced in agriculture, including crops for human consumption and animal feed. In this chapter some potential uses and benefits of nano-technology in agricultural production are mentioned and they include: nano-formulations of agrochemicals to apply pesticides and fertilizers for the improvement of crops, the application of nano-sensors and nano-biosensors in the protection of crops for the identification of diseases and agrochemical residues, nano-devices for the genetic manipulation of

Table 2.1 Recent studies on the effects of ultrasonication in food nano-material fabrication

Food product	Observations	References
Water buffalo milk	Reduction of fat globule diameter by up to 92% (sub-micron level).	Abesinghe et al. (2019)
Whipped cream	Denaturation of protein chains, fragmentation of fat globules	Amiri et al. (2018)
Whey protein	Decrease of α-helix, exposing tryptophan residues.	Cheng et al. (2018)
Milk fat / rapeseed oil	Acceleration of the crystallization process, reduction in crystal size.	Gregersen et al. (2019)
Skim milk	Less cohesive structure and more compact microgel particles.	Körzendörfer et al. (2019)
Micellar casein concentrate	Increased surface hydrophilicity, reduced particle size, changes in structure.	Zhang et al. (2018)
Soybean globulin	Reduced surface tension, increased the emulsifying activity	Liu et al. (2020)
Astaxanthin, a food colorant	Reduced particle size, ower loss of antioxidant activity, greater stability.	Flores-Miranda et al. (2020)
Meat curing	Increased salt transfer and improved sensory characteristics of pork.	Contreras-Lopez et al. (2020)
Soft cheese	Increased protein content and cheese physicochemical properties.	Carrillo-Lopez et al. (2020)
Pectin	Modified physiochemical properties, improved emulsification stability and encapsulation.	Wang et al. (2019)
Modified starch	Improved mechanochemical quality of modified starch.	Zhang et al. (2020)
Soursop fruit	Improved biocomponents extraction.	Aguilar-Hernández et al. (2020)

plants and diagnosis of plant diseases (Zhao et al. 2016; Kumar et al. 2017; Fraceto et al. 2015), postharvest handling, food processing and storage, nano-feed additives (Sekhon 2014) and longer product shelf life (Hernández-Muñoz et al. 2019), as well as applications in veterinary medicine, animal health and other areas of animal production (Scott 2005; Bollo 2007; Narducci 2007).

2.2.1 *Nano-Technology in Agriculture*

One of the keys to improve consumer acceptance is raising awareness of nanotechnology in the agri-food sector, including feed and food ingredients, smart packaging and rapid detection systems. On the basis of studies in terms of antioxidant capacity, antibacterial properties and toxicological studies (He et al. 2019), concerns have arisen regarding the safety of nano-materials. Also, the commercialization of food based on nano-particles requires more research and industries must demonstrate that these technologies do not have a negative impact on the environment (FDA 2014).

Nano-transporters such as poly (ε-caprolactone) nano-capsules are being developed to carry herbicides such as atrazine. Experimentally, the improvement in herbicidal activity has been observed in treatments of model plants such as mustard (*Brassica juncea*) compared to commercial atrazine (Fraceto et al. 2015). Other nano-transporters designed with Mesoporous silica (Torney et al. 2007) and polymer nano-particles (Kumar et al. 2017) have also been developed as a controlled release system for pesticides. Torney et al. (2007) studied mesoporous silica nano-particles (3 nm size) as transporters of DNA and chemical substances, inside plant cells. Mesoporous silica particles are chemically coated and they can serve as gene containers, that can be integrated into plants. This coating causes the capacity of the plant to capture and transport the particles through the wall and membrane of the cell. There, they are inserted and activate the biological genes in a precise and controlled way, without causing any toxic side effect. This technique has also been successfully applied to introduce nano-particles in pumpkins and DNA to tobacco and corn plants (Corredor et al. 2009).

Nano-scale carriers can be used to achieve slow release of these products and apply the principles of strategies known as "precision agriculture", observing improvements in crop yields without damaging soil and water (Duhan et al. 2017). Other research is focusing on nano-transporters that allow the transfer of genes or DNA from plants to develop insect-resistant varieties (Sekhon 2014; Khot et al. 2012). Nano-materials such as metal oxide compounds (ZnO, TiO_2 and CuO) have been studied extensively in relation to their protective effect of diseases in plants produced by pathogens, due to their potent intrinsic toxicity (Duhan et al. 2017).

Silver nano-particles (Ag-NPs) have been experimented as pesticides to reduce the burden of pests on crops. Studies of the biological synthesis of Ag-NPs from white radish (*Raphanus sativus var. Aegyptiacus*) in sizes from 6 to 38 nm, has shown a 20% mortality against the land snail (Ali et al. 2015). In another investigation using Ag-NPs from culture of *Serratia sp* (BHU-S4) in wheat plants, an effective antifungal activity against *Bipolaris sorokiniana*, a pathogen causing stain disease, was reported (Mishra et al. 2014). Similar investigation with Ag-NPs of *Serratia sp* (BHU-S4) in wheat plants demonstrated antifungal activitiy against *Bipolaris sorokiniana*, pathogen responsible of the spot disease (Mishra et al. 2014). In fenugreek seeds (*Trigonella foenum-graecum*) the application of different concentrations of Ag-NPs (0, 10, 20, 30 and 40 μg/mL) revealed a significant improve in the germination potential, mean germination time, seed germination index, seed vigor index, fresh seedling weight and dry weight (Hojjat 2015).

Zinc oxide nano-particles (ZnO-NPs) have been shown to have better antimicrobial activity than large zinc particles. The low size (less than 100 nm) and a high surface-volume ratio of nano-particles allow better interaction with bacteria. They affect the development and performance of crops and accumulate in plant tissues, including edible parts (Rajput et al. 2018). According to Capaldi Arruda et al. (2015) nano-particles could directly decompose in the soil and produce ions, which can be incorporated into the plant system. The uptake mechanism of nano-particles is generally considered as an active transport mechanism that includes several other cellular processes such as signaling, recycling and regulation of the plasma membrane (Etxeberria et al. 2009). They have also been shown to induce free radical formation in wheat, resulting in increased malondialdehyde and lower levels of reduced glutathione (Panda et al. 2003) and reduced chlorophyll content (Aarti et al. 2006).

In tomato seedlings, ZnO-NPs have been reported to induce oxidative stress by promoting the antioxidant enzyme against stress to salinity (Li et al. 2016; Rajput et al. 2015). The toxicological effect of ZnO-NPs on buckwheat (*Fagopyrum esculentum*) at high concentrations (10–2000 mg/L) revealed a biomass drop, damaged cells from the root surface and an abnormal defense induction against ROS (Lee et al. 2013). Boonyanitipong et al. (2011) observed that ZnO-NPs reduced the number of roots and atrophied the length of rice seedlings (*Oryza sativa L*) while Raskar and Laware (2014) found that ZnO-NP inhibited chlorophyll biosynthesis, as well as photosynthesis efficiency in Arabidopsis.

Another study by Zafar et al. (2016) demonstrated the effects of nano-particles on germination and growth of Brassica nigra shoots. Wang et al. (2016) investigated the effect of different doses (0, 50, 100, 200, 250, and 300 mg/L of ZnO-NP) with a particle size <50 nm on biomass accumulation and photosynthesis in Arabidopsis. Compared to the control, plants exposed to 300 mg/L ZnO-NPs showed an 80% reduction in growth along with a 50% reduction in chlorophyll content. There was also a 50% reduction in the net photosynthesis rate, leaf stomatal conductance, intercellular CO_2 concentration, and transpiration rate. ZnO-NPs and their ionic salts can be toxic during the early stages of development and growth of corn and cabbage (Pokhrel and Dubey 2013). Future research on the use of ZnO-NPs in plants, distribution and incorporation into the environment, should be within the current risk assessments associated with ZnO-NPs to safeguard plant-animal-human functioning.

Titanium dioxide is a photocatalyst used in the manufacture of pigments (Sang et al. 2014) whose function is to stimulate the production of more carbohydrates, promoting growth and the rate of photosynthesis in plants (Owolade and Ogunleti 2008; Chen et al. 2014). It also has photocatalytic activity to degrade pesticides (Pelaez et al. 2012). Titanium dioxide nano-particles (TiO_2-NPs) have been synthesized from the aqueous extract of the *Psidium guajava* leaf, spherical nano-particles with an average size of 32–58 nm (Santhoshkumar et al. 2014). These nano-particles were tested against *Aeromonas hydrophila* (MTCC-1739), *Proteus mirabilis* (MTCC-442), *Escherichia coli* (MTCC-1677), *Staphylococcus aureus* (MTCC-3160) and *Pseudomonas aeruginosa* (MTCC-4030) bacteria. The maximum zone of inhibition was observed against *Staphylococcus aureus* (25 mm) and *Escherichia coli* (23 mm) when titanium dioxide nano-particles were used at a concentration of 20 μg/ml.

Foliar application of 10 mg/L TiO_2-NPs on *Vigna radiata L.* was found to be more environmentally friendly fertilizer, and also resulted in significant increase in stem length (17.02%), root length (49.6%), root area (43%), root nodules (67.5%), chlorophyll content (46.4%) and total soluble protein (94%) (Raliya, Biswas and Tarafdar 2015). In addition, copper is characterized by being a very abundant conductor metal, which has excellent physical, chemical and antibacterial properties (Carrillo et al. 2016; Shende et al. 2015). Unlike other antimicrobial metals, it has a broad spectrum of action against fungi and phytopathogenic bacteria (Betancourt et al. 2014).

It has also been reported efficacy of antifungal and antibacterial activity in zinc nano-particles for the growth of fungi such as *Fusarium graminearum, Aspergillus flavus, A. niger, A. fumigatus, F. culmorum and F. oxysporium* (Dimkpa et al. 2013; Rajiv et al. 2013). Other products such as nano-scale micronutrients (Mn, Cu, Fe, Zn, Mo, Ni and B) have an important application in the development of nano-fertilizers, reporting an improvement in nutrient absorption efficiency and avoiding losses as it happens with mineral products when applied a conventional manner (Dimkpa and Bindraban 2018). Other nano-materials including carbon nano-onions, also known as onion-like carbon or multi-layered fullerenes, and chitosan nano-particles alleged to improve the growth and quality of the crops, however, studies are still needs to carry out to assess their biosecurity (Tripathi et al. 2017; Khalifa and Hasaneen 2018).

2.2.2 Nano-Technology in Food Packaging

In the food sector, nano-technology is focusing on the improvement of packaging design, through intelligent packaging based on nano-sensors and polymer films of antibacterial and antifungal nano-composites that help to improve the safety and quality of food (Hernández-Muñoz et al. 2019). Nano-technology in the design of food packaging is based on the use of materials whose particles have at least one dimension within the nanometric scale (10^{-9} m), conventionally between 1 and 100 nm (Jeevanandam et al. 2018).

The classification of nano-materials is complex, however, three criteria can be distinguished (Villena de Francisco and Garcia-Estepa 2018):

1. Classification according to its origin. They are classified into: (a) natural nano-materials, e.g. ocean spray (O'Dowd et al. 2004) and nano-metric materials from combustion processes such as forest fires and volcanic ash (Oberdörster et al. 2005). (b) Involuntary nano-materials generated by human activity, such as internal combustion engines, thermal power plants and other sources of thermal degradation (Oberdörster et al. 2005; Tiede et al. 2008). (c) Artificial or manufactured: inorganic, used in food and food packaging and organic, to improve nutritional value (Cameán et al. 2010; FAO/WHO 2010). Engineered nano-materials are intentionally produced using nano-technology through the approach of different methods: "top down", a mechanical and physical particle production processes, is the manufacturing method that reduces the size of larger materials; This is done through processes such as crushing or grinding; Materials such as metal oxides are pulverized using high-energy ball mills until a nano-structure has been produced (Raab et al. 2011). A major disadvantage is that this approach

requires a large amount of energy and produces waste (Mendoza and Rodríguez-López 2007). The "bottom-up" approach is self-assembly of individual components (atoms or molecules), using physical and chemical techniques or gas and liquid phase. It includes aerosol processes, sol-gel processes, precipitation reactions, and methods such as gas condensation, chemical vapor deposition, chemical vapor condensation, and solvothermic and sonochemical methods (Charitidis et al. 2014; Rajput 2015). The disadvantage of chemical synthesis of nanomaterials is that the desired crystalline forms are often not configurable and that the thermal stability of the powder product is less. The advantage is that the liquid phase allows the production of highly porous materials.

2. Classification according to the United States Environmental Protection Agency (EPA 2017). EPA recently classified engineered nano-materials according to their chemical composition and physical disposition of the material: carbon-based, either spherical, ellipsoidal, cylindrical, or nanotube; metal or metal oxide-based, usually nanoscale spherical particles consisting wholly or partially of one or more metals; dendrimers which are repeatedly branched molecules, typically symmetrical and spherical, that provide internal cavities for other molecules and quantum dots that are nano-crystalline semiconductors, usually metal complexes, selenides or sulfides.
3. Classification according to the food industry (FSAI 2008) (Table 2.2). Nanoparticles: they can be distinguished by their chemical characteristics, their ability to transport different ingredients and react against environmental conditions, whether organic or inorganic. Nanofibers: They have a diameter of approximately 5 nm and a length of more than 15 μm and are used as thickeners in food and filtering agents. Nano-emulsions: between 50 and 500 nm per drop, which gives them rheological characteristics and variable stability. They are used to stabilize some ingredients, increase viscosity, and encapsulate components for later release. Nanoclay: typically made of phosphosilicate and used primarily in food packaging, as it acts as a barrier against oxygen and carbon dioxide. With nanoclay it is possible to create lighter, thinner and stronger plastic.

Nanofibre and nano-layers materials are used as reinforcement fillers in most polymeric nano-composites, while nano-particulate materials are more used for the development of active and intelligent nano-composite such as antimicrobial, oxygen scavengers (Xiao et al. 2004; Emamifar 2011) and biosensors that can detect changes related to deterioration, the presence of pathogens and chemical contaminants, and therefore provide real-time status of the freshness of food. This reflects important changes in the packaging industry. However, many of the applications of nano-technology are currently in a stage of development and most require research to ensure safety in their application (Ranjan et al. 2014).

Table 2.2 Types of nano-materials and their application in food

Nano-materials	Application/function	Challenges	References
Nano-particles Silver (Ag) Titanium dioxide (TiO_2) Magnesium oxide (MgO) Copper oxide (CuO) Zinc oxide (ZnO)	Improved bioavailability and antimicrobial activity. Nano-particles of those metals and metal oxides are also, in general, excellent antimicrobial activity sorbents, catalysts, sensors and reducing agents	Development of novel materials designed for active and intelligent packages. Effect on consumer health	Huang et al. (2011), Du et al. (2010), Hernández-Muñoz et al. (2019)
Nano-additives	Protect animals against mycotoxicosis		Hassan et al. (2013), Gholami-Ahangaran and Zia-Jahromi (2014), Mouhamed et al. (2015)
Nano-liquid vitamins	Mixed for in poultry and livestock feed and nano-particles that act by eliminating pathogens in the gastrointestinal tract	Increase their bioavailability compared with conventional formulations	FAO/WHO (2010)
Metal nanoparticles	Added to feed (livestock and poultry) for their antimicrobial properties and positive effects on growth	More studies on the migration of Nano-particles	Fondevila et al. (2009), Andi et al. (2011), Sahoo et al. (2014), Swain et al. (2016)
Organic Nano-particles			
Protein	Nano-encapsulation of hydrophobic nutraceuticals. Improved functionalities (gelation, heat stability)		Semo et al. (2007)
Polymeric	Nano-encapsulation and improved functionalities (delivery, antimicrobial)		Chen and Subirade (2005)
Nano-fibres Globular proteins	Improved functionalities (Thermal stability, thickening agent, shelf life)	The sustainability and recycling of nano-packages also has to be considered. Regulatory authorities	Fernandez et al. (2009)
Nano-emulsions Oil in water	Nano-encapsulation and regulated release of bioactive agents and nutrients		Huang et al. (2010)

(continued)

Table 2.2 (continued)

Nano-materials	Application/function	Challenges	References
Nanoclays Montmorillonite (mmt)	Improved properties in packaging (barrier, thermal, durability)	Information to evaluate the safety of nano-composites applied to food packaging. Development of standardized procedures to determine the impact of nano-particles in human health.	Avella et al. (2005)

Adopted and modified from FSAI (2008), Ramachandraiah et al. (2015) and Hernández-Muñoz et al. (2019)

2.2.3 *Nano-Technology in Food Processing*

The use of nano-materials as ingredients or part in formulations, offers great advantages in the processing of food. These ingredients are inorganic compounds such as SiO_2, MgO and TiO_2, which provide advantages in the heterogeneity of the consistency of the ingredients, avoiding altering their physical properties and even reducing the conservation of flavors that are not appreciable by the consumer. For example, TiO_2 nano-particles are widely used as food additives, such as chewing gum, sauces, sweets and puddings (Weir et al. 2012). They also play an important role in the animal feed industry, such as nutritional supplementation with copper oxide, iron and zinc oxide recognized by the Food and Drug Administration (FDA) and the European Food Safety Authority (EFSA), without representing any subsequent risk to the consumer (EFSA 2016).

Nano-particles of inorganic compounds have important catalytic properties as a consequence of their large chemical activity of their surface. By changing their original shapes and adopting polyhedral forms, the number of edges and corners increase. This led to an increase of their solubility and consequently their absorption capacity also increases. Photocatalysis is a particular case of the catalytic behavior of nano-particles. For instance, zinc oxide (ZnO), exposes a wide spectrum of biocidal activity towards different bacteria, fungi and viruses. This activity is due to the production of reactive oxygen species and the release of zinc ions (Zn^{2+}). Furthermore, the synthesis of this metallic oxide by green chemical routes grants it with a higher bioactivity which is attributed to a larger surface area (Ma et al. 2014), higher absorption capacity (Qian et al. 2015), crystallinity and transmission. On the other hand, metallic copper nano-particles formation and stabilization are complex processes.

Copper oxide (Cu_2O) is more frequently used. These copper ions can damage the bacterial cell membrane, enter cells and modify their enzymatic function, leading to microbial death (Ren et al. 2009). The photocatalytic activity of titanium oxide (TiO_2), is an electro-chemical and photo-electrochemical reaction starting when radiation is able to excite a semiconductor, to the point of making it to behave like a conductor. When radiation hits, photons from the valence band (VB) of TiO_2, electrons move to the conduction band (CB), generating oxide-reduction reactions. The photocatalysis process is described in Fig. 2.1.

Nano-particles and nanotubes are used as gelling and foaming agents, with the particularity that silver nano-particles help eliminate pathogens and chemicals (Kumar 2015) from surfaces in contact with food and kitchen utensils made of stainless steel (Chen et al. 2010). Nano-particles are also used in other processes such as nano-filtration, the main technology for water purification, where they are capable of eliminating heavy metals, organic matter and organic and inorganic substances (Sekhon 2014). Also, in drinking water treatment plants materials such as

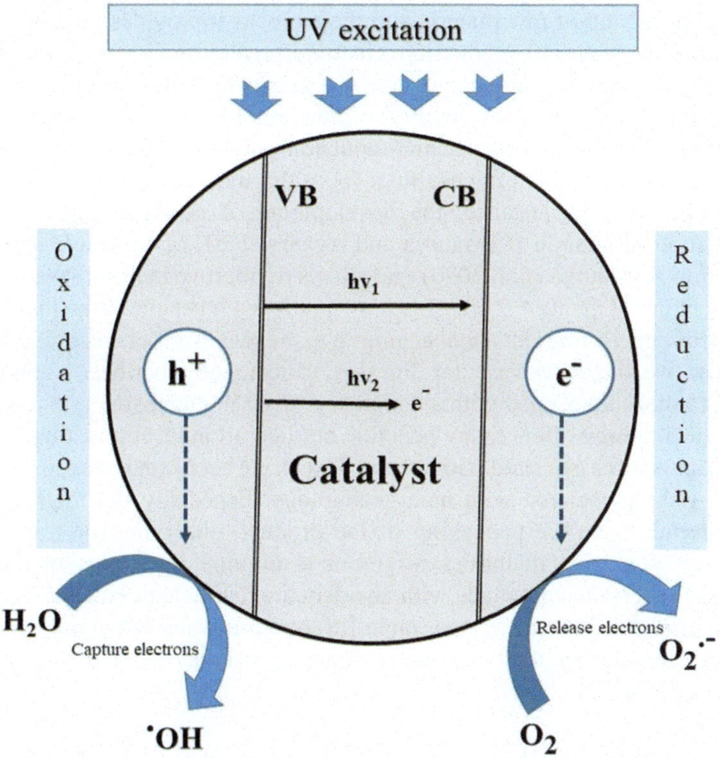

Fig. 2.1 Photo-catalysis process begins with the excitation of a semiconductor particle (Catalyst) by UV rays. Under these stimulation conditions, electron-hole pairs are created by the excitation of electrons from valence band (VB) to conduction band (CB). Electron-hole pairs average life ranges in some picoseconds. During this time, they must migrate to the surface and generate highly reactive free radicals that react with the surrounding species through oxidation-reduction processes. Electron-hole pairs that fail to separate and react with species on the surface recombine and the energy dissipates. Electron-hole pairs are able to break some molecular bonds and reducing or oxidizing them to make them less complex species. (Adopted and modified from Ashkarran et al. (2014) and Betancur et al. (2016))

carbon nanotubes and alumina fibers are used in combination with activated carbon, to remove organic matter from municipal wastewater effluent (Kazner et al. 2008).

In the food industry, nano-filtration has multiple applications. Fruit juices have traditionally been concentrated by vacuum evaporation, which results in a loss of fresh juice aroma, color changes and a cooked flavor due to thermal effects. Nano-filtration techniques allow obtaining products very similar to fresh ones, reducing and simplifying the clarification process (Sotoft et al. 2012). These technologies are also used in the dairy industry for the concentration of serum and demineralization (Cuartas-Uribe et al. 2007; Suárez et al. 2009), separation of lactic acid (Li et al. 2008) and recovery of lactose (Cuartas-Uribe et al. 2010). Another application is the use of nano-silica to filter and eliminate substances that produce a sour taste in some plant extracts (Noormans 2010).

The use of nano-materials in food provides many benefits along the food chain, from the production of raw materials to the table, as it provides greater security in the intermediate stages of production, ensuring greater quality control of the products mainly through the detection of external agents by nano-sensors. It also allows to innovate products, with the creation of new ingredients or food supplements by means of nano-encapsulation or nano-emulsions, achieving a slow release of some compounds and even obtaining healthier foods through the improvement of organoleptic properties. For instance, the development of new techniques for micro-encapsulation of vitamin D (Maurya and Aggarwal 2017a, b; Maurya et al. 2019) and Vitamin A (Maurya et al. 2020) that allows to improve their bio-availability and the nutrient enrichment of food. This may guarantee a benefit in the human health, derived from micro-nutrients intake, aiming to prevent disorders resulting from neurodegenerative and cardiovascular illnesses, cancer, and other health conditions, in addition to those associated with a deficiency in the metabolism.

Nano-technology offers many benefits, but like all innovations, there are disadvantages and risks associated with its use. Tests have been conducted, evaluating the potential risks associated with nano-technology. Especially the migration of the nano-materials from the packaging of the product, observing the transfer to the food; however, in small quantities, migration is minimal. In conclusion, the changes in the food sector must be made with an adequate risk-benefit balance in the use of nano-materials, and in most cases, more information is needed about the risks and an optimal regulation that guarantees food security (Villena de Francisco and Garcia-Estepa 2018).

2.2.4 Nano-Technology in Animal Production

The applications of nano-technology in animals health are identified around four areas: (1) administration of medicines, nutrients, probiotics, supplements and other substances; (2) diagnosis and treatment of diseases with nanoparticles that allow the detection and elimination of the causal agent of the disease; (3) identity registration that allows the traceability of an animal and its products; and (4) management of reproduction with hormonal immunosensors (Kuzma 2010; Scott 2005). In the area of pathogen detection many sensors have been developed to detect bacteria. The microfluidic system has been widely used for bacterial analysis because it has shown many advantages, such as analyzing a sample with small reagent volumes in a short time and processing multiple samples in a single device (Wibowo et al. 2018). On the other hand, Shaibani et al. (2016) reported the detection of colibacteries by electrochemical method that uses a sensor with polyvinyl alcohol hydrogel (PVA) nanofibers that acts as a protective layer. Changes in the pH of the media indicate the presence of *E. coli* in a water sample.

The company Illuminaria has developed a system called NanoDetect for the rapid detection and portable analysis of DNA. This system is based on nanotechnology that combines PCR to rapidly detect pathogens in real time and in situ (Kuzma 2010). Other nanoscale projects have evaluated the immunomagnetic capacity of *Salmonella typhimirium* in the skin of chickens (Duncanson 2004), concluding that the integrated system with both the ability to detect and eliminate pathogens before or during food processing could bring great benefits in reducing the risk of foodborne diseases.

In the detection of viruses such as foot-and-mouth disease, which generated severe consequences in countries such as the United Kingdom, the use of gold film nano-structures (nano-materials are linked in a portable detector) has been investigated to increase sensitivity to detection of the virus before presenting the symptoms of the disease. This could have great benefits for animal health and the economic security of farmers (Israel 2002). Other nano-materials such as chitosan nano-particles have antimicrobial capacity for the treatment of bovine mastitis (*Staphylococcus aureus*), causing damage to the membrane of bacterial cells without affecting the viability of bovine cells (Orellano et al. 2019).

In the management of animal feed, compounds such as zinc oxide prevent diarrhea in piglets, ensuring minimal weight loss and better performance. However, high doses of this compound result in a high level of excretion in the environment. The application of nano-technology from zinc oxide nano-products guarantees minimal weight loss at lower doses, with less environmental excretion (Sekhon 2014). In another study, silver nano-particles were evaluated as additives in diets for weaned pigs, and their effect on digestive microbiota and intestinal morphology, productive yields and silver retention in tissues; the results showed that the effect of silver is mediated according to its antimicrobial properties, acting against certain bacterial groups or simply reducing the microbial load of the small intestine (Fondevila et al. 2009). Applications of magnetic nano-particles have been found for the recovery of aflatoxin B_1 and zearalenone from food, using monoclonal antibodies (Kim et al. 2012).

In the area of genetic engineering, silica nano-particles have been evaluated, showing an ability to improve DNA absorption in mammalian cells compared to other transfer systems that are not viruses (Luo et al. 2004). The use of nanotechnology for the transference of DNA could provide benefits to animal health, however, the issue involves social responsibility, ethics and probably subject to the same laws as transgenic animals (Luo et al. 2004).

Ensuring the traceability of animals prevents the spread of diseases, preserve identity and track the product throughout the supply chain. The detection by means of nano-sensors, with the combination of probes of oligononucloetides using photonano-lithography, can detect genes specific for cytochrome b to identify multiple species in a sample. The application has been destined to the feed and food industries (Kuzma 2010). It has also been proposed the use of nanobarcodes, designed from particles that are made of metals such as platinum, gold, silver and nickel, to track animal byproducts at points of sale and ensure that they do not end up in animal feed (Jayarao et al. 2009).

In animal reproduction, the development of nano-biosensors pretends to improve the technical management. Nano-biosensors are created by nano-materials such as nano-particles, nano-tubes, nano-wires and nano-fibers (Silva 2014). Nanotubes implanted under the skin of animals have the ability to bind and help to detect estradiol antibody at estrus, by near-infrared fluorescence. The signal from this sensor is integrated into a monitoring central, as a small part of a more complex control system to monitor and activate a reproductive program of an herd (Kuzma 2010; Scott 2005). The development and validation of these nano-biosensors is important as a promising tool for reproductive management. However, these advances must ultimately come to the real chain production. This will help researchers and professionals in the development of new food products for the demanding market (Silva 2014).

2.2.5 Nanotechnology Future Trends in Food and Agriculture

In animal production, the most important benefits of nano-technology are reported in the efficiency for the use of nutrients, health management, traceability and management of animal reproduction. Nano-technology in animal reproduction is an emerging field that offers opportunities to provide new solutions to old problems and has the potential to demonstrate continued progress in the years to come. In the food sector, nano-technologies surpass conventional technologies in food processing, avoiding contamination, providing advantages in the design of smart packaging, food preservation, improvement in product quality and favoring its shelf life. The use of nano-sensors to control the quality of crops, food and some commonly used practices in managing animal production will continue to be investigated. The development of nano-materials in the agricultural sector and in animal production considering the production chain from handling, processing, packaging, security and storage improves the bioavailability of food.

Future prospects for nanotechnology in agriculture and animal production should focus on continuing to investigate the possible effects of toxicity, the mechanisms of action of nano-materials and their possible effect as an environmental pollutant. It is essential to emphasize the potential effects in terms of nano-toxicology and nano-security. With the aim of improving public acceptance and compliance with health regulations to guarantee its application at all levels of the production chain.

2.3 Ultrasound and Nano-Technology Application to Improve Meat Quality

Despite there is a huge gap of research in the combination of both technologies, high-intensity ultrasound and nano-technology applied directly in meat, there are clear examples of potential uses of both technologies to improve the sanitary, sensorial and technological quality of meat. Some of the most relevant applications of nano-emulsions into the food industry include their use for decontamination of equipment, packaging and food itself. One of the most promising area for nanotechnology application has been in meat packaging production (Ranjan et al. 2014).

2.3.1 Ultrasound in Food Systems

High-intensity ultrasound applied in food science has been used to cause mechanical, physical or chemical changes in the exposed food (Chemat and Zill-E-Huma 2011). The most studied phenomenon of ultrasonicating food is the cavitation. A production of gas bubbles in liquid media, as a result of compression and decompression forces that over as implosion of bubbles, generating physical forces and increase of temperature in the liquid (Luque-Garcia and Luque de Castro 2001). Multiple effects of cavitation on foods are described, from molecular to microscopic structural changes (Ozuna et al. 2015; Suslick and Flannigan 2008). The nutrients in food that are more studied under high intensity ultrasound forces are the proteins. Animal protein have been modified structurally and functionally under particular conditions of ultrasonication (Chandrapala et al. 2012a, b). Molecular changes promoted by cavitation may lead to denaturation, aggregation, increase of hydrophobicity and emulsion stability (Arzeni et al. 2012).

On the other side, the use of nano-technology in foods is impacting the industry from food safety to synthesis of new products and ingredients (Chen et al. 2006). The applications are classified into four main groups; products, processing technology, food safety and security, and materials (Fig. 2.2). Nano-emulsions production for encapsulation and delivery of compounds, and nano-products for incorporation in food packaging, have been reported to be some of the major fields of nanotechnology applied to food industry, and that includes meat industry (Ranjan et al. 2014; Nile et al. 2020).

2.3.2 Nano-Technology and Ultrasound in Meat

The use of high intensity ultrasound for nano-emulsions is an emerging field of study. High intensity ultrasound has shown to improve the stability of nanoemulsions during storage and the functionality of the emulsions in the foods. One of

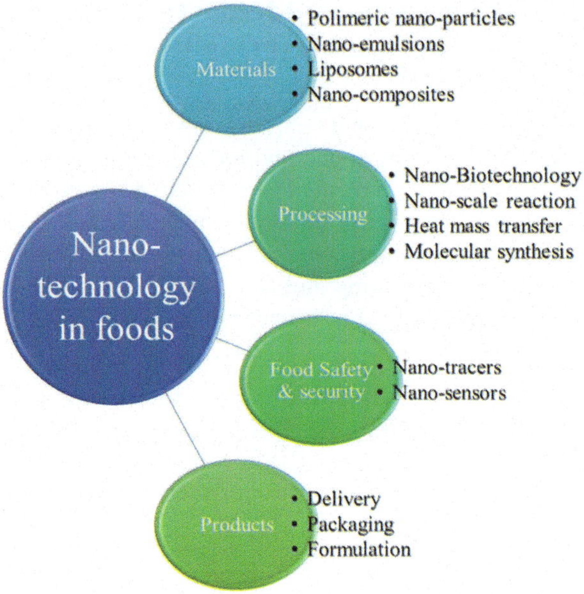

Fig. 2.2 Overview of nano-structures in food and their application in food science. (Adopted and modified with permission Pathakoti et al. (2017) and Nile et al. (2020))

the most notable study applying both technologies on meat is described by Ojha et al. (2017). They aimed to modify the fatty acid profile of pork. Hence, they combined the two novel technologies such as nano-encapsulation and ultrasound to investigate the ability of high intensity ultrasound to enhance the diffusion of micro-encapsulated fatty acids into the meat. Muscle *Semitendinousus* was submerged in a suspension of nano-vesicles of fish oil, and ultrasonicated at 25 kHz for either 30 or 60 min. Ultrasonication increased long chain omega-3 polyunsaturated fatty acids (PUFAn3) eicosapentaenoic acid (C20:5n3), docosapentaenoic acid (C22:5n3), and docosahexaenoic acid C22:6n3) into meat. They also observed that iltrasonication (60 min) of meat can not only reduce the thrombogenic index (tendency to form clots into vessels) from 1.07 to 0.81 as well as omega-6/-3 ratio which resulted in the improvement of fatty acid profile in the meat.

High intensity ultrasound has been considered as an important alternative for reducing nano-size of animal proteins. Particularly, bovine gelatin and egg white protein. O'Sullivan et al. (2016), ultrasonicated 50 ml aliquots of both animal proteins solutions for up to 2 min at an intensity of ~34 W/cm^2, using a 12 mm diameter probe attached to the ultrasonic processor. Later, they measured the size of molecules by dynamic light scattering and characterized the molecular structure by sodium dodecyl sulfate polyacrylamide gel electrophoresis. Their findings indicated that high intensity ultrasound significantly reduces ($P < 0.05$) protein size as sonication time increases with no reduction on the primary structure. After a sonication of 1 min there is minimal further reduction in protein size. They attributed this to disruption of the hydrophobic and electrostatic interactions which maintain untreated protein aggregates from the high hydrodynamic shear forces associated with ultrasonic cavitation. Further, emulsions with the ultrasonicated proteins had smaller droplet size in concentrations >1% (W/V) in comparison with untreated proteins.

Mahdi Jafari et al. (2006) tested the efficiency of high intensity ultrasound to produce nano-emulsions and compared against microfluidization, one of the best recognized methods to produce emulsions. They produced an oil-in water nano-emulsion of d-limonene for microencapsulation, finding the same size of emulsion (150–700 nm) between treatments. However, size was reduced as time of sonication was increased and high intensity ultrasound was more convenient in terms of operations and cleaning. D-limonene has been shown to be an excellent antimicrobial, it maintains oxidation stability and its dispersion in water is still maintained through microencapsulation. Besides, D-limonene has shown to reduce dramatically bacterial populations in foods. Particularly, D-limonene has reduced *Listeria monocytogenes* thermal resistance up to hundred times (Maté et al. 2016). In beef, D-limonene has been tried as an antimicrobial in packaging. When D-limonene proportion increases in the packs, the vapour permeability and oxygen transmission rate were reduced. Beef shelf-life was also increased by D-limonene. Particularly, total viable count, total coliform, *Pseudomonas spp.* and *Staphylococcus aureus* were reduced by limonene. The shelf life of the control sample and the sample packed with poly (lactic acid)-limonene (4%) was approximately 6 days while the samples packed with poly (lactic acid)-limonene at the concentration of 6 and 8% were assured for at least 9 and 12 days of storage (Sangkasanya et al. 2018). As the last example, many potential combinations of ultrasound and nano-technology may result on improvement of quality in beef.

The use of high intensity ultrasound for the production of nano-materials with potential integration in meat packaging is an evolving field of research. Active packaging is a current path to increase the shelf life of foods. One of the most problematic issues to attend while designing active packaging is to reduce the bacterial spoilage during the process and storage of food (Yildirim et al. 2018). Particularly in meat, some metallic nano-particles such as zinc oxide (ZnO nano-particles) have been prepared by ultrasonication (0.5; amplitude: 20%; time: 10 min). They showed to reduce microbial counts of mesophilic and psychotropic bacterial cells in cod fillets, when fillets were modified atmosphere packed with the ZnO nano-particles enclosed in the coating of the film for packaging. ZnO nano-particles had shown bactericidal effects for Gram-positive and Gram-negative bacteria. However, they also increased the functionality of the packs by improved quality parameters of the fillets such as; reduction of gumminess and adhesiveness, and increase of water retention during 72 and 144 h of storage (Mizielińska et al. 2018).

Other recent use of high intensity ultrasound in the food industry is the synthesis of nano-particles for application in the detection of contaminants in meat. Muthumariyappan et al. (2019), developed an ultrasound based sonochemical method to incorporate Perovskite-type barium titanate ($BaTiO_3$) nano-particles inside a layered and reduced graphene oxide sheets (rGOs). The ultrasound reduced the graphene oxide matrix and offered a sensor with an excellent response to detect ractopamine in meat. Ractopamine is a contaminant and toxic ingredient for human, which has been used as an animal growth promotor in many countries. Further, the sensor of ractopamine is also food toxic. Hence, the synthesis of the BaTiO3@rGOs, through sonochemistry, implies a double benefit for the meat industry.

More recently, Kehinde et al. (2020) published a broad review on the use of high-intensity ultrasound as nano, micro and macro application in the food industry. Their review includes a section on the limitations of the ultrasound technology in the food industry, which agrees with our own opinion. The high intensity ultrasound has a wide range of applications and benefits in the food industry. However, the major difficulty for adoption on an industrial scale is the lack of ultrasonication equipment for all the food processes with potential application (Nile et al. 2020).

On one hand, the scalability of ultrasonication equipment for the industrial use can be problematic due to the high cost of components and the scalability of the components in the equipment. Further, it implies a high cost of maintenance for an adequate functioning and for the damage control (Kehinde et al. 2020). Patist and Bates (2008) analysed the key learnings of escalating the ultrasonication from the laboratory to commercial production. They presented some business case examples of ultrasonication applications for defoaming, emulsification, extrusion, extraction, and waste treatment including; the investment and benefit (US k$/yr), and the payback time. They concluded that despite the high interest in the high intensity ultrasound technology and the benefits such as higher product yields, shorter processing times, and reduced operating and maintenance cost, the development of commercial ultrasonic equipment is slow and manufacturers are not willing to develop new designs.

On the other hand, there are some technical issues such as nutrient damaging during ultrasonication, that are a big concern for the food industry. At least three technological problems are reported with the use of high intensity ultrasound in foods; generation of free radicals and the subsequent oxidation of nutrients such as lipids or proteins, and proteins denaturation. Lipid oxidation in meat by high intensity ultrasound application has been recently reported. Thiobarbituric acid reactive substances value, an indicator of lipid oxidation, increases when beef muscles are ultrasonicated (11 W/cm^2), after 14 d of display (Peña-González et al. 2017). Furthermore, by high intensity ultrasound application (2.39, 6.23, 11.32 and 20.96 W/cm^2) during the curing process of beef, lipid oxidation can increase the double (from 0.6 to 1.2 mg of malonaldehyde acid/kg meat), compared to control samples (Kang et al. 2016). High intensity ultrasound has also shown to promote lipid oxidation in beef and pork. The oxidation of myosin, may increase the formation of cross-linking and production of free radicals that accelerate the oxidation of other proteins or meat components (Kang et al. 2016, 2017; Wang et al. 2018).

2.3.3 Ultrasonication Future Trends in Food and Agriculture

Nano-technology and high-intensity ultrasonication are two very encouraging technologies that are already used at different levels in the food industry. They both have been applied separately with a remarkable success in some processes of the meat industry. Nano-technology has been more widely applied in industrial processes, while high-intensity ultrasonication has shown promising results in laboratory trials and basic applications like material decontamination. Nevertheless, the combined application of both technologies remains limited, even at experimental levels. There is a gap of knowledge on their combined effect on meat and meat products. The emerging combination of the two technologies is centred around three main fields; nano-materials, food safety and security, and nano-products. Examples of successful combined applications are; a decrease in the size of animal proteins, the production of nano-emulsions for microencapsulation of antimicrobial components, the production of metallic nano-particles for improving the meat packaging, and the production of nano-particles of $BATiO_3$, as nano-sensors. Yet, there are technological and economical limitations related to the single application of each of these technologies, that could become major drawbacks when implementing a combination of two. Furthermore, there are practically no worldwide regulations or safety trials for the use of these technologies, which could be the most important concern when the number of implementations in the field or industry increases.

Despite the advances in the development of nano-technology and the application of ultrasound in the meat industry, as well as the favourable results and the promising expectations of both technologies applied in general in the food industry, attention should be given to the quickly increasing concern about the safety and health risks, and lack of experimental trials on the use of nano-technology in foods. The use of nano-technology in foods for human consumption must be validated, because this represents the largest knowledge gap. Another possible trend that may help to reduce the risk for human health is the development of bio-nano-products or bio-nanomaterials, resulting in an innocuous alternative for application in foods. A change in the way that biosynthesis for nano-technologies is utilized, at least in the food industry is another priority. However, if there are no direct implications of potential risk, the range of possibilities of the combined technologies in meat production and processing is unlimited. Combined technologies may help to increase efficiency in the meat production from the farm to the fork.

2.4 Ultrasound and Nano-Materials in the Dairy Industry

Ultrasound and the application of nano-materials in milk and milk products industry have evolved as two separate technologies. The ultrasound produces changes in the structural and functional properties of milk and its components due to the phenomenon of acoustic cavitation (Chandrapala et al. 2011, 2012a, 2013; Shanmugam et al. 2012; Nguyen and Anema 2017; Liu et al. 2014; Dahroud et al. 2016; Durnikin et al. 2016) while the application of nano-materials improves the quality and shelf life of milk, thanks to the development of packaging materials and, especially, to the encapsulation of bioactive compounds that can be released at specific sites (Ivanov and Rashevskaya 2011; Riley et al. 1999; Graveland-Bikker and de Kruif 2006; Dong et al. 2006; Ke and Yongping 2005; Akbari et al. 2006; Otte et al. 2005; Xiao et al. 2004; Moraru et al. 2003; Brody 2007; Seo et al. 2011; Ahn et al. 2013; Ahn and Kwak 2012; Ko 2012; Choi et al. 2012, 2014; Kim et al. 2014; Lee et al. 2015; Park et al. 2007, 2008, 2010). Although both technologies produce benefits in terms of the improvement in physical, chemical, sensory, structural and functional characteristics and properties of food, there are radical differences between them.

Ultrasound is a non-invasive physical technology, whose main advantages are that it does not cause secondary changes or unfavorable impacts associated with conventional thermal treatments, and it does not represent any risk to health (Dong et al. 2019; Alarcon-Rojo et al. 2018; Leong et al. 2017). On the other hand, nano-materials constitute materials whose synthesis can be by physical, chemical and / or biological route; only a few have the potential to be applied in dairy systems as there are controversy and consumer concern about possible negative effects, coupled with the limited research that exists on nano-structured materials in biological systems (in vivo) and their impact on the environment and in the long-term ecosystems (Jokar and Abdul Rahman 2014; Zhang et al. 2015; Carrillo-Lopez et al. 2014, 2016).

2.4.1 Ultrasound and Nano-Materials

The convergence of both technologies (ultrasound and nano-materials) is well recognized for many years, where the synthesis of nano-materials is carried out through the use of ultrasound as assisted technology, known as sonochemistry (Fig. 2.3). The advantage of sonochemistry for the production of nano-materials is that the extreme reaction conditions include extremely high temperatures and pressures (5000 °K and 1000 bar) during too short times (Suslick 1990), whose physical foundations are caused by the phenomenon of acoustic cavitation which consists of the formation, growth and collapse of bubbles and nebulization (Bang and Suslick 2010). On the other hand, the chemical effects of the ultrasound in water include the generation of free radicals (Ḥ and OḤ) that can recombine to form H_2 and H_2O_2.

The application of ultrasound in nanometric-sized food systems includes the development of nano-emulsions, smart packaging with nanoparticulate materials,

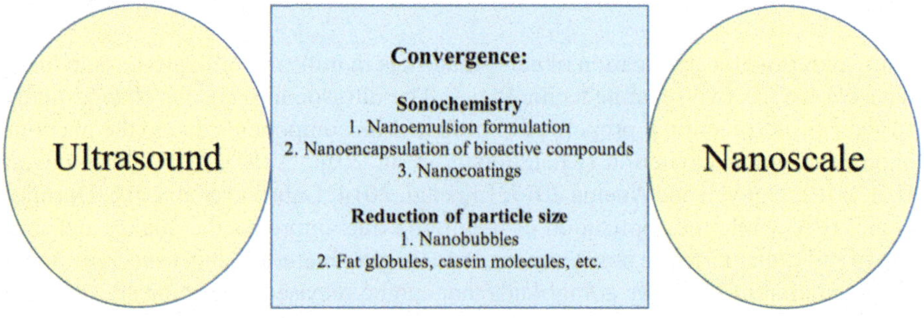

Fig. 2.3 Convergence of ultrasound and nano-technology as technologies with application in food

nano-polymers, nano-lipids, and nano-capsules that make nutrient bioavailability efficient (Jokar and Abdul Rahman 2014; Zhang et al. 2015). In this regard, nano-liposomes have been synthesized by ultrasonication as carriers for vitamin release (Bochicchio et al. 2016), the biocompatibility of curcumin nanoparticles as carriers of cancer drugs (Zhang et al. 2015), coatings based on zinc oxide nanoparticles for bacterial control of cod fillets (Mizielinska et al. 2018), and euemol and chitosan nano-emulsions have been formulated by ultrasound with antimicrobial and antioxidant functionalities (Shao et al. 2018).

A potential application of ultrasound is the reduction of particle size down to the nanometric level, Shabana et al. (2019) produced starch nanoparticles by applying ultrasound on potato starch. Nano-encapsulation of metabolites of interest for the development of functional foods continues to be a novel and interesting topic, such is the case of encapsulation of fatty acids for the improvement of the fatty acid profile in pork (Ojha et al. 2017). Finally, films with antioxidant and antimicrobial properties have been developed from essential oil clove and hazelnut meal protein emulsions (Gul et al. 2018). Regarding the joint nanotechnology and ultrasound application in milk and dairy products, Adhikari et al. (2019) reported the application of ultrasound (20 kHz, 20 s, 1 °C) in apple juice concentrate and whole milk to generate dissolved CO_2 nanobubbles, in order to improve freezing parameters. The results showed that at 2000 ppm CO_2 after 20 s, the nucleation time and freezing time decreased from 11.1 to 5.2 min and from 39.2 to 35.5 min, respectively.

2.4.2 *Effects on Milk and Dairy Products*

In the first instance, ultrasound has multiple potential applications in milk and milk products, most important are the emulsification and homogenization of milk beverages, including the fractionation of milk and the removal of layers of fat for the production of dairy products with lower fat content (Shanmugam et al. 2012; Nguyen and Anema 2017). The alteration of the casein micelles produces milk with smaller particle sizes, and improves the curd firmness (Chandrapala et al. 2011, 2013; Shanmugam et al. 2012; Liu et al. 2014). No less important are the fermented milk products, where the inoculation of milk with specific strains (mainly lactic acid bacteria) lowers the pH producing lactic acid and other metabolites that affect the taste of beverages (yogurt and probiotic beverages) and cheeses during the process of maturation (Dahroud et al. 2016; Durnikin et al. 2016). Table 2.3 summarizes the ultrasound applications of greatest relevance in milk and dairy products according to the modification of their components.

Nano-materials that have potential for application in food science and technology include nanoparticles, nano-emulsions, nanocomposites and nano-structured materials (Moraru et al. 2003), while nanosensors and nano-trades are used as part of food safety. In this regard, Maurya and Aggarwal (2019b), Maurya et al. (2019 and 2020) have documented various studies on encapsulated nano-particles as a tool to formulate effective vitamin D delivery systems, detailing the mode of action to

Table 2.3 Relevant applications of ultrasound in milk and dairy products

Modified component	Processing conditions	Results	References
Whey proteins	20 kHz, 450 W, 50% amplitude, 1–60 min	Greater denaturation during long sonication times (> 5 min). Minor changes in secondary structure and protein hydrophobicity.	Chandrapala et al. (2011)
Whey proteins, caseins and fat	20 kHz, 90 y 180 W, 15–60 min.	Denaturation of serum proteins, formation of micellar aggregates and disruption of serum proteins. Reduction of size of fat globule and casein molecules.	Shanmugam et al. (2012)
(-lactoalbumin and ®-lactoglobulin	20 kHz, 31 W, 50% amplitude, 1–60 min.	Exposure of thiol groups of β-lactoglobulin and interaction with α-lactalbumin disulfide bonds. Decrease in hydrophobicity and increase in the size of aggregates.	Chandrapala et al. (2012b)
Proteins	20 kHx, 31 W, 5 min.	Sonication before the addition of sodium pyrophosphate to casein systems forms a firm gel with low syneresis; and sonication after the addition of sodium pyrophosphate produces a weak gel with high syneresis.	Chandrapala et al. (2013)
Fat	22.5 kHz, 50 W	Homogenization of fat globules, its surface is stabilized by proteins, produces functional protein / fat complexes. Acidified and sonicated milk at <60 °C produces firm gels.	Nguyen and Anema (2017)
Proteins	20 kHz, 101 kW/m^2, 15 min., 30 °C	Ultrasonicated milk at pH 8.0 and readjusted to pH 6.7 before curing forms firm gels in less time.	Liu et al. (2014)
Metabolic activity of *Lactobacillus casei* subsp. Casei	20–60% amplitude, 15–60 s every 2 h	Greater production of lactic acid, cell reproduction and consumption of substrate.	Dahroud et al. (2016)
Lactococcus lactis, *Lactobacillus plantarum* and *Propionibacterium acidipropionici*	880 kHz, 0.1–0.7 W/cm^3, 100–120 s, 10 mL/s	Increase in cell biomass and in the production of lactic and propionic acid.	Durnikin et al. (2016)

improve bioavailability. Release systems reported in these reviews include those derived from lipids (liposomes, niosomes, nano-particles, and nano-emulsions) and polymers (micelles, hydrogels, nano-emulsions, nano-spheres, and nano-capsules). The composition of the matrix includes lipids such as phosphatidylcholine, methylparaben and propylparaben, lecithin, fatty acids, gums and oils, while emulsion systems include protein and polymer components such as protein isolates, chitosan, casein and whey proteins, cellulose, β-cyclodextrin, polyvinylpyrrolidone and amylose and amylopectin.

Particularly in the dairy industry there have been reported three potential applications: nano-particulated delivery systems such as nano-capsules and supply of biologically active substances with release properties, solubility and absorption through the cells, ingredients and additives that improve texture, taste and sensory and functional properties, and finally, antibacterial and intelligent packaging (with nano-sensors and microbial activators that stop deterioration and prolong shelf life), all of them as part of food safety and biosafety (Chen et al. 2006; Richardson and Piehowski 2008). Regarding nano-particulate delivery systems, Maurya and Aggarwal (2019a) developed a phase inversion based nano-emulsion process to encapsulate vitamin D_3. Of all the combinations of components used for nanoparticle formation, the researchers found that using 30% (v/v) of Kolliphor, 20% (v/v) of caprylic−/capric triglyceride, and 50% (v/v) aqueous phase (NaCl) produced a stable emulsion with high encapsulation efficiency and high bioavailability of vitamin D, so that the nano-emulsion had high sensory acceptability in fortified buttermilk. In another study, these same researchers (Maurya and Aggarwal 2019b) encapsulated vitamin D again using a phase inversion-based cold water dilution method based on Kolliphor, caprylic/capric triglyceride and water. The nanostructured lipid vehicle formed by this technique was used to fortify a milk-based drink, which had high sensory acceptability and high physicochemical stability against various environmental stresses (temperature, pH, and ionic strength).

Table 2.4 shows some studies where nano-materials have been applied in milk and dairy products, emphasizing the type of nano-structured material and its synthesis method (as indicated by the research work) as well as the field of application.

2.4.3 Summary and Future Trends

There are very few studies that combine ultrasound and nanotechnology as technologies applied to milk and dairy products. This is due to the fact that ultrasound is a physical technology that modifies the components and structure of food, so its application in industry and convergence with other technologies such as the application of heat and pressure is more appropriate without representing any risk to health. Nano-technology requires multiple disciplines for the synthesis of materials at the nanometric level; it regularly needs polymers, chemicals and solvents, so further studies are needed to ensure that they pose no risk to health and the environment.

The research on the application of ultrasound and nano-technology in milk and dairy products is increasing. The convergence of both technologies is still in process, with few studies focused on the synthesis of nano-materials using ultrasound. In the near future, ultrasound may be implemented in the dairy industry due to the multiple benefits that this technology has when combined with heat and pressure.

Table 2.4 Nano-materials in milk and dairy products

Nano-material	Synthesis method	Aplication/results	References
Nano-nutraceuticals (nano-structured butter)	Addition of herbal supplements with surfactant property.	Additives. The addition of polysaccharides and cryo-powders reduced the size of the nano-structural elements of the butter (5–25 times), its architecture and morphology.	Ivanov and Rashevskaya (2011)
Biopolymeric nano-particles (co-polymers of polylactic acid and polyethylene glycol).	Precipitation / solvent evaporation	Nano-particulate delivery systems.	Riley et al. (1999)
Nano-tubes of α-lactalbumin.	Hydrolysis (incubation) of α-lactalbumin with Bacillus licheniformis protease, at 323 K.	Nano-particulate delivery systems. Production of self-assembling blocks in stable nano-tubes. Applications as viscosifier, in gelation and encapsulation.	Graveland-Bikker and de Kruif (2006)
Electronic nose with zinc oxide nanowires.	Immunosensor of Staphylococcus enterotoxin B in milk.	Sensors (0.5 ng * mL − 1). Detection of Staphylococcus enterotoxin in milk.	Dong et al. (2006)
Packings with polymer-nano-clay.	Inter-layer polymerization in situ with montmorillonite whose natural structure of nano-wires limits gas permeation.	Smart packaging coatings of dairy products, cheese packaging. The polymers used are polyamides (PA), nylon, polyofelins, polystyrene (PS), ethylene-vinylacetate (EVA), epoxy resins, polyurethane, polyimides and polyethylene terephthalate (PET).	Ke and Yongping (2005), Akbari et al. (2006)
Nano-fibers of α-lactalbumin.	Proteolysis (incubation) of α-lactalbumin with Bacillus licheniformis protein at pH 7.5 and 50 °C	Nano-particulate delivery systems. After the hydrolysis of α-lactalbumin, dimers were formed which subsequently were added in fibrillar strands with a diameter of 5 nm. They have the potential to bind with vitamins and enzymes, or to encapsulate nutraceuticals and mask undesirable flavors and aromas.	Otte et al. (2005)
Nano-crystalline TiO_2 films.	TiO_2 nano-particles synthesized by aqueous hydrolysis.	Smart packaging. Films that achieve deoxygenation driven by light in closed environments.	Xiao et al. (2004)
Nano-composite nylon MXD6	Incorporation of nano-clays (montmorillonite) in nylon 6.	Smart packaging. Potential for use in PET bottles as an oxygen barrier layer for dairy products and in multilayer cheese films.	Moraru et al. (2003), Brody (2007)

(continued)

Table 2.4 (continued)

Nano-material	Synthesis method	Aplication/results	References
Nano-chitosan	Dry grinding at room temperature.	Additives. A milk product with nano-chitosan powder reduced total cholesterol, LDL cholesterol and triglycerides in rats. The nano-chitosan in yogurt produced hypocholesterolemic and hypoglycaemic effects in rats.	Park et al. (2010), Seo et al. (2011)
Nano-peanuts	Dry grinding at room temperature.	Additives. Milk supplemented with nano-peanuts increases its antioxidant activity without affecting the acceptability or physicochemical properties. Yogurt added with nano-peanuts decreases its pH after 16 days of storage; the antioxidant activity increases. Caciocavallo cheese added with nano-peanuts could delay and / or prevent collagen-induced arthritis in mice.	Ahn et al. (2013), Ahn and Kwak (2012), Ko (2012), Choi et al. (2012), Kim et al. (2014)
Oyster shell nanopoly	Dry grinding at room temperature.	Additives. The milk showed no sediment after 16 days of storage at 4 °C; no physicochemical or sensory properties were affected.	Lee et al. 2015
Nano-calcio	30–900 nm commercial nano-calcium (NanoTechWorld).	Additives. Milk supplemented with nano-calcium helped reform the trabecular bone in osteoporotic rats.	Park et al. (2007, 2008)
Nano-ginseng powder	Dry grinding at room temperature with Apexel Co. spray.	The red ginseng in Asiago cheeses produced hard texture, yellow color and holes, astringency and bitterness increased, so concentrations lower than 0.1% of ginseng are recommended.	Choi et al. (2014)
Nano-emulsion (vitamin D)	Phase inversion temperature	Yogurt fortified with vitamin D and supplemented with goji polyphenol berry extract (Lycium barbarum) had a greater ability to inhibit vitamin D degradation without affecting consumer palatability during shelf life.	Maurya and Aggarwal (2017a, b)
Nano-emulsion containing encapsulated vitamin D nano-particles	Phase inversion based on nano-emulsion manufacturing process	Buttermilk sensory acceptability fortified with vitamin D3 nano-emulsion; the nano-emulsion showed high physicochemical stability against environmental stresses (temperature, pH and salt).	Maurya and Aggarwal (2019a)

(continued)

Table 2.4 (continued)

Nano-material	Synthesis method	Aplication/results	References
Nano-structured lipid carrier for encapsulation of vitamin D3	Phase inversion based on the manufacturing process of a nano-structured lipid carrier	The fortification of Lassi (milk-based drink) with encapsulated vitamin D had high sensory acceptability; the nano-structured lipid carrier had high physicochemical stability against environmental stresses (temperature, pH and ionic strength).	Maurya and Aggarwal (2019b)

However, the application of nano-materials in food requires studies on toxicity and safety in their use, including regulations in legislation.

2.5 Disadvantages of Nano-Technology in Food

The use of nano-technology in food has its own disadvantages and restrictions. There are described toxicological aspects of nano-materials (Teow et al. 2011), as well as the safety concerns and the lack of regulatory laws around the world concerning the use of nano-technology (Nile et al. 2020). There is evidence on nano-particle cytotoxicity and primary and secondary genotoxicity when they access to the animal system through skin penetration, ingestion, inhalation, injections or medical implantations. Once in the cells, they interact with the molecules, causing reactive oxygen species production, degeneration of mitochondria, DNA, chromosomal abnormalities, gene/protein expression failure, and apoptosis, among other negative effects. Most of these effects have been observed *in vitro* (i.e. stem cells, monocites, lymphocytes, human epitelium and endothelium) and some have been confirmed in animals (i.e. rats, mice, zebrafish embryos) with silver, titanium and ZnO nano-particles, but there is still a lack of studies and knowledge of negative effects in human health (Nile et al. 2020; Teow et al. 2011). Even so, nano-particles used in packaging materials remain not harmful for humans as soon as they are not integrated or translocated into the food (Teow et al. 2011; Valdiglesias et al. 2013).

2.6 Conclusions

In the food industry ultrasound and nano-technology have evolved as two distinct technologies. The convergence between the two technologies is the result of changes at the nanoscale that ultrasound causes on food components, including the development of nano-materials using ultrasound as an assisted technology such as: nano-liposomes, nano-emulsions, nano-encapsulates, nano-structured lipids and nano-particles. Ultrasound causes structural changes that modify the components and properties in meat, milk and their products. However, more research is needed regarding the standardization of ultrasound parameters such as frequencies, intensities, times and temperatures, which would facilitate the optimal design of equipment for industrial scale-up. Additionally, the use of accompanying technologies, such as the application of heat and pressure to induce improvements in microbiological and sensory quality, could be a good complement to improve the performance of ultrasound. Regarding the application of nanotechnology in food, studies focused on the development of nano-fertilizers, nano-pesticides, nano-transporters, and nano-sensors in agricultural production will continue to be investigated.

In spite of the big number of studies on the use of nano-particles as food additives, the safety of their use in food is still debated, especially in metallic nano-particles and oxide as antibacterial and antifungal in packaging. However, the encapsulation and development of nano-emulsions for the controlled release of compounds constitutes the application with the greatest potential in food, including the use of nano-technology for the administration of drugs, nutrients and supplements in animals and the diagnosis and treatment of diseases. Studies on the toxicity of nano-materials in animals and the long-term effects on human health and the environment are the main restriction that limit their use in the short term. For this reason, future studies should focus on evaluating the safety in the use of nano-materials, including the regulation of environmental and commercial legislation.

2.7 Future Prospects

As discussed in this chapter many potential combinations of ultrasound and nano-technology may result in improvement of quality in meat. The most important applications that need to be further investigated are the use of ultrasound for the production of nano-materials with potential integration in meat packaging, the synthesis of nano-particles for application in the detection of contaminants in meat, the application of ultrasound as an assistant technology in nano-emulsions, and the use of ultrasound for reducing nano-size of animal proteins and induce meat tenderization among others. However, provided the lack of ultrasonication equipment, as the major limitation for adoption of the ultrasound technology an industrial scale, is overcome the application of ultrasound technology in nano-material science will be satisfactory and efficiently utilized.

In the dairy industry both technologies, ultrasound and nano-materials, would continue being studied since the results have been very promising in terms of product quality improvement. The positive changes ultrasound causes in the structural and functional properties of milk and the application of nano-materials focused to new packaging materials and the encapsulation of bioactive compounds will lead, in the short and long term, diverse applications in dairy technology. Furthermore, the application of ultrasound in nanometric-sized food systems such as the development of nano-emulsions, smart packaging with nano-particulate materials, nano-polymers, nano-lipids, and nano-capsules that make nutrient bioavailability efficient will continue to drive and further develop innovations for the dairy industry.

Finally, regarding regulatory laws, Nile et al. (2020) established clearly that apart from the efforts made by the United States' Drug and Food Administration, the European Union Novel Foods Regulation, and the Australia and New Zealand Food Standards, there is a compulsory and urgent need for an international regulatory system for the nano-particles used in the food industry. Especially for those countries considered leaders in the nano-particle production such as China and Japan.

References

Aarti PD, Tanaka R, Tanaka A (2006) Effects of oxidative stress on chlorophyll biosynthesis in cucumber (Cucumis sativus) cotyledons. Physiol Plant 128(1):186–197. https://doi.org/10.1111/j.1399-3054.2006.00720.x

Abesinghe AMNL, Vidanarachchi JK, Islam N, Prakash S, Silva KFST, Bhandari B, Karim MA (2019) Effects of ultrasonication on the physicochemical properties of milk fat globules of Bubalus bubalis (water buffalo) under processing conditions: a comparison with shear-homogenization. Innovative Food Sci Emerg Technol 59:102237. https://doi.org/10.1016/j.ifset.2019.102237

Adhikari BM, Tung VP, Truong T, Bansal N, Bhandari B (2019) Impact of in-situ CO_2 nano-bubbles generation on freezing parameters of selected liquid foods. Food Biophys 15:97–112. https://doi.org/10.1007/s11483-019-09604-z

Aguilar-Hernández G, Vivar-Vera MÁ, García-Magaña ML, González-Silva N, Pérez-Larios A, Montalvo-González E (2020) Ultrasound-assisted extraction of total acetogenins from the soursop fruit by response surface methodology. Molecules 25(5):1139. https://doi.org/10.3390/molecules25051139

Ahn YJ, Kwak HS (2012) Comparison of nanopowdered and powdered peanut sprout-added yogurt on its physicochemical and sensory properties during storage. Korean J Food Sci Anim Resour 32:553–560. https://doi.org/10.5851/kosfa.2012.32.5.553

Ahn YJ, Ganesan P, Kwak HS (2013) Effect of nanopowdered peanut sprouts on physico- chemical and sensory properties of milk. Korean J Food Sci Anim Resour 33:9–15. https://doi.org/10.5851/kosfa.2013.33.1.9

Akbari Z, Ghomashchi T, Aroujalian A (2006) Potential of nanotechnology for food packaging industry. Paper presented at "Nano and Micro Technologies in the Food Health Food Industries". In: Conference organised by Institute of Nanotechnology, Amsterdam, 25–26 October 2006

Alarcón-Rojo AD, Janacua H, Rodríguez JC, Paniwnyk L, Mason TJ (2015) Power ultrasound in meat processing. Meat Sci 107:86–93. https://doi.org/10.1016/j.meatsci.2015.04.015

Alarcon-Rojo AD, Peña-Gonzalez EP, Garcia-Galicia IA, Carrillo-Lopez LM, Huerta-Jimenez M, Reyez-Villagrana RA, Vidales HJ (2018) Ultrasound application to improve meat quality. In: Descriptive food science. InTech Open, London, pp 153–172. https://doi.org/10.5772/intechopen.77973

Ali SM, Yousef NMH, Nafady NA (2015) Application of biosynthesized silver nanoparticles for the control of land snail *Eobania vermiculataand* some plant pathogenic fungi. J Nanomater 2015:1–10. https://doi.org/10.1155/2015/218904

Amiri A, Mousakhani-Ganjeh A, Torbati S, Ghaffarinejhad G, Esmaeilzadeh Kenari R (2018) Impact of high-intensity ultrasound duration and intensity on the structural properties of whipped cream. Int Dairy J 78:152–158. https://doi.org/10.1016/j.idairyj.2017.12.002

Andi MA, Hashemi M, Ahmadi F (2011) Effects of feed type with/without nanosil on cumulative performance, relative organ weight and some blood parameters of broilers. Glob Vet 7:605–609

Arzeni C, Martínez K, Zema P, Arias A, Pérez OE, Pilosof AMR (2012) Comparative study of high intensity ultrasound effects on food proteins functionality. J Food Eng 108(3):463–472. https://doi.org/10.1016/J.JFOODENG.2011.08.018

Ashkarran AA, Hamidinezhad H, Haddadi H, Mahmoudi M (2014) Double-doped TiO_2 nanoparticles as an efficient visible-light-active photocatalyst and antibacterial agent under solar simulated light. Appl Surf Sci 301:338–345. https://doi.org/10.1016/j.apsusc.2014.02.074

Avella M, De Vlieger JJ, Errico ME, Fischer S, Vacca P, Volpe MG (2005) Biodegradable starch/clay nanocomposite films for food packaging applications. Food Chem 93:467–474. https://doi.org/10.1016/j.foodchem.2004.10.024

Bang JH, Suslick KS (2010) Applications of ultrasound to the synthesis of nanostructured materials. Adv Mater 22:1039–1059. https://doi.org/10.1002/adma.200904093

Behrend O, Ax K, Schubert H (2000) Influence of continuous phase viscosity on emulsification by ultrasound. Ultrason Sonochem 7(2):77–85. https://doi.org/10.1016/s1350-4177(99)00029-2

Betancourt R, Reyes P, Puente B, Ávila C, Rodríguez O, Cadenas G, Lira R, García L (2014) Synthesis of copper nanoparticles by thermal decomposition and their antimicrobial properties. J Nanomater 2014:1–5. https://doi.org/10.1155/2014/980545

Betancur HCP, Hernández MV, Buitrago SR (2016) Nanoparticles for antibacterial materials and titanium dioxide applications. Rev Cuba Investig Biomed 35(4):387–402

Bochicchio S, Barba AA, Grassi G, Lamberti G (2016) Vitamin delivery: carriers based on nanoliposomes produced via ultrasonic irradiation. LWT Food Sci Technol 69:9–16. https://doi.org/10.1016/j.lwt.2016.01.025

Bollo E (2007) Nanotechnologies applied to veterinary diagnostics. Vet Res Commun 3:145–147. https://doi.org/10.1007/s11259-007-0080-x

Boonyanitipong P, Kositsup B, Kumar P, Baruah S, Dutta J (2011) Toxicity of ZnO and TiO_2 nanoparticles on germinating rice seed Oryza sativa L. Int J Biosci Biochem Bioinform 1(4):282–285

Brody L (2007) Nanocomposite technology in food packaging. Food Technol 61(10):80–83

Cameán AM, Cacho JF, Cepeda A, Farré R, Vidal MC, Jos A, López R (2010) Informe del Comité Científico de la Agencia Española de Seguridad Alimentaria y Nutrición (AESAN) en relación al uso de la nanotecnología en la industria alimentaria. Revista del Comité Científico de la AESAN 11:29–46. https://dialnet.unirioja.es/servlet/articulo?codigo=3438776

Capaldi Arruda SC, Diniz Silva AL, Moretto Galazzi R, Antunes Azevedo R, Zezzi Arruda MA (2015) Nanoparticles applied to plant science: a review. Talanta 131:693–705. https://doi.org/10.1016/j.talanta.2014.08.050

Carrillo J, Meléndez H, Puente B, Padrón G, Ledezma A, Betancourt R (2016) Composite based on poly (acrylic acid co itaconic acid) hydrogel with antibacterial performance. Polym Compos 39(1):171–180. https://doi.org/10.1002/pc.23917

Carrillo-López LM, Zavaleta-Mancera HA, Vilchis-Néstor A, Soto-Hernández RM, Arenas-Alatorre J, Trejo-Téllez LI, Gómez-Merino F (2014) Biosynthesis of silver nanoparticles using *Chenopodium ambrosioides*. J Nanomater 2014:1–9. https://doi.org/10.1155/2014/951746

Carrillo-López LM, Soto-Hernández RM, Zavaleta-Mancera HA, Vilchis-Néstor AR (2016) Study of the performance of the organic extracts of *Chenopodium ambrosioides* for Ag nanoparticle synthesis. J Nanomater 2016:1–13. https://doi.org/10.1155/2016/4714162

Carrillo-Lopez LM, Juarez-Morales MG, Garcia-Galicia IA, Alarcon-Rojo AD, Huerta-Jimenez M (2020) The effect of high intensity ultrasound on physicochemical and microbiological properties of Mexican panela cheese. Foods 9:313. https://doi.org/10.3390/foods9030313

Chandrapala J, Zisu B, Palmer M, Kentish S, Ashokkumar M (2011) Effects of ultrasound on the thermal and structural characteristics of proteins in reconstituted whey protein concentrate. Ultrason Sonochem 18:951–957. https://doi.org/10.1016/j.ultsonch.2010.12.016

Chandrapala J, Oliver C, Kentish S, Ashokkumar M (2012a) Ultrasonics in food processing. Ultrason Sonochem 19(5):975–983. https://doi.org/10.1016/j.ultsonch.2012.01.010

Chandrapala J, Zisu B, Kentish S, Ashokkumar M (2012b) The effects of high-intensity ultrasound on the structural and functional properties of α-Lactalbumin, β-Lactoglobulin and their mixtures. Food Res Int 48:940–943. https://doi.org/10.1016/j.foodres.2012.02.021

Chandrapala J, Zisu B, Kentish S, Ashokkumar M (2013) Influence of ultrasound on chemically induced gelation of micellar casein systems. J Dairy Res 80(2):138–143. https://doi.org/10.1017/S0022029912000696

Charitidis CA, Georgiou P, Koklioti MA, Trompeta A-F, Markakis V (2014) Manufacturing nanomaterials: from research to industry. Manuf Rev 1:11. https://doi.org/10.1051/mfreview/2014009

Chemat F, Zill-E-Huma KMK (2011) Applications of ultrasound in food technology: processing, preservation and extraction. Ultrason Sonochem 18(4):813–835. https://doi.org/10.1016/j.ultsonch.2010.11.023

Chen L, Subirade M (2005) Chitosan/β-lactoglobulin core–shell nanoparticles as nutraceutical carriers. Biomaterials 26(30):6041–6053. https://doi.org/10.1016/j.biomaterials.2005.03.011

Chen H, Weiss J, Shahidi F (2006) Nanotechnology in neutraceuticals and functional food technology. Food Technol 60:30–36

Chen L, Zheng L, Lv Y, Liu H, Wang G, Ren N, Liu D, Wang J, Boughton RI (2010) Chemical assembly of silver nanoparticles on stainless steel for antimicrobial applications. Surf Coat Technol 204(23):3871–3875. https://doi.org/10.1016/j.surfcoat.2010.05.003

Chen H, Seiber JN, Hotze M (2014) ACS select on nanotechnology in food and agriculture: a perspective on implications and applications. J Agric Food Chem 62(6):1209–1212. https://doi.org/10.1021/jf5002588

Cheng Y, Donkor PO, Ren X, Wu J, Agyemang K, Ayim I, Ma H (2018) Effect of ultrasound pretreatment with mono-frequency and simultaneous dual frequency on the mechanical properties and microstructure of whey protein emulsion gels. Food Hydrocoll. https://doi.org/10.1016/j.foodhyd.2018.11.007

Choi KH, Kim DH, Mijan MA, Kwak HS (2012) Effect of nanopowdered peanut sprout-added Caciocavallo cheese on collagen-induced arthritis (CIA) mouse. In: Abstract of Annual Meeting of Korean Society for Food Science of Animal Resources. https://doi.org/10.5851/kosfa.2014.34.1.49

Choi KH, Yoo SH, Kwak HS (2014) Comparison of the physicochemical and sensory properties of Asiago cheeses with added nano-powdered red ginseng and powdered red ginseng during ripening. Int J Dairy Technol 67(3):348–357. https://doi.org/10.1111/1471-0307.12136

Contreras-Lopez G, Carnero-Hernandez A, Huerta-Jimenez M, Alarcon-Rojo AD, Garcia-Galicia IA, Carrillo-Lopez L (2020) High intensity ultrasound applied on cured pork: sensory and physicochemical characteristics. Food Sci Nutr 8(2):786–795. https://doi.org/10.1002/fsn3.1321

Corredor E, Testillano P, Coronado M, González P, Fernández P, Marquina C, de la Fuente IR, Rubiales D, Pérez A, Risueño M (2009) Nanoparticle penetration and transport in living pumpkin plants: in situ subcellular identification. BMC Plant Biol 9(1):1–11. https://doi.org/10.1186/1471-2229-9-45

Cuartas-Uribe B, Alcaina-Miranda MI, Soriano-Costa E, Bes-Pia A (2007) Comparison of the behavior of two nanofiltration membranes for sweet whey demineralization. J Dairy Sci 90(3):1094–1101. https://doi.org/10.3168/jds.S0022-0302(07)71596-5

Cuartas-Uribe B, Vincent-Vela MC, Álvarez-Blanco S, Alcaina-Miranda MI, Soriano Costa E (2010) Application of nanofiltration models for the prediction of lactose retention using three modes of operation. J Food Eng 99(3):373–376. https://doi.org/10.1016/j.jfoodeng.2010.03.023

Dahroud BD, Mokarram RR, Khiabani MS, Hamishehkar H, Bialvaei AZ, Yousefi M, Kafil HS (2016) Low intensity ultrasound increases the fermentation efficiency of Lactobacillus casei subsp. casei ATTC 39392. Int J Biol Macromol 86:462–467. https://doi.org/10.1016/j.ijbiomac.2016.01.103

Dimkpa CO, Bindraban PS (2018) Nanofertilizers: new products for the industry? J Agric Food Chem 66:6462–6473. https://doi.org/10.1021/acs.jafc.7b02150

Dimkpa CO, McLean JE, Britt DW, Anderson AJ (2013) Antifungal activity of ZnO nanoparticles and their interactive effect with a biocontrol bacterium on growth antagonism of the

plant pathogen *Fusarium graminearum*. Biometals 26(6):913–924. https://doi.org/10.1007/s10534-013-9667-6
Dong Y, Phillips KS, Cheng Q (2006) Immunosensing of Staphylococcus exterotoxin B (SEB) in milk with PDMS microfluidic systems using reinforced supported bilayer membranes (r-SBMs). Lab Chip 6:675–681
Dong W, Stomackin G, Lin X, Martin GK, Jung TT (2019) Distortion product otoacoustic emissions: sensitive measures of tympanic -membrane perforation and healing processes in a gerbil model. Hear Res 378:3–12. https://doi.org/10.1016/j.heares.2019.01.015
Du M, Guo B, Jia D (2010) Newly emerging applications of halloysite nanotubes: a review. Polym Int 59:574–582. https://doi.org/10.1002/pi.2754
Duhan JS, Kumar R, Kumar N, Kaur P, Nehra K, Duhan S (2017) Nanotechnology: the new perspective in precision agriculture. Biotechnol Rep 15:11–23. https://doi.org/10.1016/j.btre.2017.03.002
Duncanson P (2004) Is there a bug on board? Microbiologist 5(1):34–35
Durnikin D, Silantyeva M, Ereshchenko O (2016) Ultrasound-enhanced cell production of lactic and propionic acid bacteria under submerged cultivation for industrial purposes. Biol Bull Bogdan Chmelnitskiy Melitopol State Pedagogical Univ 6:287–293. https://doi.org/10.15421/201659
EFSA (2016) Panel on additives and products or substances used in animal feed (FEEDAP). Safety and efficacy of dicopper oxide as feed additive for all animal specie. ESFA J 14:4509. https://doi.org/10.2903/j.efsa.2016.4509
Emamifar A (2011) Applications of antimicrobial polymer nanocomposites in food packaging. In: Hashim A (ed) Advances in nanocomposite technology. InTech Open Ltd, London. https://doi.org/10.5772/18343
EPA (Environmental Protection Agency, US) (2017) Exposure assessment tools by chemical classes. Nanomaterials. https://www.epa.gov/expobox/exposure-assessmenttools-chemical-classes-nanomaterials. Accessed 27 Apr 2020
Etxeberria E, Gonzalez P, Pozueta J (2009) Evidence for two endocytic transport pathways in plant cells. Plant Sci 177:341–348. https://doi.org/10.1016/j.plantsci.2009.06.014
FAO/WHO (Food and Agriculture Organization of the United Nations/World Health Organization) (2010) FAO/WHO expert meeting on the application of nanotechnologies in the food and agriculture sectors: potential food safety implications: meeting report. FAO, Rome, p 130
FDA (2014) Guidance for industry, assessing the effects of significant manufacturing process changes, including emerging technologies, on the safety and regulatory status of food ingredients and food contact substances, including food ingredients that are color additives. Office Of food additive safety, HFS-205 center for food safety and applied nutrition Food and Drug Administration, College Park. Accessed 26 Feb 2019
Fernandez A, Giner ST, Lagaron JM (2009) Novel route to stabilization of bioactive antioxidants by encapsulation in electrospun fibers of zein prolamine. Food Hydrocoll 23(5):1427–1432. https://doi.org/10.1016/j.foodhyd.2008.10.011
Flores-Miranda G, Yáñez-Fernández J, San Martin Martinez E (2020) Effect of processing parameters on astaxanthin nanoemulsions with stearic acid using ultrasonic emulsification. Rev Mex Ing Chim 19(3):1301–1313. https://doi.org/10.24275/rmiq/Alim936
Fondevila M, Herrer R, Casallas MC, Abecia L, Ducha JJ (2009) Silver nanoparticles as a potential antimicrobial additive for weaned pigs. Anim Feed Sci Technol 150(3–4):259–269. https://doi.org/10.1016/j.anifeedsci.2008.09.003
Fraceto LF, Grillo R, Oliveira HC et al (2015) Nanoencapsulation enhances the post-emergence herbicidal activity of atrazine against mustard plants. PLoS One 10:e0132971. https://doi.org/10.1371/journal.pone.0132971
FSAI (Food Safety Authority of Ireland) (2008) The relevance for food safety of applications of nanotechnology in the food and feed industries. Food Safety Authority of Ireland, Dublin. https://doi.org/10.5281/zenodo.807218. Accessed 7 March 2019
Gallego-Juarez JA (2010) High-power ultrasonic processing: recent developments and prospective advances. Phys Procedia 3(1):35–47. https://doi.org/10.1016/j.phpro.2010.01.006

Gholami-Ahangaran M, Zia-Jahromi N (2014) Effect of nanosilver on blood parameters in chickens having aflatoxicosis. Toxicol Ind Health 30(2):192–196. https://doi.org/10.1177/0748233712452611

Graveland-Bikker JF, de Kruif CG (2006) Unique milk protein-based nanotubes: food and nanotechnology meet. Trends Food Sci Technol 17(5):196–203. https://doi.org/10.1016/j.tifs.2005.12.009

Gregersen SB, Wiking L, Hammershøj M (2019) Acceleration of acid gel formation by high intensity ultrasound is linked to whey protein denaturation and formation of functional milk fat globule-protein complexes. J Food Eng 254:17–24. https://doi.org/10.1016/j.jfoodeng.2019.03.004

Gul O, Saricaoglu FT, Besir A, Atalar I, Yazici F (2018) Effect of ultrasound treatment on the properties of nano-emulsion films obtained from hazelnut meal protein and clove essential oil. Ultrason Sonochem 41:466–474. https://doi.org/10.1016/j.ultsonch.2017.10.011

Hassan AA, Howayda ME, Mahmoud HH (2013) Effect of zinc oxide nanoparticles on the growth of mycotoxigenic mould. Stud Chem Process Technol 1(4):66–74

He X, Deng H, Hwang HM (2019) The current application of nanotechnology in food and agriculture. J Food Drug Anal 27:1–21. https://doi.org/10.1016/j.jfda.2018.12.002

Hernández-Muñoz P, Cerisuelo JP, Domínguez I, López-Carballo G, Catalá R, Gavara R (2019) Nanotechnology in food packaging. In: Lopez Rubio A, Fabra Rovira MJ, Martinez Sanz M, Gomez GML (eds) Nanomaterials for food applications, 1st edn. Elsevier, Amsterdam, pp 205–232

Hojjat SS (2015) Impact of silver nanoparticles on germinated fenugreek seed. Int J Agric Crop Sci 8:627–630

Huang Q, Yu H, Ru Q (2010) Bioavailability and delivery of nutraceuticals using nanotechnology. J Food Sci 75:50–57. https://doi.org/10.1111/j.1750-3841.2009.01457.x

Huang J, Zhan G, Zheng B, Sun D, Lu F, Lin Y, Chen H, Zheng Z, Zheng Y, Li Q (2011) Biogenic silver nanoparticles bycacumen platycladiextract: synthesis, formation mechanism, and antibacterial activity. Ind Eng Chem Res 50(15):9095–9106. https://doi.org/10.1021/ie200858y

Israel B (2002) Detection of FMDv by anchoring transitions of liquid crystals. USDA CRIS database 0192234

Ivanov SV, Rashevskaya TA (2011) The nanostructure's management is the basis for a functional fatty food's production. Proc Food Sci 1:24–31. https://doi.org/10.1016/j.profoo.2011.09.005

Jayarao B, Wolfgang DR, Keating CD, Van Saun RJ, Hovingh E (2009) Medicine nanobarcodes-based bioassays for tracing consignments of meat and bone meat. Available at http://vbs.psu.edu/ext/research/projects/nanobarcodes-based-bioassays-for-tracing-consignmentsof-meat-and-bone-meal/?searchterm=None. Accessed 27 Feb 2019

Jeevanandam J, Barhoum A, Chan YS, Dufresne A, Danquah MK (2018) Review on nanoparticles and nanostructured materials: history, sources, toxicity and regulations. Beilstein J Nanotechnol 9:1050–1074. https://doi.org/10.3762/bjnano.9.98

Jokar M, Adbul Rahman R (2014) Study of silver ion migration from melt-blended and layered deposited silver polyethylene nanocomposite into food simulants and apple juice. Food Addit Contam: Part A 31(4):734–742. https://doi.org/10.1080/19440049.2013.878812

Kang D, Zou Y, Chen Y, Xing L, Zhou G, Zhang W (2016) Effects of power ultrasound on oxidation and structure of beef proteins during curing processing. Ultrason Sonochem 33(2016):47–53. https://doi.org/10.1016/j.ultsonch.2016.04.024

Kang D, Gao X, Ge Q, Zhou G, Zhang W (2017) Effects of ultrasound on the beef structure and water distribution during curing through protein degradation and modification. Ultrason Sonochem 38:317–325. https://doi.org/10.1016/j.ultsonch.2017.03.026

Kazner C, Wintgens T, Melin T, Baghoth S, Sharma S, Amy G (2008) Comparing the effluent organic matter removal of direct NF and powdered activated carbon/NF as high quality pretreatment options for artificial groundwater recharge. Water Sci Technol 57(6):821–827. https://doi.org/10.2166/wst.2008.164

Ke Z, Yongping B (2005) Improve the gas barrier property of PET film with montmorillonite by *in situ* interlayer polymerisation. Mater Lett 59:3348–3351. https://doi.org/10.1016/j.matlet.2005.05.070

Kehinde BA, Sharma P, Kaur S (2020) Recent nano-, micro- and macrotechnological applications of ultrasonication in food-based systems. Crit Rev Food Sci Nutr. https://doi.org/10.1080/10408398.2020.1740646

Khalifa NS, Hasaneen MN (2018) The effect of chitosanePMAAeNPK nanofertilizer on Pisum sativum plants. 3 Biotech 8(4):193. https://doi.org/10.1007/s13205-018-1221-3

Kharissova OV, Kharisov BI, Valdés JJR, Méndez UO (2011) Ultrasound in nanochemistry: recent advances. Synth React Inorg Met-Org Nano-Met Chem 41(5):429–448

Khot LR, Sankaran S, Maja JM, Ehsani R, Schuster EW (2012) Applications of nano-materials in agricultural production and crop protection: a review. Crop Prot 35:64–70. https://doi.org/10.1016/j.cropro.2012.01.007

Kim HJ, Kim SH, Lee JK et al (2012) A novel mycotoxin purification system using magnetic nanoparticles for the recovery of aflatoxin B1 and zearalenone from feed. J Vet Sci 13(4):363–369. https://doi.org/10.4142/jvs.2012.13.4.363

Kim DH, Chang YH, Kwak HS (2014) The preventive effect of nanopowdered peanut sprout-added Caciocavallo cheese on collagen-induced arthritis mice. Korean J Food Sci Anim 34(1):49–56. https://doi.org/10.5851/kosfa.2014.34.1.49

Ko EJ (2012) Physicochemical properties of nanopowdered peanut sprout-added Caciocavallo cheese during ripening. Dissertation, Sejong University, Seoul, Korea

Körzendörfer A, Schäfer J, Hinrichs J, Nöbel S (2019) Power ultrasound as a tool to improve the processability of protein-enriched fermented milk gels for Greek yogurt manufacture. J Dairy Sci 102:7826–7837. https://doi.org/10.3168/jds.2019-16541

Kumar LY (2015) Role and adverse effects of nano-materials in food technology. J Toxicol Health 2:1–11. https://doi.org/10.7243/2056-3779-2-2

Kumar S, Kumar D, Dilbaghi N (2017) Preparation, characterization, and bio-efficacy evaluation of controlled release carbendazim-loaded polymeric nanoparticles. Environ Sci Pollut Res 24:926–937. https://doi.org/10.1007/s11356-016-7774-y

Kuzma J (2010) Nanotechnology in animal production-upstream assessment of applications. Livest Sci 130:14–24. https://doi.org/10.1016/j.livsci.2010.02.006

Lee S, Chung H, Kim S, Lee I (2013) The genotoxic effect of ZnO and CuO nanoparticles on early growth of buckwheat, Fagopyrum esculentum. Water Air Soil Pollut 224:1668–1678. https://doi.org/10.1007/s11270-013-1668-0

Lee YK, Ahn SI, Chang YH, Kwak HS (2015) Physicochemical and sensory properties of milk supplemented with dispersible nanopowdered oyster shell during storage. J Dairy Sci 98(9):5841–5849. https://doi.org/10.3168/jds.2014-9105

Leong T, Juliano P, Knoerzer K (2017) Advances in ultrasonic and megasonic processing of foods. Food Eng Rev 93:237–256. https://doi.org/10.1007/s12393-017-9167-5

Li Y, Shahbazi A, Williams K, Wan C (2008) Separate and concentrate lactic acid using combination of nanofiltration and reverse osmosis membranes. Appl Biochem Biotechnol 147:1–9. https://doi.org/10.1007/s12010-007-8047-5

Li M, Ahammed GJ, Li C, Bao X, Yu J, Huang C, Yin H, Zhou J (2016) Brassinosteroid ameliorates zinc oxide nanoparticles-induced oxidative stress by improving antioxidant potential and redox homeostasis in tomato seedling. Front Plant Sci 7:615. https://doi.org/10.3389/fpls.2016.00615

Liu Z, Juliano P, Williams RP, Niere J, Augustin MA (2014) Ultrasound improves the renneting properties of milk. Ultrason Sonochem 21(6):2131–2137. https://doi.org/10.1016/j.ultsonch.2014.03.034

Liu L, Zeng J, Sun B, Zhang N, He Y, Shi Y, Zhu X (2020) Ultrasound-assisted mild heating treatment improves the emulsifying properties of 11S globulins. Molecules 25:875. https://doi.org/10.3390/molecules25040875

Luo D, Han E, Belcheva N, Saltzman WM (2004) A self-assembled, modular DNA delivery system mediated by silica nanoparticles. J Control Release 95:333–341. https://doi.org/10.1016/j.jconrel.2003.11.019

Luque-Garcia JL, Luque de Castro MD (2001) Extraction of fat-soluble vitamins. J Chromatogr A 935(1–2):3–11. https://doi.org/10.1016/s0021-9673(01)01118-9

Ma G, Liang X, Li L, Qiao R, Jiang D, Ding Y, Chen H (2014) Cu-doped zinc oxide and its polythiophene composites: preparation and antibacterial properties. Chemosphere 100(2):146–151. https://doi.org/10.1016/j.chemosphere.2013.11.053

Mahdi Jafari S, He Y, Bhandari B (2006) Nano-emulsion production by sonication and microfluidization – a comparison. Int J Food Prop 9(3):475–485. https://doi.org/10.1080/10942910600596464

Maté J, Periago PM, Palop A (2016) When nanoemulsified, d-limonene reduces Listeria monocytogenes heat resistance about one hundred times. Food Control 59:824–828. https://doi.org/10.1016/J.FOODCONT.2015.07.020

Maurya VK, Aggarwal M (2017a) Enhancing bio-availability of vitamin D by Nano-engineered based delivery systems-An overview. Int J Curr Microbiol App Sci 6(7):340–353. https://doi.org/10.20546/ijcmas.2017.607.040

Maurya VK, Aggarwal M (2017b) Impact of aqueous/ethanolic goji berry (Lycium barbarum) fruit extract supplementation on vitamin D stability in yoghurt. Int J Curr Microbiol App Sci 6(8):2016–2029. https://doi.org/10.20546/ijcmas.2017.608.240

Maurya VK, Aggarwal M (2019a) A phase inversion based nanoemulsion fabrication process to encapsulate vitamin D3 for food applications. J Steroid Biochem Mol Biol 190:88–98. https://doi.org/10.1016/j.jsbmb.2019.03.021

Maurya VK, Aggarwal M (2019b) Fabrication of nano-structured lipid carrier for encapsulation of vitamin D3 for fortification of 'Lassi'; a milk based beverage. J Steroid Biochem Mol Biol 193:105429. https://doi.org/10.1016/j.jsbmb.2019.105429

Maurya VK, Bashir K, Aggarwal M (2019) Vitamin D microencapsulation and fortification: trends and technologies. J Steroid Biochem Mol Biol 196:105489. https://doi.org/10.1016/j.jsbmb.2019.105489

Maurya VK, Aggarwal M, Ranjan V, Gothandam KM (2020) Improving bioavailability of vitamin A in food by encapsulation: an update. In: Nanoscience in medicine, vol 1. Springer, Cham, pp 117–145. https://doi.org/10.1007/978-3-030-29207-2_4

Mendoza G, Rodríguez-López JL (2007) La nanociencia y la nanotecnología: una revolución en curso. Perfiles Latinoamericanos 29:161–186. http://www.redalyc.org/pdf/115/11502906.pdf

Mishra S, Singh BR, Singh A, Keswani C, Naqvi AH, Singh HB (2014) Biofabricated silver nanoparticles act as a strong fungicide against Bipolaris sorokiniana causing spot blotch disease in wheat. PLoS One 9:e97881. https://doi.org/10.1371/journal.pone.0097881

Mizielińska M, Kowalska U, Jarosz M, Sumińska P (2018) A comparison of the effects of packaging containing nano ZnO or polylysine on the microbial purity and texture of cod (*Gadus morhua*) fillets. Nanomaterials 8:158. https://doi.org/10.3390/nano8030158

Moraru CI, Panchapakesan CP, Huang Q, Takhistov P, Liu S, Kokini JL (2003) Nanotechnology: a new frontier in food science. Food Technol 57(12):24–29

Mouhamed AE, Hassan AA, Hassan MA, El Hariria M, Refaia M (2015) Effect of metal nanoparticles on the growth of ochratoxigenic moulds and Ochratoxin A production isolated from food and feed. Int J Res Stud Biosci 3(9):38–52. http://scholar.cu.edu.eg/?q=hanem/files/03v3i904-6.pdf

Muthumariyappan A, Rajaji U, Chen SM, Baskaran N, Chen TW, Jothi Ramalingam R (2019) Sonochemical synthesis of perovskite-type barium titanate nanoparticles decorated on reduced graphene oxide nanosheets as an effective electrode material for the rapid determination of ractopamine in meat samples. Ultrason Sonochem 56:318. https://doi.org/10.1016/j.ultsonch.2019.04.005

Narducci D (2007) An introduction to nanotechnologies: what's in it for us? Vet Res Commun 31:131–137. https://doi.org/10.1007/s11259-007-0082-8

Nguyen HA, Anema G (2017) Ultrasonication of reconstituted whole milk and its effect on acid gelation. Food Chem 217:593–601. https://doi.org/10.1016/j.foodchem.2016.08.117

Nile SH, Baskar V, Selvaraj D, Nile A, Xiao J, Kai G (2020) Nanotechnologies in food science: applications, recent trends, and future perspectives. In: Nano-micro letters, vol 12. Springer, Singapore. https://doi.org/10.1007/s40820-020-0383-9

Noormans AG (2010) Impact of nanotechnology in food production. Lámpsakos 4:28–35

O'Sullivan J, Murray B, Flynn C, Norton I (2016) The effect of ultrasound treatment on the structural, physical and emulsifying properties of animal and vegetable proteins. Food Hydrocoll 53:141–154. https://doi.org/10.1016/j.foodhyd.2015.02.009

Oberdörster G, Oberdörster E, Oberdörster J (2005) Nanotoxicology: an emerging discipline evolving from studies of ultrafine particles. Environ Health Perspect 113(7):823–839. https://doi.org/10.1289/ehp.7339

O'Dowd CD, Aalto PP, Yoon YY, Hämeri K (2004) The use of the pulse height analyser ultrafine condensation particle counter (PHA-UCPC) technique applied to sizing of nucleation mode particles of differing chemical composition. J Aerosol Sci 35(2):205–216. https://doi.org/10.1016/j.jaerosci.2003.08.003

Ojha KS, Perussello CA, García CÁ, Kerry JP, Pando D, Tiwari BK (2017) Ultrasonic-assisted incorporation of nano-encapsulated omega-3 fatty acids to enhance the fatty acid profile of pork meat. Meat Sci 132:99–106. https://doi.org/10.1016/j.meatsci.2017.04.260

Orellano MS, Isaac P, Breser ML, Bohl LP, Conesa A, Falcone RD, Porporatto C (2019) Chitosan nanoparticles enhance the antibacterial activity of the native polymer against bovine mastitis pathogens. Carbohydr Polym 213:1–9. https://doi.org/10.1016/j.carbpol.2019.02.016

Otte J, Ipsen R, Bauer R, Bjerrum MJ, Waninge R (2005) Formation of amyloid-like fibrils upon limited proteolysis of bovine α-lactalbumin. Int Dairy J 15(3):219–229. https://doi.org/10.1016/j.idairyj.2004.07.004

Owolade O, Ogunleti D (2008) Effects of titanium dioxide on the diseases, development and yield of edible cowpea. J Plant Prot Res 48(3):329–335. https://doi.org/10.2478/v10045-008-0042-5

Ozuna C, Paniagua-Martínez I, Castaño-Tostado E, Ozimek L, Amaya-Llano SL (2015) Innovative applications of high-intensity ultrasound in the development of functional food ingredients: production of protein hydrolysates and bioactive peptides. Food Res Int 77:685–696. https://doi.org/10.1016/j.foodres.2015.10.015

Panda S, Chaudhury I, Khan M (2003) Heavy metals induce lipid peroxidation and affect antioxidants in wheat leaves. Biol Plant 46:289–294. https://doi.org/10.1023/A:1022871131698

Park HS, Jeon BJ, Ahn J, Kwak HS (2007) Effects of nanocalcium supplemented milk on bone calcium metabolism in ovariectomized rats. Asian Australas J Anim Sci 20:1266–1271. https://doi.org/10.5713/ajas.2007.1266

Park HS, Ahn J, Kwak HS (2008) Effect of nano-calcium-enriched milk on calcium metabolism in ovariectomized rats. J Med Food 11:454–459. https://doi.org/10.1089/jmf.2007.0086

Park JH, Hong EK, Ahn J, Kwak HS (2010) Properties of nanopowdered chitosan and its cholesterol lowering effects in rats. Food Sci Biotechnol 19:1457–1462. https://doi.org/10.1007/s10068-010-0208-6

Pathakoti K, Manubolu M, Hwang HM (2017) Nanostructures: current uses and future applications in food science. J Food Drug Anal 25(2):245–253. https://doi.org/10.1016/j.jfda.2017.02.004

Patist A, Bates D (2008) Ultrasonic innovations in the food industry: from the laboratory to commercial production. Innovative Food Sci Emerg Technol 9(2):147–154. https://doi.org/10.1016/j.ifset.2007.07.004

Pelaez M, Nolan NT, Pillai SC et al (2012) A review on the visible light active titanium dioxide photocatalysts for environmental applications. Appl Catal B 125:331–349. https://doi.org/10.1016/j.apcatb.2012.05.036

Peña-González EM, Alarcón-Rojo AD, Rentería A, García I, Santellano E, Quintero A, Luna L (2017) Quality and sensory profile of ultrasound-treated beef. Ital J Food Sci 29(3):463–475. https://doi.org/10.14674/1120-1770/ijfs.v604

Pokhrel LR, Dubey B (2013) Evaluation of developmental responses of two crop plants exposed to silver and zinc oxide nanoparticles. Sci Total Environ 452–453:321. https://doi.org/10.1016/j.scitotenv.2013.02.059

Qian Y, Yao J, Russel M, Chen K, Wang X (2015) Characterization of green synthesized nano-formulation (ZnO-A. vera) and their antibacterial activity against pathogens. Environ Toxicol Pharmacol 39(2):736–746. https://doi.org/10.1016/j.etap.2015.01.015

Raab C, Simkó M, Fiedeler U, Nentwich M, Gazsó A (2011) Production of nanoparticles and nano-materials. NanoTrust-Dossier 6:1–4. epub.oeaw.ac.at/ita/nanotrust-dossiers/dossier006en.pdf

Rajiv P, Rajeshwari S, Venckatesh R (2013) Bio-fabrication of zinc oxide nanoparticles using leaf extract of Parthenium hysterophorus L. and its size-dependent antifungal activity against plant fungal pathogens. Spectrochim Acta A 112:384–387. https://doi.org/10.1016/j.saa.2013.04.072

Rajput N (2015) Methods of preparation of nanoparticles – a review. IJAET 7(4):1806–1811

Rajput VD, Chen Y, Ayup M (2015) Effects of high salinity on physiological and anatomical indices in the early stages of Populus euphratica growth. Russ J Plant Physiol 62(2):229–236. https://doi.org/10.1134/S1021443715020168

Rajput VD, Minkina TM, Behal A, Sushkova SN, Mandzhieva S et al (2018) Effects of zinc-oxide nanoparticles on soil, plants, animals and soil organisms: a review. Environ Nanotechnol Monit Manage 9:76–84. https://doi.org/10.1016/j.enmm.2017.12.006

Raliya R, Biswas P, Tarafdar JC (2015) TiO2 nanoparticle biosynthesis and its physiological effect on mung bean (*Vigna radiata* L.). Biotechnol Rep 5:22–26. https://goo.gl/ZgbMBZ

Ramachandraiah K, Han SG, Chin KB (2015) Nanotechnology in meat processing and packaging: potential applications—a review. Asian Australas J Anim Sci 28(2):290–302. https://doi.org/10.5713/ajas.14.0607

Ranjan S, Chakraborty AR, Ramalingam C, Kumar A, Dasgupta N, Melvin Samuel S, Shanker R (2014) Nanoscience and nanotechnologies in food industries: opportunities and research trends. J Nanopart Res. https://doi.org/10.1007/s11051-014-2464-5

Raskar SV, Laware SL (2014) Effect of zinc oxide nanoparticles on cytology and seed germination in onion. Int J Curr Microbiol App Sci 3(2):467–473

Ren G, Hu D, Cheng EWC, Vargas-Reus MA, Reip P, Allaker RP et al (2009) Characterisation of copper oxide nanoparticles for antimicrobial applications. Int J Antimicrob Agents 33(6):587–590. https://doi.org/10.1016/j.ijantimicag.2008.12.004

Richardson NSM, Piehowski KE (2008) Nanotechnology in nutritional sciences. Minerva Biotechnol 20:17–126

Riley T, Govender T, Stolnik S, Xiong CD, Garnett MC, Illum L, Davis SS (1999) Colloidal stability and drug incorporation aspects of micellarlike PLA-PEG nanoparticles. Colloids Surf B 16:47–159. https://doi.org/10.1016/S0927-7765(99)00066-1

Sahoo A, Swain R, Mishra SK (2014) Effect of inorganic, organic and nano zinc supplemented diets on bioavailability and immunity status of broilers. Int J Adv Res 2(11):828–837. https://www.semanticscholar.org/paper/ISSN-2320-5407-International-Journal-of-Advanced-2%2C-Sahoo-Swain/19904ec74dd98432677ccc156f58f293d42ac404

Sang L, Zhao Y, Burda C (2014) TiO_2 nanoparticles as functional building blocks. Chem Rev 114:9283–9318. https://doi.org/10.1021/cr400629p

Sangkasanya S, Naknaen P, Petchwattana N (2018) Feasibility application of biodegradable active films produced by poly(lactic acid) incorporating with limonene as an antimicrobial packaging for fresh beef meat. In: Proceedings of the 2018 8th international conference on bioscience, biochemistry and bioinformatics. ACM, New York, pp 60–64. https://doi.org/10.1145/3180382.3180395

Santhoshkumar T, Rahuman AA, Jayaseelan C, Rajakumar G, Marimuthu S et al (2014) Green synthesis of titanium dioxide nanoparticles using Psidium guajava extract and its antibacterial and antioxidant properties. Asian Pac J Trop Med 7(12):968–976. https://doi.org/10.1016/s1995-7645(14)60171-1

Scott NR (2005) Nanotechnology and animal health. Rev Sci Tech OIE 24:425–432. https://doi.org/10.20506/rst.24.1.1579

Sekhon BS (2014) Nanotechnology in agri-food production: an overview. Nanotechnol Sci Appl 7:31–53. https://doi.org/10.2147/NSA.S39406

Semo E, Kesselman E, Danino D, Livney YD (2007) Casein micelle as a natural nano-capsular vehicle for nutraceuticals. Food Hydrocoll 21:936–942. https://doi.org/10.1016/j.foodhyd.2006.09.006

Seo MH, Chang YH, Lee S, Kwak HS (2011) The physicochemical and sensory properties of milk supplemented with ascorbic acid-soluble nano chitosan during storage. Int J Dairy Technol 64:57–63. https://doi.org/10.1111/j.1471-0307.2010.00630.x

Shabana S, Prasansha R, Kalinina I, Potoroko I, Bagale U, Shirish SH (2019) Ultrasound assisted acid hydrolyzed structure modification and loading of antioxidants on potato starch nanoparticles. Ultrason Sonochem 51:444–450. https://doi.org/10.1016/j.ultsonch.2018.07.023

Shaibani PM, Jiang K, Haghighat G, Hassanpourfard M, Etayash H, Naicker S, Thundat T (2016) The detection of Escherichia coli with the pH sensitive hydrogel nanofiber-light addressable potentiometric sensor (NF-LAPS). Sensors Actuators B Chem 226:176–183. https://doi.org/10.1016/j.snb.2015.11.135

Shanmugam A, Chandrapala J, Ashokkumar M (2012) The effect of ultrasound on the physical and functional properties of skim milk. Innovative Food Sci Emerg Technol 16:251–258. https://doi.org/10.1016/j.ifset.2012.06.005

Shao Y, Wu C, Wu T, Li Y, Chen S, Yuan C, Hu Y (2018) Eugenol-chitosan nanoemulsions by ultrasound-mediated emulsification: formulation, characterization and antimicrobial activity. Carbohydr Polym 193:144–152. https://doi.org/10.1016/j.carbpol.2018.03.101

Shende S, Ingle A, Gade A, Rai M (2015) Green synthesis of copper nanoparticles by *Citrus medica* Linn. (Idilimbu) juice and its antimicrobial activity. World J Microbiol Biotechnol 31(6):865–873. https://doi.org/10.1007/s11274-015-1840-3

Silva LP (2014) Potential practical implications of nanotechnology in animal reproductive biotechnologies. Anim Reprod 11(3):278–280

Sotoft LF, Christensen KV, Andrésen R, Norddahl B (2012) Full scale plant with membrane based concentration of blackcurrant juice on the basis of laboratory and pilot scale tests. Chem Eng Process Process Intensif 54:12–21. https://doi.org/10.1016/j.cep.2012.01.007

Suárez E, Lobo A, Álvarez S, Riera FA, Álvarez R (2009) Demineralization of whey and milk ultrafiltration permeate by means of nanofiltration. Desalination 241:272–280. https://doi.org/10.1016/j.desal.2007.11.087

Suslick KS (1990) Sonochemistry. Science 247:1439–1445. https://doi.org/10.1126/science.247.4949.1439

Suslick KS, Flannigan DJ (2008) Inside a collapsing bubble: sonoluminescence and the conditions during cavitation. Annu Rev Phys Chem 59(1):659–683. https://doi.org/10.1146/annurev.physchem.59.032607.093739

Swain PS, Rao SBN, Rajendran D, Dominic G, Selvaraju S (2016) Nano zinc, an alternative to conventional zinc as animal feed supplement: a review. Anim Nutr. https://doi.org/10.1016/j.aninu.2016.06.003

Teow Y, Asharani PV, Hande MP, Valiyaveettil S (2011) Health impact and safety of engineered nanomaterials. Chem Commun 47(25):7025–7038. https://doi.org/10.1039/c0cc05271j

Tiede K, Boxall ABA, Tear SP, Lewis J, David H, Hassellöv M (2008) Detection and characterization of engineered nanoparticles in food and the environment. Food Addit Contam 25(7):795–821. https://doi.org/10.1080/02652030802007553

Torney F, Trewyn BG, Lin VS-Y, Wang K (2007) Mesoporous silica nanoparticles deliver DNA and chemicals into plants. Nat Nanotechnol 2(5):295–300. https://doi.org/10.1038/nnano.2007.108

Tripathi KM, Bhati A, Singh A, Sonker AK, Sarkar S, Sonkar SK (2017) Sustainable changes in the contents of metallic micronutrients in first generation gram seeds imposed by carbon nano-onions: life cycle seed to seed study. ACS Sustain Chem Eng 5:2906–2916. https://doi.org/10.1021/acssuschemeng.6b01937

Valdiglesias V, Costa C, Sharma V, Kiliç G, Pásaro E, Teixeira JP, Dhawan A, Laffon B (2013) Comparative study on effects of two different types of titanium dioxide nanoparticles on human neuronal cells. Food Chem Toxicol 57:352–361. https://doi.org/10.1016/j.fct.2013.04.010

Villena de Francisco E, García-Estepa RM (2018) Nanotechnology in the agrofood industry. J Food Eng 238:1–11. https://doi.org/10.1016/j.jfoodeng.2018.05.024

Wang X, Yang X, Chen S, Li Q, Wang QW, Hou C, Gao X, Wang L, Wang S (2016) Zinc oxide nanoparticles affect biomass accumulation and photosynthesis in Arabidopsis. Front Plant Sci 6:1243. https://doi.org/10.3389/fpls.2015.01243

Wang A, Kang D, Zhang W, Zhang C, Zou Y, Zhou G (2018) Changes in calpain activity, protein degradation and microstructure of beef M. semitendinosus by the application of ultrasound. Food Chem 245:724–730. https://doi.org/10.1016/J.FOODCHEM.2017.12.003

Wang W, Feng Y, Chen W, Wang Y, Wilder G, Liu D, Yin Y (2019) Ultrasonic modification of pectin for enhanced 2-furfurylthiol encapsulation: process optimization and mechanisms. J Sci Food Agric 100:110. https://doi.org/10.1002/jsfa.10000

Weir A, Westerhoff P, Fabricius L, Hristovski K, Von Goetz N (2012) Titanium dioxide nanoparticles in food and personal care products. Environ Sci Technol 46(4):2242–2250. https://doi.org/10.1021/es204168d

Wibowo KM, Sahdan MZ, Ramli NI, Muslihati A, Rosni N, Tsen VH et al (2018) Detection of Escherichia coli bacteria in wastewater by using graphene as a sensing material. J Phys Conf Ser 995:012063. https://doi.org/10.1088/1742-6596/995/1/012063

Xiao EL, Gres ANM, Hague SA, Millis A, Durrant JR (2004) Light driven oxygen scavenging by Titania polymer nanocomposite films. J Photochem Photobiol A 162:253–259. https://doi.org/10.1016/j.nainr.2003.08.010

Yildirim S, Röcker B, Pettersen MK, Nilsen-Nygaard J, Ayhan Z, Rutkaite R, Radusin T, Suminska P, Marcos B, Coma V (2018) Active packaging applications for food. Compr Rev Food Sci Food Saf 17(1):165–199. https://doi.org/10.1111/1541-4337.12322

Zafar H, Ali A, Ali JS, Haq IU, Zia M (2016) Effect of ZnO nanoparticles on Brassica nigra seedlings and stem explants: growth dynamics and antioxidative response. Front Plant Sci 7(32):535. https://doi.org/10.3389/fpls.2016.00535

Zhang J, Li S, An FF, Liu J, Jin S, Zhang JC, Wang PC, Zhang X, Lee CS, Liang XJ (2015) Self-carried curcumin nanoparticles for in vitro and in vivo cancer therapy with real-time monitoring of drug release. Nanoscale 7(32):13503–13510. https://doi.org/10.1039/C5NR03259H

Zhang R, Pang X, Lu J, Liu L, Zhang S, Lv J (2018) Effect of high intensity ultrasound pre-treatment on functional and structural properties of micellar casein concentrates. Ultrason Sonochem 47:10–16. https://doi.org/10.1016/j.ultsonch.2018.04.011

Zhang Y, Dai Y, Hou H, Li X, Dong H, Wang W, Zhang H (2020) Ultrasound-assisted preparation of octenyl succinic anhydride modified starch and its influence mechanism on the quality. Food Chem 5:100077. https://doi.org/10.1016/j.fochx.2020.100077

Zhao L, Ortiz C, Adeleye AS, Hu Q, Zhou H, Huang Y, Keller A (2016) Metabolomics to detect response of lettuce (*Lactuca sativa*) to $Cu(OH)_2$ nanopesticides: oxidative stress response and detoxification mechanisms. Environ Sci Technol 50:9697–9707. https://doi.org/10.1021/acs.est.6b02763

Chapter 3
Nanotechnology in Food Industry-Applications and Future Perspectives

Yogita Lugani, Simmi Oberoi, and Gurdeep Rattu

Abstract Nanotechnology is one of the emerging technologies involving the use of engineered nanomaterials ranging in size from 1–100 nanometers. It has promising applications in different sectors including pharmacy, health care, textiles, pulp and paper, energy, transport, agriculture, food processing, and information technology. Currently, there is a rapid increase in global population which leads to enhanced food demand. However, traditional technologies of food production are not sufficient to meet such demand. Hence, major focus of governments, and economists are running towards the development of novel technologies to avoid the situation of food crisis in future. Food companies are implementing nanotechnology in number of ways; smart packaging, nanocapsules, smart food, and nano-robot food production. Most of the company claims that nanotechnology applications in food will make the food safe for consumption. Different engineered nanomaterials such as nano-tubes, nano-fibers, and metal/metal oxide nanoparticles are being used for food processing and preservation, food packaging, detection of pathogens in food samples, and production and controlled delivery of nutraceuticals. Nanodevices, nanoswitches, electronic nose, nanochips, and biosensor have emerged into food sector for smart sensing and unique delivery system. However, there are various adverse effects of engineered nanomaterials on environment and human health. In view of this, attention is paid by research groups on toxicological studies of nanomaterials for assessment of risks to environment and human health from nanotechnology derived food products. The current chapter focuses on the applications of

Y. Lugani
Department of Biotechnology, Punjabi University, Patiala, Punjab, India

S. Oberoi
Department of Community Medicine, Government Medical College, Patiala, India

G. Rattu (✉)
Basic and Applied Science, National Institute of Food Technology Entrepreneurship and Management (NIFTEM), Kundli, Haryana, India

V. K. Maurya et al. (eds.), *Sustainable Agriculture Reviews 55*, Sustainable Agriculture Reviews 55, https://doi.org/10.1007/978-3-030-76813-3_3

engineered nanomaterials in food sector, their health hazards, and safety regulations for their safe use in food industries.

Keywords Nanotechnology · Nanomaterials · Food industry · Nanosensors · Food safety regulations

3.1 Introduction

Agricultural science and food safety are important disciplines for dietary health and longevity. With increased globalization and consumer outlook towards food safety, the need for overall quality assessment and acceptability, paved its role in the supply chain management from farm to fork (Ahumada and Villalobos 2009). In the past several decades, nanotechnology has emerged to be an attractive element in the food processing and preservation sector. Nanotechnology is an emerging field in material, and life sciences which involves the use of nanoscale materials with unique physical, chemical, electrical, optical, and magnetic properties (NSTC 2007). There are two major classes of nanoparticles i.e. organic (carbohydrate-based, protein-based, and lipid-based) (Shin et al. 2015), and inorganic (metals, and metal oxides like silver, titanium dioxide, zinc dioxide, silicon dioxide, and iron oxide) nanoparticles (He and Hwang 2016; Rattu et al. 2020). The nanomaterials used for different industrial applications are metallic nanoparticles, carbon nanotubes, quantum dots, nanowires, nanocermics, dendrimers, liposomes, and fullerenes (Lugani et al. 2018; Ealias and Saravanakumar 2017; Abobatta 2018).

Nanotechnology has shown applications in different industrial sectors such as food, cosmetics, energy, paints and coatings, textiles and clothings, medicines and drugs, and defense and security (Viswanathan and Radecki 2008; Bryksa and Yada 2012; Arora et al. 2017; Lugani et al. 2018). Presence of toxicants/contaminants in food products lead to economic loss in food industry, which would be a global public concern in a scenario of rapidly increasing global population. Therefore, food, and bioprocessing industries are facing challenges for developing, and applying systems which promises safe, efficient, and high-quality foods. Nanotechnology is one of the evolving fields which involves use of different nanomaterials in food sector due to their unique properties like improvement of texture, consistency, physical performance, and nutritional value of food products, enhanced shelf-life of products, controlled release at the target site, pathogen detection, fortification of vitamins and minerals in food, anti-microbial properties, and removal of food contaminants.

The use of some advanced techniques like micro electromechanical systems, DNA microarrays, and microfluidics along with nanotechnology enhance its use in delivery of active ingredients, separation of contaminants from food, and encapsulation of nutraceuticals (Ravichandran 2010). The major players of nanotechnology in food sector are NanoShel, NanoXpert Technologies, NanoBio Chemicals,

Velbionanotech, Sisco Research Laboratories, Meda Biotech, Quantum Corporations, Dabur Pharma, Aveka Group, Aveka Inc., Balchem Corporation, Firmenich SA, Taste Tech Ltd., Encapsys LLC, LycoRed Ltd., Adnano Technologies, Sensient Technologies Corporation, Cargill Inc., Coating Place Inc., Maxx Performance Inc., ABCO Laboratories, Inc., Advances BioNutrition Corporation, Royal DSM N.V, Friesland Campina Kievit (Food Encapsulation Market: 2018–2024). Table 3.1 shows the nano-products from food industry available in the market. Although there are various benefits of use of nanotechnology in food sector, their prolonged use can lead to serious complications such as environmental poisoning, toxicity in various human organs, altered cell morphology, allergic reactions, hypersensitivity reactions, and carcinogenic effects (Bumbudsanpharoke and Ko 2015). Hence, many food agencies have recommended both *in vivo*, and *in vitro* toxicity studies of nanomaterials before their commercial use. The current chapter is aimed at revealing potential applications of nanomaterials in food sector, mechanism of action of nanomaterials, their safety issues, and regulatory guidelines for safe use of nanotechnology.

Table 3.1 Nano products from food industry available in the market (Bumbudsanpharoke and Ko 2015; Hamad et al. 2018)

S.No.	Trademark/ Commercial name of product	Manufacturer	Nanomaterial	Improved product functionality
1.	Nano silver baby mug	Baby dream	Silver nanoparticles (Ag NPs)	Enhanced antibacterial properties
2.	Everin Food Containers Nanosilver Airtight	NewLife Co., Ltd.	Ag NPs	Possesses antibacterial property which keeps food fresher for longer time
3.	Sina Antibacterial Food Storages	Dai Dong Tien Co.	Ag NPs	Prevents food from dirt, remove foul smell, and inhibits germ growth
4.	Mycrohydrin powder	RBC Lifesciences	Silica-mineral hydride complex	Increased potency and bioavailability, and acts as powerful antioxidant
5.	Zeomic	Sinanen Zeomic Co., Ltd.	Silver-base zeolite	Antimicrobial (bacterial, yeasts, and molds) property
6.	Oat chocolate Nutritional drink mix	Toddler health	Iron oxide nanoparticles (Fe_3O_4 NPs)	Increased reactivity and bioavailability
7.	Imperm Nylon Nanocomposite	Mitsubishi Gas Chemical Company, Inc.	Nanoclay	Cost effective material with easy processing, and maintaining barrier properties
8.	Durethan KU 2-2601 plastic wrapping	Bayer	Silica nanoparticles in polymer-based nanocomposite	Enhanced shelf life of product by preventing the penetration of oxygen

3.2 Nanotechnology in Food Industries

It has been considered that conventional agricultural techniques are not sufficient to meet the food demand for future generations, and restore damaged ecosystem. There is an immediate need to develop, and adapt new technologies which can overcome this problem. Nanotechnology has gained tremendous impetus in food sector to achieve this goal. There is loss of major nutritional supplements during production, and processing of food products, which generates the need of seeking more nutritional supplements for producing better quality food. Nanotechnology plays a major role in increasing food yield, enhancing shelf-life of food products, and decreasing depletion of nutrients (He et al. 2019). Nanomaterials are used in food sector for food preservation, food packaging (Wesley et al. 2014), nutritional drinks (Miller and Senjen 2008), nutritional supplements (Skalickova et al. 2017). It is also used to test quality of food (Coles and Frewer 2013; Paul et al. 2017), and detection of pathogens (Mousavi and Rezaei 2011; Arora et al. 2017; Aly et al. 2018) in foods. Nanomaterials are used in agricultural industries in different forms such as biosensors for aqua culture (Kumar et al. 2017), nano-pesticide (Corradini et al. 2010), nano-fertilizer (Abobatta 2018), plant growth regulators (Choy et al. 2007), nanosensors (Viswanathan and Radecki 2008), waste management (Bharathi et al. 2016), post-harvest technology (Meetoo 2011), animal husbandry (Eguchi et al. 2013), and agricultural engineering aspects (Melendi et al. 2008). The applications of Nanotechnology in food industries are summarized in Fig. 3.1 (He et al. 2019).

3.2.1 Food Processing

Nanomaterials are well designed as color or flavor additives, preservatives, or carriers for food supplement (nanoencapsulation and nanoemulsion), including animal feed products. The unique properties of engineered nanomaterials offer great advantages for food processing as ingredients or supplement. The conventional methods used for food processing are ohmic heating, irradiation, and high hydrostatic pressure (Neethirajan and Jayas 2011). Addition of nanomaterials with the conventional methods results in various improvements (Mohammed et al. 2011). Nanoparticles are used in food processing to improve the color, flavor, stability, nutritional quality, processing yield, and flow properties. SiO_2 (amorphous silica) and TiO_2 oxides have been recommended by European Food and Safety Authority (EFSA) for use in food additives (E551) (Qi et al. 2004; Skocaj et al. 2011). Titanium dioxide (TiO_2) is considered as an inert and safe material and has been used in many applications (Skocaj et al. 2011). TiO_2 is permitted as an additive (E171) in food and pharmaceutical products (Rowe et al. 2003). TiO_2 (E171) use in various food products for opacity (mozzarella and cottage cheeses, lemon curd and sauces) cross linking, packaging (capsules), also in sweets where it provides a barrier between different colors (Skocaj et al. 2011). Food additive E551 contains SiO_2 NPs as anticaking

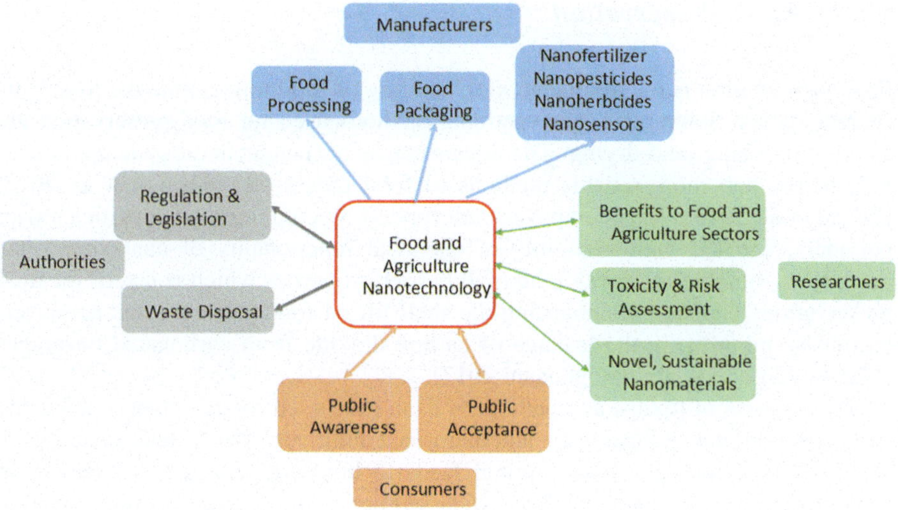

Fig. 3.1 Schematic illustration of food nanotechnology from scientific research to commercialized product (He et al. 2019)

agents that keep powders such as tea, powdered sugar, coffee, milk powder and table salt, free flowing (Bouwmeester et al. 2014). The commonly used methods of food processing with nanomaterials are mineral and vitamin fortification, nutraceuticals incorporation, addition of viscosifying agents, and nutrient delivery (Huang et al. 2010). Nanoencapsulation is one of the methods of food processing, and it is used for delivery of minerals, vitamins, and lipophilic health supplements (Dreher 2004). The six basic ways for preparation of nanocapsules are nanoprecipitation, emulsion-diffusion, double emulsification, emulsion-coacervation, polymer coating, and layer-by-layer (Maynard et al. 2006). Nanochelates are nanocoils which composed of soy based phospholipids which are phosphatidyl serine, phosphatidic acid, dioleoylnphosphatidyl serine, diphosphatidyl glycerol, phosphatidylethanolamine, phosphatidylinositol, phosphatidyl glycerol, phosphatidyl choline, dioleoyl phosphatidic acid, dipalmitoyl phosphatidyl glycerol, distearoyl phosphatidylserine, and dimyristoyl phosphatidyl serine which wrap around the micronutrients that result in their stability and the enhancement of nutrient content of the food (Abbas et al. 2009). Nanoemulsions, made from tributyl phosphate, soyabean or nonionic surfactants, are used in food processing to prevent food spoilage from Gram-positive bacteria (Wang et al. 2012). Nanoemulsions are small in size, and thermally stable, therefore, they are used in preparation of various food products like flavored oils, sweeteners, and salad dressing beverages (Hogan et al. 2001; Wang et al. 2012).

3.2.2 Food Preservation

Food preservation is the treatment, and handling of food to preclude the loss of its characteristics. Some of the conventional methods used for food preservation are canning, freezing, and drying. The advancement of nanotechnology helps to provide better, and more reliable methods of food preservation (Davis et al. 2013; Hamad et al. 2018). Nanocomposites are formed by combining nanoparticles with polymers, and the high versatility of chemical functionality of nanocomposites make them suitable for developing high barrier properties which is useful for food preservation. They aid in enhancing the shelf life of food products, and act as gas barrier by minimizing the leakage of carbon dioxide from carbonated beverages (Mallakpour and Rashidimoghadam 2017).

The removal of toxins, and pathogens from processed foods is succeeded using surface-functionalized nanoclay, and nanosized additives to yield better nano feed. Nanoclay is incorporated into animal feeds to bind with mycotoxins present in feeds, to improve its shelf life. The processed nano feed encourages the activation of animal's immune system to maintain healthy cell activity and overall animal health, improve phosphate utilization, improve bone growth, and reduce mortality rate (Sekhon 2014). The commercial nanoclays available in the market are Imperm, Durethan, and Aegis. Imperm is nanoclay based polymer made up of nylon and nanoclay, and is used in food sector to scavenge oxygen (Sekhon 2014). Durethan is made up of polyamide, and it gives toughness to paperboard containers for fruit juices. Aegis is used in carbonated beverages because it acts as oxygen scavenger.

Nanoparticles are used in food preservation due to their ability in adhering food color, stability, and property of flow. However, their effectiveness relies on their bioavailability (Hamad et al. 2018). Silver nanoparticles are observed to extend the shelf life of vegetables, and fruits by absorbing and decomposing ethylene, and they are more effective as bactericide against Gram negative bacteria due to their easy penetration through thin cell wall (Zhao et al. 2008). Titanium dioxide is another nanoparticle which has showed antimicrobial activity, but its usage is limited because it easily gets photocatalyzed (Arora and Padua 2010). Other nanoparticles which have been reported for antimicrobial activity are cadmium, copper and copper oxide, chitosan, magnesium oxide, single walled carbon nanotube, selenium, and telluride (Arshak et al. 2007).

3.2.3 Food Packaging

Food packaging is one of the largest commercial application of nanotechnology in food sector. Food industries are already making packaging materials using nanotechnology for enhancing the shelf life of food products, and improving food safety. An edible antibacterial nano-coating was developed by U.S. company Sono-Tec Corporation which has been directly applied to bakery goods (Amin 2007). Kodak company has developed nanotechnology based antimicrobial packaging, and active packaging for absorbing oxygen (Asadi and Mousavi 2006). The nanotech company pSiNutria has already developed nano-based tracking technologies by introducing edible BioSilicon in foods for pathogen detection (Miller and Senjen 2008). Chemical sensors are used by Nestle, British Airways, MonoPrix Supermarkets for detecting color change in food products (Pal 2017).

Nanoparticles are used in food packaging to improve the mechanical, barrier, thermal, chemical, and antimicrobial properties of foods. Among many novel nanomaterials, nanoclay is one of the most widely used and studied for food packaging due to their mechanical, thermal, and barrier properties, and low cost. For instance, 1% (w/w) bentonite clay/poly (vinyl alcohol) loaded nanocomposite membrane significantly enhanced permeance (Jose et al. 2014). Nanoparticles such as titanium oxide, silicate nanoparticles, and zinc oxide are used to reduce leakage of moisture for keeping the food fresh for long duration, and flow of oxygen inside the packaging containers (Mihindukulasuriya and Lim 2014; Hamad et al. 2018). Nanocor are used in packaging materials to enhance several properties like light weight, better recyclability, and avoid spoilage and flavor issues. The shelf life of beer bottles has been increased using nanocomposite materials (Pereda et al. 2019). The commonly used biodegradable nanocomposites for packaging application are polylactic acid (PLA), polybutylene succinate (PBS), polyhydroxybutyrate (PHB), starch and derivates, and aliphatic polyesters (Wesley et al. 2014). The use of nanocomposites in contact with foods has been approved by United States Food and Drug Administration (USFDA) (Badgley et al. 2007; Sozer and Kokini 2009; FDA issues 2015). The other nanomaterials used in antimicrobial food packaging are carbon nanotubes, nanocopper oxide, nano magnesium oxide, and nano titanium dioxide (Chaudhry et al. 2008). The development of chemical sensors, and biosensors results in use of sensing devices to monitor quality, integrity, wholeness, and safety of food, and it may be incorporated into food packaging technology, which is called as smart or intelligent packaging (Sahoo et al. 2007). The detection of several food borne pathogens such as anthrax, *E.coli*, tularemia bacteria, Ebola, and severe acute respiratory syndrome (SARS) virus has been done using fluorescent nanobarcode detection system by observing different color codes in a computer scanner. For the detection of presence of mycotoxins, bacteria, viruses, and other pathogens in foods, biomimetic sensors and smart biosensors have been developed (Coles and Frewer 2013). In another study, the smart packaging of foods has been reported using compatible luminescence oxygen biosensor (Kelly 2017). Other applications in food contact packaging include pesticides detection, pathogens detection and toxins detection and are also under active research and development due to the ultra-sensitive properties of nanomaterials (Sahoo et al. 2018; Sun et al. 2018). Table 3.2 summarizes some of the potent optical sensors for detection of foodborne or waterborne pathogens in food sample using nanomaterials. It gives the reported analytes, food samples, the nanomaterial or matrix used and the limit of detection (Khansili et al. 2018).

Table 3.2 Some important optical sensors for detection foodborne or waterborne pathogens (Khansili et al. 2018)

Analyte	Nanomaterial or matrix used	Sample	Limit of detection	Detection time per assay (minutes)	Reference(s)
Escherichia coli	Silica particles	Water	3–5 cells	–	Kalele et al. (2006)
Salmonella typhimurium	PBS	Chicken meat samples	10–20 cells/mL	12	Salam et al. (2013)
Mycobacterium tuberculosis	Sputum	Bovine Milk	2×10^2 cells/mL	30	He et al. (2002)
Mycobacterium avium	Au NPs	Milk	10^3 cells/mL	42	Yakes et al. (2008)
Listeria. monocytogenes	Tris buffer	Uncooked foods	10^7 cells/mL	30	Schlundt (2002)
Pseudomonas aeruginosa	Nutrient broth	Meat samples	1.3×10^7 cells/mL	20	Kim et al. (2004)
Salmonella enteritidis	Saline solution	Milk	10^5 cells/mL	35	Si et al. (2001)
Salmonella typhi	QDs	Chicken carcass wash water	10^3 cells/mL	15	Yang and Li (2005)
Salmonella paratyphi	PBS	Water	5×10^6 cells/mL	50	Fung and Wong (2001)

Au NPs gold nanoparticles, *NPs* nanoparticles, *QDs* quantum dots, *PBS* phosphate buffer saline

3.2.4 Encapsulation and Delivery of Active Ingredients in Food

Nanotechnology has the potential to detect gene expression under different stress conditions, delivery of genes, pesticides and drugs to specific sites in plants and animals with minimal side effects. This technology provides new opportunities for development of bio-pesticides in the form of nanoencapsulation, nanoformulation, and functionalized nanoparticles (He et al. 2019). Nanoencapsulation system offers profuse benefits in food sector such as enhanced stability and integrity, pH-triggered and moisture-triggered release, enhanced food stability and integrity, protection against rancidity and oxidation, taste masking, retention of volatile ingredients, long lasting organoleptic perception, and consecutive delivery of multiple active ingredients (Aigbogun et al. 2017). Nanocapsules have been used as nutritional supplements, and nano-food additives to enhance the bioavailability, and allow better dispersion of insoluble additives. The commonly used nano-sized carriers are micelles, liposomes, and protein-based carriers (Duran et al. 2007). The use of lipid based nanoencapsulation in the form of nanococheleates, nanoliposomes, and archaeosomes has also been reported for nano-delivery of antimicrobials, enzymes, food additives, and nutraceuticals (Mozafari et al. 2008). Nanosilicates are used for encapsulating enzymes which can be used in nutrient release, and drug release systems (Neethirajan et al. 2009). The nutraceuticals incorporated in carriers to prevent the accumulation of cholesterol are β-carotenes, phytosterols, and lycopene (Mozafari et al. 2006). Nutraceuticals, and bioactive compounds available in functional foods (omega-3-fatty acid from salmon oil, β -carotene from carrots, lycopene from tomato, isoflavones from soyabean, conjugated linoleic acid from cheese, and β-glucan from oats) are delivered using nanotechnology (Chen et al. 2006). α-lactalbumin is used for designing engineered nanotubes (ENT), and ENT acts as nanoencapsulation for pharmaceuticals, nutrients, and bioactive compounds (Graveland and Kruif 2006).

Nanocapsules were integrated into bread by George Weston Foods, Australia to promote controlled release of probiotics for improving gut health (Neethirajan and Jayas 2007). The health promoting ingredient i.e. vitamin D_3 is delivered using nanostructured lipid carrier (NLC) (Maurya and Aggarwal 2019). Here, a phase inversion based NLC fabrication process for Vitamin D_3 encapsulation was studied and using this, NLC fortified Lassi (milk-based beverage) was developed (Maurya and Aggarwal 2019; Maurya et al. 2020). The viability of probiotics like *Bifidobacterium* sp., *Lactobacillus casei, Lb. acidophilus*, and *Lb. rhamnosus* can be improved in yogurt by their encapsulation with calcium alginate (Duncan 2011). Some of the commonly used nano-formulations which are used as food supplements are solid-lipid nanoparticles, core-shell nanoparticles, layered double hydroxides, mesoporous silica nanoparticles, nanocapsules, nanogels, nanosponges, nanoliposomes, nanoemulsions, micelles, and cyclodextrin complexes (Jampilek et al. 2019).

3.2.5 *Nanodevices*

Nanotechnology is used to improve current agricultural practices by enhancing the management, and conservation of inputs in crops, fisheries, and animal production (Pramanik and Pramanik 2016; Singh 2016). Nanosensors can be used in agriculture for detection of pesticides on the surface of fruits and vegetables, and identification of carcinogens in food materials (Meetoo 2011; Srivastava et al. 2017). Nanosensors have high sensitivity, and selectivity to detect subtle changes in food quality and color, and gases released due to spoilage by pathogens. Table 3.3 shows the usage of nanosensors in different sectors (Khansili et al. 2018). Nanosensors are found to be more efficient than conventional chemical sensors for quantification of small number of contaminants in food (Mannino and Scampicchio 2007). The integration of micro and nano-structured elements within the biosensing systems (magnetic micro- or nanoparticles, graphite microparticles, gold nanocomposites, nanowires, carbon nanotubes, nanorods, and bioreactors) has provided enhanced analytical improvements and performances in the detection of various food-borne pathogens, allergens (gliadin), food additives (folic acids), and food residues (antibiotics, pesticides) (Rattu and Krishna 2017). Gold, platinum, and palladium are used in gas sensors, and gold nanoparticles are used for detection of aflatoxin B_1 in milk (Kumar et al. 2017; Khansili et al. 2020). Among all the metal nanoparticles,

Table 3.3 Nanosensors used in food and biological sensor applications (Khansili et al. 2018)

Biosensor type	Label free	Commercialization	Multiplexing	Specific biological Applications	Reference(s)
SPR	Yes	+++	++	Xenobiotics and toxins in food-carbohydrate-specific interactions-protein & antigens in biological and clinical samples-	Pennacchio et al. (2014), Choi et al. (2014) Safina (2012) and Bornehag et al. (2014)
LSPR	Yes	+	++	Cancer biomarker Toxin detection in food samples-detection of DNA hybridization-screening of antigen–antibody interactions-	Lee et al. (2013), Piliarik et al. (2012) and Endo et al. (2006)
Evanescent wave fluorescence	No	+++	+++	Clinical biomarkers-Clinical diagnostics, biodefence, food testing-	Yildirim et al. (2012) and Taitt et al. (2015)
Bioluminescent optical fibre	No	+	++	Multidetection of genotoxins by live cell array-response of cells to genotoxic agents-	Jia et al. (2012) and Biran et al. (2003)
Ellipsometric	Yes	+	++	Detection of serum tumour biomarker-characterizing viral receptor profiles-	Fei et al. (2015) and Zhang et al. (2011)
SERS	Yes	+	+	Protein biomarker in environment-detection of cancer proteins-	Srivastava et al. (2014)

+ defines **small-scale,** ++ defines **fine-scale,** +++ defines **broad-scale**
SPR Surface plasmon resonance
LSPR Localized surface plasmon resonance
SERS Surface-enhanced Raman spectroscopy

copper nanoparticles are observed to have broad spectrum antimicrobial properties against bacteria, and fungi with minimum phytotoxic effects.

Electronic nose or e-nose is a specific type of sensor arrays. It is an odour mapper which can discriminate different volatile compounds due to the electronic response resulting from the various gas sensors, typically metal-oxide based chemosensors

(Rattu and Krishna 2017). Electronic nose has been reported to classify cereal grains, to discriminate strongly musty and weakly musty oat samples effectively (Schaller et al. 1998). On the other side, electronic tongue or e-tongue comprising of 30 chemical based sensors and pattern recognition elements for processing of data. Principle of the electronic tongues function in a similar way to the "electronic nose". A pattern of signals is generated, that can be correlated to certain features or qualities of the sample. It is used for analysis of soft drinks, coffee, mineral water and flesh food (Vidic et al. 2006).

3.3 Nanotechnology and Food Safety

Nanotechnology has shown tremendous applications in agriculture, and food industry. The major topics which need to be considered with growth, and application of this technology are risk evaluation and consumer perception. The detailed studies such as nutritional value, metabolism, and possible contaminants including allergens are required to be conducted before altering the food composition. The key determinants and source of potential adverse health effects are physico-chemical characteristics of nanomaterials. Organization for Economic Co-operation and Development (OECD 2013) has defined a list of physico-chemical properties, and the major properties for nanotoxicity issues are size, chemical composition aggregation/agglomeration state, and surface coating of nanomaterials (Bar-Ilan et al. 2009). The EU Scientific Committee on Emerging and Newly Identified Health Risks (SCENIHR) has reported that free and low solubility nanomaterials are of prior concern for human, and environmental safety (European Commission 2004; Commission 2005). Nanomaterials have unique physical, and chemical properties, which may be responsible for their hazardous effects on environment as well as human health.

Several nanoparticles may disrupt the normal functioning of cellular components by attaching to receptors of cells which further inhibit the immune system (Jordan et al. 2005). Carbon nanotubes are commonly used in food packaging, and toxic effects of these carbon nanotubes on human skin, and lungs has been reported (Mills and Hazafy 2009). There are also some reports on toxic effects of cobalt, iron, silver, titanium, and tungsten nanoparticles. The nanoparticles can lead to enhanced oxidative stress by forming free radicals which may induce cancer, DNA mutations, and even cell death. Previously, the increased airway fibrosis with allergic asthma was found in mice when exposed to carbon nanotubes (Rasmussen et al. 2009). A previous *in vivo* study of female BALB/c mice exposed to nanoparticles has reported the induction of allergen-specific Th2-type immune responses. This study also showed the induction of high level of OVA-specific immunoglobulin (IgE, IgG1) anti-bodies during intranasal exposure of ovalbumin (OVA) plus SiO_2 nanoparticles (Yoshida et al. 2011). Similarly, Hirai et al. (2014) also showed the induction of nanoparticle-specific immune responses when exposed to Ag nanoparticles. The carbon black nanoparticles with small particle size, high surface area, and high purity are associated with enhanced gene expression of allergy-associated Th-2 cytokines, interleukin-4 (IL-4), IL-10, and IL-13 (Lefebvre et al. 2014). The extensive use of nanomaterials in various food products by food industries result in release of nanomaterials in soil, and water bodies which lead to their accumulation in food chain, and alteration of their normal microbiota. Hence, both pelagic, and benthic species are affected in marine bodies. Different metal-based nanoparticles like ZnO, Ag, and CuO are reported as metal-leaching nanomaterials, and these metal nanomaterials are associated with increased intracellular level of reactive oxygen species (ROS), which may lead to DNA damage, and lipid peroxidation (McShan et al. 2014). The induction of ROS levels by NPs leads to the activation of defense pathway to combat the oxidative stress (Fig. 3.2). When the rate of ROS generation overweighs the rate of ROS scavenging, it leads to a harmful imbalance in the anti-oxidative system. This imbalance (often called as oxidative burst) results in widespread damage in cells including peroxidation of membrane lipids, oxidative damage to vital biomolecules such as nucleic acids and proteins and also the activation of programmed cell death (PCD) pathway (Gratao et al. 2005).

Some of the factors required for evaluating the risk assessment for use of nanomaterials in food products are type and amount of food consumed, their osmotic

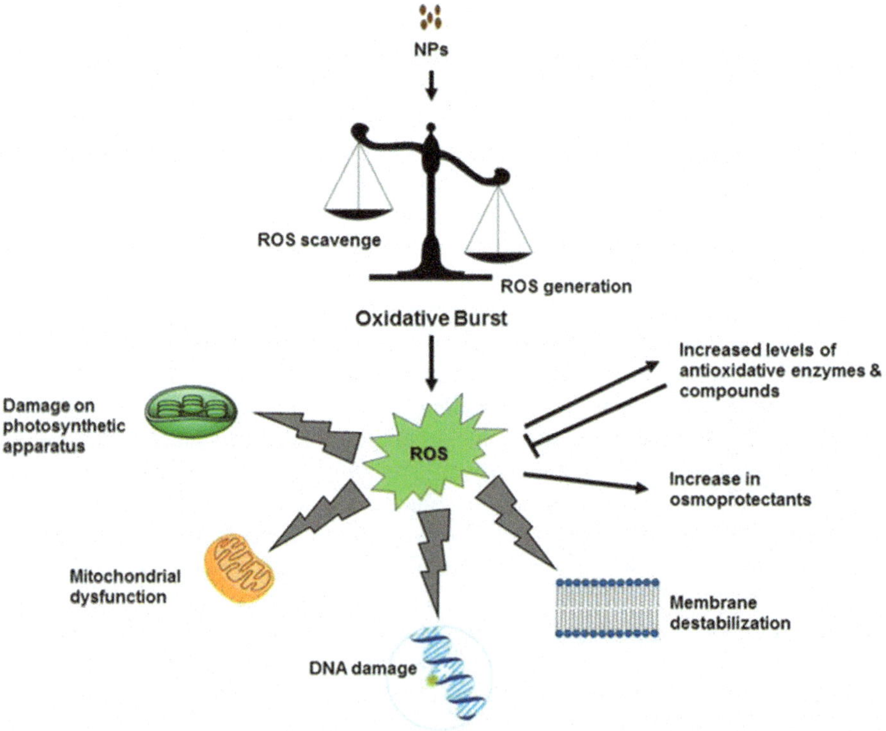

Fig. 3.2 Graphical illustration of ROS-mediated impacts of NPs on the intracellular environment

concentration, absorption, distribution, metabolism, excretion, physical factors, chemical factors, and biological molecules (He et al. 2015; Wani and Kothari 2018). It is essential to pay attention on studies for interactions between nanomaterials, and biological systems to understand actual toxicity of nanomaterials using *in silico, in vivo*, and *in vitro* studies. The nanomaterials enter the human body through ingestion, and reaches GIT (gastrointestinal tract). GIT is one of the protective covering of mucus (complex network of highly branched glycoproteins, and macromolecules) which makes interaction with nanomaterials. The physico-chemical properties of nanomaterials may alter in GIT due to their interaction with digestive enzymes, food, electrolytes, and intestinal microbiota. The reactivity and toxicity of nanomaterials may change with change in pH in different segments of GIT. These nanomaterials can be absorbed in epithelial cells like M-cells of Peyer's Patches in GALT (gut-associated lymphoid tissue) through absorption (Powell et al. 2010). The action mechanism of nanomaterials in human body is shown in Fig. 3.3. The most relevant route for uptake of nanomaterials is transcellular route due to elimination of macromolecules from tight junctions of epithelial cells (Tang and Goodenough 2003). It has been reported previously that chitosan nanoparticles promote paracellular transport of macromolecules due to loosening of epithelial tight junctions (Sonaje et al. 2011). The nanomaterials may form corona of adsorbed proteins, small molecules, and ions in the biological fluids, which may lead to decreased cytotoxicity due to decrease in uptake of nanoparticles (Martirosyan and Schneider 2014).

It has also been observed that titanium dioxide nanoparticles can induce epithelium impairment through ileum epithelium at Peyer's patches. The toxic effects of titanium dioxide nanoparticles, which have been administered orally (at a dose of 1000 mg/Kg body weight per day), was investigated using conventional approaches, and metabolomics analysis (Bu et al. 2010). Further, nanomaterials are translocated to internal body compartments with internalization through gut epithelium. These nanomaterials may enter the bloodstream into different organs through portal circulation to the liver or through mesenteric lymph nodes into the lympho-reticular

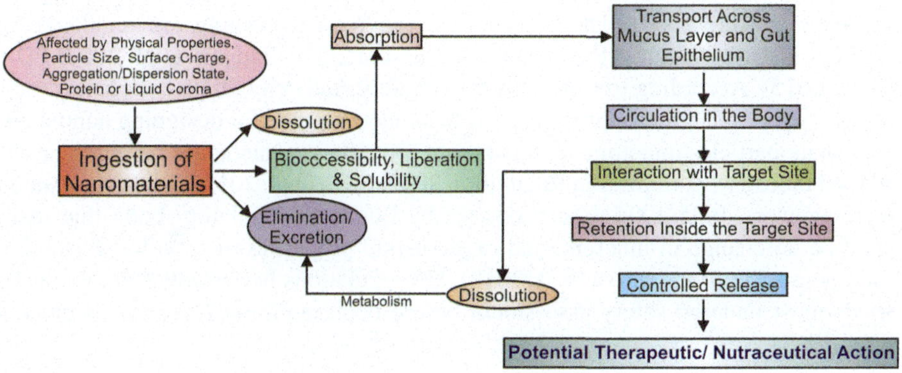

Fig. 3.3 Mechanism of action of nanomaterials in human body

system (Martirosyan and Schneider 2014). Previously, gold nanoparticles of different size (1.4–200 nm), and opposite surface charges were passed through intestinal membranes of adult female rats, and it has been observed that small sized nanoparticles (2.8 nm) passed easily across the intestinal barrier compared to large once, and negatively charged particles were absorbed more readily than positively charged particles (Schleh et al. 2012). Teow et al. (2011) reported the health impact, and safety issues with use of nanoparticles through absorption, and distribution in human body with emphasis on genotoxicity and cytotoxicity. It has been revealed from the modern techniques that nanoparticles have high reactivity, and ability to cross the blood capillaries, and membrane barriers, which may lead to their toxicodynamic, and toxico-kinetic properties. The current information regarding metabolism of engineered nanomaterials in human model on oral administration is very limited. Hence, government and non-government firms should focus on extensive research on use of nanotechnology for practical and industrial applications.

3.4 Safety Regulations on Use of Nanomaterials

The great public concern for use of nanotechnology is due to health implications of nano-particles after entering inside the body. Hence, assessments and evaluations are essential to check the potential risks of nanomaterials on human health. Safety regulations which have been developed by regulatory bodies for use of nanomaterials in food, and agriculture industries to be followed for safe use of nanotechnology. The major regulatory bodies in world are European Food and Safety Authority (EFSA), National Institute for Occupational Safety and Health (NIOSH), Environmental Protection Agency (EPA), Food and Drug Administration (FDA) US Patent and Trademark Office (USPTO), Consumer Product Safety Commission (CPSC), US Department of Agriculture (USDA), and Occupational Safety and Health Administration (OSHA) (Qi et al. 2004). European Union regulations for food and food packaging has recommended that nano-foods should meet the recommended specific risk assessment, and safety standards before their introduction to market (Halliday 2007). The nano-foods, and food packaging are regulated by USFDA in United States (European Commission 2004; Badgley et al. 2007; FDA issues 2015). According to European Food Safety Authority regulation; heavy metals and mycotoxins free approach needs to be incorporated for designing nanomaterials (nanoparticles/quantum dots/ nanotubes/ nanowires/nanoclay) before their use in food industry (Commission Regulation 2011; Silva et al. 2012). It has been stated in Framework 1935/2004 regulations set by European regulatory body that there shall be no change in inherent, and organoleptic properties of food by substances incorporated in foods (Silva et al. 2012). EU regulations has established that nano-foods must undergo safety assessment before being authorized for use (Cubadda et al. 2013).

3.5 Conclusions and Future Perspectives

Nanotechnology is emerging technology which is gaining tremendous impetus due to its potential applications in agriculture, and food sector which will play an important role in future to meet the increasing food demand of growing population. It is used in agriculture, and food sectors in many aspects such as disease treatment, food security, bioavailability, packaging material, diagnostic kits, cellular and molecular biology tools. Nanotechnology has the potential to provide smart, intelligent, and active packaging system, and food quality tracking-tracing-monitoring system. The nano-formulated agrochemicals like fertilizers, pesticides, antimicrobials, detoxifying compounds, veterinary medicine, and biosides can be developed by using encapsulated nanoparticles. Most of the nanosystems are still at developing stage, and researchers are trying to develop better, and efficient nanocarriers with enhanced bioavailability without compromising quality, and taste of food products. The nanofoods should be labeled properly to give the customer freedom for choosing the products based on their need. A little information is available on absorption, distribution, metabolism, and excretion of nanoparticles, and hence food regulatory bodies stresses on analysis of risk assessment of nanomaterials. The availability of incomplete food safety regulations in many countries encourages the need for developing international regulation for use of nanoparticles. There is an immediate need for developing standardized approaches to assess the hazardous effects of nanomaterials on human body, and environment. Further, the quantitative analysis of nanomaterials can provide the scientific basis for their risk assessment that can also be used for safe use of nanomaterials in food sector.

References

Abbas KA, Saleh AM, Mohamed A, MohdAzhan N (2009) The recent advances in the nanotechnology and its applications in food processing: a review. J Food Agric Environ 7:14–17. https://agris.fao.org/agris-search/search.do?recordID=US201301728140

Abobatta WF (2018) Nanotechnology applications in agriculture. Acta Sci Agric 2:99–102. https://actascientific.com/ASAG/pdf/ASAG-02-0108.pdf

Ahumada O, Villalobos JR (2009) Application of planning models in the agri-food supply chain: a review. Eur J Oper Res 195:1–20. https://doi.org/10.1016/j.ejor.2008.02.014

Aigbogun IE, Mohammed SSD, Orukotan AA, Tanko JD (2017) The role of nanotechnology in food industries-a review. Adv Appl Microbiol 7:1–9. https://doi.org/10.9734/jamb/2017/38175

Aly MA, Domig KJ, Kneifel W, Reimhult E (2018) Immunogold nanoparticles for rapid plasmonic detection of *Croobacter sakazakii*. Sensors 18:1–18. https://doi.org/10.3390/s18072028

Amin AE (2007) Nanoscale particles designed to block UV light. FoodProductionDaily.com Europe. 18 October. Available at: http://foodproductiondaily.com/news/ng.asp?id=80676

Arora A, Padua GW (2010) Review: nanocomposites in food packaging. J Food Sci 75:R43–R49. https://doi.org/10.1111/j.1750-3841.2009.01456.x

Arora S, Ahmed N, Sucheta SS (2017) Detecting food borne pathogens using electrochemical biosensors: an overview. Int J Chem Stud 6:1031–1039. https://www.semanticscholar.org/paper/Detecting-food-borne-pathogens-using-biosensors%3A-An-Arora-Ahmed/d511e8411fc2403a00226e67885c25df4587d859

Arshak K, Adley C, Moore C, Cunniffe C, Campion M, Harris J (2007) Characterization of polymer nanocomposite sensors for quantification of bacterial cultures. Sensor Actuat B Chem 126:226–231. https://doi.org/10.1016/j.snb.2006.12.006

Asadi G, Mousavi M (2006) Applications of nanotechnology in Food packaging. Available: http://iufost.edpsciences.org

Badgley C, Moghtader J, Quintero E, Zakem E, Chappel LM, Vazquez KA, Salon A, Perfecto I (2007) Organic agriculture and the global food supply. Renew Agric Food Sys 22(2):86–108. https://doi.org/10.1017/S1742170507001640

Bar-Ilan O, Albrecht RM, Fako VE, Furgeson DY (2009) Toxicity assessments of multisized gold and silver nanoparticles in zebrafish embryos. Small 5:1897–1910. https://doi.org/10.1002/smll.200801716

Bharathi P, Balasubramanian N, Anitha S, Vijayabharathi V, Bhuvenswari (2016) Improvement of membrane system for water treatment by synthesized gold nanoparticles. J Environ Biol 37:1407–1414. https://www.researchgate.net/publication/313057057_Improvement_of_membrane_system_for_water_treatment_by_synthesized_gold_nanoparticles

Biran I, Rissin DM, Ron EZ, Walt DR (2003) Optical imaging fiber-based live bacterial cell array biosensor. Anal Biochem 315:106–113. https://doi.org/10.1016/s0003-2697(02)00700-5

Bornehag CG, Sundell J, Weschler CJ, Sigsgaord T, Lundgren B, Hasselgren M, Hagerhed-Engman L (2014) The association between asthma and allergic symptoms in children and phthalates in house dust: a nested case–control study. Environ Health Perspect 112:1393–1397. https://doi.org/10.1289/ehp.7187

Bouwmeester H, Brandhoff P, Marvin HJP, Weigel S, Peters RJB (2014) State of the safety assessment and current use of nanomaterials in food and food production. Trends Food Sci Technol 40:200–210. https://doi.org/10.1016/j.tifs.2014.08.009

Bryksa BC, Yada RY (2012) Challenges in food nanoscale science and technology. J Food Drug Anal 20:418–421. https://www.fda.gov.tw/upload/189/Content/2014012910321861898.pdf

Bu Q, Yan G, Deng P et al (2010) NMR-based metabonomic study of the sub-acute toxicity of titanium dioxide nanoparticles in rats after oral administration. Nanotechnology 21:125105. https://doi.org/10.1088/0957-4484/21/12/125105

Bumbudsanpharoke N, Ko S (2015) Nano-food packaging: an overview of market, migration research, and safety regulations. J Food Sci 80:910–922. https://doi.org/10.1111/1750-3841.12861

Chaudhry Q, Scotter M, Blackburn J, Ross B, Boxall A, Castle L, Aitken R, Watkins R (2008) Applications and implications of nanotechnologies for the food sector. Food Addit Contam 25:241–258. https://doi.org/10.1080/02652030701744538

Chen H, Weiss J, Shahidi F (2006) Nanotechnology in nutraceuticals and functional foods. Food Technol 60:30–36. https://doi.org/10.1201/9781315370859-14

Choi Y, Kwak H, Hong S (2014) Quantification of arsenic (III) in aqueous media using a novel hybrid platform comprised of radially porous silica particles and a gold thin film. Anal Methods 6:7054–7061. https://doi.org/10.1039/c4ay01297f

Choy JH, Choi SJ, Oh JM, Park T (2007) Clay minerals and double layered hydroxides for novel biological applications. Appl Clay Sci 36:122–132. https://doi.org/10.1016/j.clay.2006.07.007

Coles D, Frewer LJ (2013) Nanotechnology applied to European food production- a review of ethical and regulatory issues. Trends Food Sci Technol 34:32–43. https://doi.org/10.1016/j.tifs.2013.08.006

Commission E (2005) Scientific committee on emerging and newly (SCENIHR) Opinion on the safety of human-derived products with regard to variant Creutzfeldt-Jakob disease. Rev Lit Arts Am. https://ec.europa.eu/health/archive/ph_risk/committees/04_scenihr/docs/scenihr_o_005.pdf

Commission Regulation (EU) No 10/2011 of 14 January 2011 on plastic materials and articles intended to come into contact with food. Official J European Union 15.1.2011. https://eur-lex.europa.eu/LexUriServ/LexUriServ.do?uri=OJ:L:2011:012:0001:0089:EN:PDF

Corradini E, Moura MR, Mattoso LHC (2010) A preliminary study on the incorporation of NPK fertilizer into chitosan nanoparticles. Express Polym Lett 4:509–515. https://doi.org/10.3144/expresspolymlett.2010.64

Cubadda F, Aureli F, D'Amato M, Raggi A, Mantovani A (2013) Nanomaterials in the food sector: new approaches for safety assessment Rapporti ISTISAN:13/48. https://www.researchgate.net/publication/281444188_Conference_Nanomaterials_in_the_food_sector_new_approaches_for_safety_assessment_Rome_Istituto_Superiore_di_Sanita_September_27_2013_Proceedings

Davis D, Guo X, Musavi L, Lin CS, Chen SH, Wu VC (2013) Gold nanoparticle-modified carbon electrode biosensor for the detection of *Listeria monocytogenes*. Ind Biotechnol 9:31–36. https://doi.org/10.1089/ind.2012.0033

Dreher KL (2004) Health and environmental impact of nanotechnology: toxicological assessment of manufactured nanoparticles. Toxicol Sci 77:3–5. https://doi.org/10.1093/toxsci/kfh041

Duncan TV (2011) Applications of nanotechnology in food packaging and food safety: barrier materials, antimicrobials and sensors. Colloid Interface Sci 363:1–24. https://doi.org/10.1016/j.jcis.2011.07.017

Duran N, Marcarto PD, Souza GIH, Alves OL, Esposito E (2007) Antibacterial effect of silver nanoparticles produced by fungal process on textile fabrics and their effluent treatment. J Biomed Nanotechnol 3:203–208. https://doi.org/10.1166/jbn.2007.022

Ealias AM, Saravanakumar MP (2017) A review on the classification of nanoparticles and their application. Mater Sci Eng 263:1–15. https://doi.org/10.1088/1757-899x/263/3/032019

Eguchi E, Cecato U, Silva SL (2013) The way of nanotechnology in Brazil animal production. Pubvet 7:1528. https://doi.org/10.1111/asj.12313

Endo T, Kerman T, Nagatani K, Hiepa NM, Kim DK, Yonezawa Y (2006) Multiple label-free detection of antigen – antibody reaction using localized surface plasmon resonance-based core – shell structured nanoparticle layer nanochip. Anal Chem 78:6465–6475. https://doi.org/10.1021/ac0608321

European Commission (2004) Community Health and Consumer Protection. Nanotechnologies: A preliminary risk analysis. Workshop organized in Brussels on 1–2 march 2004 by The Health and Consumer Protection Directorate General of the European Commission. http://europa.eu.int/comm/health/ph_risk/events_risk_en.htm

FDA (2015) Guidance on the use of nanomaterials in food for animals by Food and Drug Administration, U.S..http://www.fda.gov/AnimalVeterinary/NewsEvents/CVMUpdates/ucm457112.htm

Fei Y, Sun YS, Li Y, Yu H, Lau K, Landry JP (2015) Characterization of receptor binding profiles of influenza a viruses using an ellipsometry-based label-free glycan microarray assay platform. Biomol Ther 5:1480–1498. https://doi.org/10.3390/biom5031480

Fung YS, Wong YY (2001) Self-assembled monolayers as the coating in a quartz piezoelectric crystal immunosensor to detect salmonella in aqueous solution. Anal Chem 73:5302–5309. https://doi.org/10.1021/ac010655y

Gratao PL, Polle A, Lea PJ, Azevedo RA (2005) Making the life of heavy metal-stressed plants a little easier. Funct Plant Biol 32:481–494. https://doi.org/10.1071/fp05016

Graveland JF, Kruif CG (2006) Unique milk protein-based nanotubes: food and nanotechnology meet. Trends Food Sci Technol 7:196–203. https://doi.org/10.1016/j.tifs.2005.12.009

Halliday J (2007) EU parliament votes for tougher additives regulation. FoodNavigator.com

Hamad AF, Han JH, Kim BC, Rather IA (2018) The intertwine of nanotechnology with food industry. Saudi J Biol Sci 25:27–30. https://www.ncbi.nlm.nih.gov/pmc/articles/PMC5775102/

He X, Hwang HM (2016) Nanotechnology in food science: functionality, applicability, and safety assessment. J Food Drug Anal 24:671–681. https://doi.org/10.1016/j.jfda.2016.06.001

He FJ, Zhang LD, Zhao JW, Hu BL, Lei JT (2002) A TSM immunosensor for detection of *M. tuberculosis* with a new membrane material. Sensors Actuators B Chem 85:284–290. https://doi.org/10.1016/s0925-4005(02)00144-2

He X, Aker WG, Fu PP, Hwang HM (2015) Toxicity of engineered metal oxide nanomaterials mediated by nano-bio-eco-interactions: a review and perspective. Environ Sci Nano 2:564–582. https://doi.org/10.1039/c5en00094g

He X, Deng H, Hwang H (2019) The current application of nanotechnology in food and agriculture. J Food Drug Anal 27:1–21. https://doi.org/10.1016/j.jfda.2018.12.002

Hirai T, Yoshioka Y, Ichihashi KI, Mori T, Nishijima N, Handa T, Takahashi H, Tsunoda SI, Higashisaka K, Tsutsumi Y (2014) Silver nanoparticles induce silver nanoparticle-specific allergic responses (HYP6P). J Immunol 92:118–119. https://www.semanticscholar.org/paper/Silver-nanoparticles-induce-silver-allergic-Hirai-Yoshioka/649897674d828c0a6cd8eee3cc4ab21fb32f7722

Hogan SA, McNamee BF, O'Riordan ED, O'Sullivan M (2001) Microencapsulating properties of sodium caseinate. J Agric Food Chem 49:1934–1938

http://www.foeeurope.org/activities/nanotechnology/Documents/Nano_food_report.Pdf

Huang Q, Yu H, Ru Q (2010) Bioavailability and delivery of nutraceuticals using nanotechnology. J Food Sci 75:R50–R57. https://doi.org/10.1111/j.1750-3841.2009.01457.x

Jampilek J, Kos J, Kralova K (2019) Potential of nanomaterial applications in dietary supplements and foods for special medical purposes. Nano 9:1–42. https://doi.org/10.3390/nano9020296

Jia K, Eltzov E, Toury T, Marks RS, Ionescu RE (2012) A lower limit of detection for atrazine was obtained using bioluminescent reporter bacteria via a lower incubation temperature. Ecotoxicol Environ Saf 84:221–226. https://doi.org/10.1016/j.ecoenv.2012.07.009

Jordan J, Jacob KI, Tannenbaum R, Sharaf MA, Jasiuk I (2005) Experimental trends in polymer nanocomposites-a review. Mater Sci Eng 393:1–11. https://doi.org/10.1016/j.msea.2004.09.044

Jose T, George SC, Maria HJ, Wilson R, Thomas S (2014) Effect of bentonite clay on the mechanical, thermal, and pervaporation performance of the poly (vinyl alcohol) nanocomposite membranes. Ind Eng Chem Res 53:16820–16831. https://doi.org/10.1021/ie502632p

Kalele SA, Kundu AA, Gosavi SW, Deobagkar DN, Deobagkar DD, Kulkarni SK (2006) Rapid detection of Escherichia coli by using antibody-conjugated silver nanoshells. Small 2:335–338. https://doi.org/10.1002/smll.200500286

Kelly CA (2017) Novel luminescent oxygen sensor systems for smart food packaging. Ph.D. Thesis, University College Cork, Ireland. https://cora.ucc.ie/handle/10468/3685

Khansili N, Rattu G, Krishna PM (2018) Label-free optical biosensors for food and biological sensor applications. Sens Actuators B Chem 265:35–49. https://doi.org/10.1016/j.snb.2018.03.004

Khansili N, Rattu G, Kumar A, Krishna PM (2020) Development of colorimetric sensor with zinc oxide nanoparticles for rapid detection of aflatoxin B1 in rice. Materials Today: Proceedings 21:1846–1855. https://doi.org/10.1016/j.matpr.2020.01.240

Kim N, Park IS, Kim DK (2004) Characteristics of a label-free piezoelectric immounosensor detecting *Pseudomonas aeruginosa*. Sensors Actuators B Chem 100:432–438. https://doi.org/10.1016/j.snb.2004.02.014

Kumar V, Guleria P, Mehta SK (2017) Nanosensors for food quality and safety assessment. Environ Chem Lett 15:165–177. https://www.x-mol.com/paper/1225124398925135881

Lee JH, Kim BC, Oh BK, Choi JW (2013) Highly sensitive localized surface plasmon resonance immunosensor for label-free detection of HIV-1. Nanomedicine 9:1018–1026. https://doi.org/10.1016/j.nano.2013.03.005

Lefebvre DE, Pearce B, Fine JH, Chomyshyn E, Ross N, Halappanavar S, Tayabali AF, Curran I, Bondy GS (2014) In vitro enhancement of mouse T helper 2 cell sensitization to ovalbumin allergen by carbon black nanoparticles. Toxicol Sci 138:322–332. https://doi.org/10.1093/toxsci/kfu010

Lugani Y, Kaur G, Oberoi S, Sooch BS (2018) Nanotechnology: current applications and future prospects. World J Adv Healthc Res 2:137–139. https://www.researchgate.net/publication/327369049_Nanotechnology_Current_Applications_and_Future_Prospects

Mallakpour S, Rashidimoghadam S (2017) 8- Recent developments in the synthesis of hybrid polymer/clay nanocomposites. Hybrid Polymer Composite Materials Applications 227–265. doi:https://doi.org/10.1016/B978-0-08-100785-3.00008-5

Mannino S, Scampicchio M (2007) Nanotechnology and food quality control. Veterin Res Commun 31:149–151. https://doi.org/10.1007/s11259-007-0081-9
Martirosyan A, Schneider YJ (2014) Engineered nanomaterials in food: implications for food safety and consumer health. Int J Environ Res Pub Health 11:5720–5750. https://doi.org/10.3390/ijerph110605720
Maurya VK, Aggarwal M (2019) Fabrication of nano-structured lipid carrier for encapsulation of vitamin D3 for fortification of 'Lassi'; a milk based beverage. J Steroid Biochem Mol Biol 193:105429. https://doi.org/10.1016/j.jsbmb.2019.105429
Maurya VK, Bashir K, Aggarwal M (2020) Vitamin D microencapsulation and fortification: trends and technologies. J Steroid Biochem Mol Biol 196:105489. https://doi.org/10.1016/j.jsbmb.2019.105489
Maynard AD, Aitken RJ, Butz T et al (2006) Safe handling of nanotechnology. Nature 444:267–269. https://doi.org/10.1038/444267a
McShan D, Ray PC, Yu H (2014) Molecular toxicity mechanism of nanosilver. J Food Drug Anal 22:116–127. https://doi.org/10.1016/j.jfda.2014.01.010
Meetoo DD (2011) Nanotechnology and the food sector: from the farm to the table. Emirates J Food Agric 23:387–407. https://www.researchgate.net/publication/286054841_Nanotechnology_and_the_food_sector_From_the_farm_to_the_table
Melendi PG, Pacheco RF, Coronado MJ, Corredor E, Testillano PS, Risueno MC, Marquina C, Ibarra MR, Rubiales D, Luque AP (2008) Nanoparticles as smart treatment-delivery systems in plants: assessment of different techniques of microscopy for their visualization in plant tissues. Ann Bot 101:187–195. https://doi.org/10.1093/aob/mcm283
Mihindukulasuriya SDF, Lim LT (2014) Nanotechnology development in food packaging: a review. Trends Food Sci Technol 40:149–167. https://doi.org/10.1016/j.tifs.2014.09.009
Miller G, Senjen R (2008) Out of the laboratory and on to our plates- nanotechnology in food and agriculture. Available: https://1bps6437gg8c169i0y1drtgz-wpengine.netdna-ssl.com/wp-content/uploads/2017/legacy/Nanotechnology_in_food_and_agriculture_-_web_resolution.pdf
Mills A, Hazafy D (2009) Nanocrystalline SnO_2-based, UVB-activated, colourimetric oxygen indicator. Sens Actuators B Chem 136:344–349. https://doi.org/10.1016/j.snb.2008.12.048
Mohammed NA, Ahmed IAM, Babiker EE (2011) Nutritional evaluation of sorghum flour (*Sorghum bicolor L. Moench*) during processing of injera. World Acad Sci Eng Technol 51:72–76. https://doi.org/10.31274/rtd-180814-5025
Mousavi SR, Rezaei M (2011) Nanotechnology in agriculture and food production. J Appl Environ Biol Sci 1:414–419. https://www.researchgate.net/publication/216346568_Nanotechnology_in_Agriculture_and_Food_Production
Mozafari MR, Flanagan J, Matia-Merino L (2006) Recent trends in the lipid-based nanoencapsulation of antioxidants and their role in foods. J Sci Food Agricult 86:2038–2045. https://doi.org/10.1002/jsfa.2576
Mozafari MR, Johnson C, Hatziantoniou S, Demetzos C (2008) Nanoliposomes and their applications in food nanaotechnology. J Liposome Res 18:309–327. https://doi.org/10.1080/08982100802465941
Neethirajan S, Jayas DS (2007) Sensors for grain storage. ASABE annual international meeting, pp. 17–20. https://doi.org/10.13031/2013.23510
Neethirajan S, Jayas DS (2011) Nanotechnology for the food and bioprocessing industries. Food Bioproc Tech 4:39–47. https://doi.org/10.1007/s11947-010-0328-2
Neethirajan S, Freund MS, Shafai C, Jayas DS, Thomson DJ (2009) Development of carbon dioxide sensor for agri-food industry. Science 5(8):453–471. https://doi.org/10.1007/s11947-008-0154-y
NSTC (2007) The national nanotechnology initiative-strategic plan, December 2007. Executive Office of the President of the United States. https://www.nano.gov/sites/default/files/pub_resource/nni_strategic_plan_2007.pdf

OECD (2013) Guidance manual for the testing of manufactured nanomaterials: OECD's sponsorship programme. [(accessed on 20 December 2013)]. Available online.: http://www.oecd.org/science/nanosafety/publicationsintheseriesonthesafetyofmanufacturednanomaterials.htm

Pal M (2017) Nanotechnology: a new approach in food packaging. J Food Hyg Saf 2:2. https://doi.org/10.4172/2476-2059.1000121

Paul IE, Kumar DN, Rajeshwari A, Alex SA, Karthiga D, Raichur AM, Chandrasekaran N, Mukherjee A (2017) Detection of food contaminates by gold and silver nanoparticles. In: Grumezescu AM (ed) Nanobiosensors: nanotechnology in the agri-food industry 8. Elsevier Inc, pp 129–165. https://doi.org/10.1016/b978-0-12-804301-1.00004-7

Pennacchio G, Ruggiero M, Staiano G, Piccialli G, Oliviero A, Lewkowicz A (2014) Surface plasmon resonance based biochip for the detection of patulin toxin. Opt Mater 36:1670–1675. https://doi.org/10.1016/j.optmat.2013.12.045

Pereda M, Marcovich NE, Ansorena MR (2019) Nanotechnology in food packaging applications: barrier materials, antimicrobial agents, sensors, and safety assessment. In: Handbook of Ecomaterials. Springer, Cham, pp 1–22. https://doi.org/10.1007/978-3-319-68255-6_30

Piliarik M, Šípová H, Kvasnička P, Galler N, Krenn JR, Homola J (2012) High-resolution biosensor based on localized surface plasmons. Opt ˇExpress 20:672–680. https://doi.org/10.1364/oe.20.000672

Powell JJ, Faria N, Thomas-McKay E, Pele LC (2010) Origin and fate of dietary nanoparticles and microparticles in the gastrointestinal tract. J Autoimmun 34:226–233. https://doi.org/10.1016/j.jaut.2009.11.006

Pramanik S, Pramanik G (2016) Nanotechnology for sustainable agriculture in India. In: Rajan S, Dasgupta N, Lichtfouse E (eds) Nanoscience in food and agriculture 3, Sustainable agriculture reviews, vol 23. Springer, Cham, pp 243–280. https://doi.org/10.1007/978-3-319-48009-1_10

Qi LF, Xu ZR, Jiang X, Hu C, Zou X (2004) Preparation and antibacterial activity of chitosan nanoparticles. Carbohydr Res 339:2693–2700. https://doi.org/10.1016/j.carres.2004.09.007

Rasmussen JPR, Tewksbury EW, Moss OR, Cesta MF, Wong BA, Bonner JC (2009) Inhaled multiwalled carbon nanotubes potentiate airway fibrosis in murine allergic asthma. Am J Respir Cell Mol Biol 40:349–358. https://doi.org/10.1165/rcmb.2008-0276oc

Rattu G, Krishna PM (2017) Label-free electrochemical biosensors for food and drug application. Int J Bio-Inorg Hybrid Nanomater 6:185–203. http://ijbihn.iauvaramin.ac.ir/article_660055.html

Rattu G, Khansili N, Krishna PM (2020) Polyacrylic acid modified cerium oxide nanoparticles: synthesis and characterization as a peroxidase mimic for non-enzymatic H2O2 sensor. Curr Nanosci 16:816–828. https://doi.org/10.2174/1573413715666191204124329

Ravichandran R (2010) Nanotechnology applications in food and food processing: innovative green approaches, opportunities and uncertainties for global market. Int J Green Nanotechnol 1:72–96. https://doi.org/10.1080/19430871003684440

Rowe RC, Sheskey PJ, Weller PJ (2003) Fourth ed. London: Pharmaceutical Press, London, United Kingdom, and the American Pharmaceutical Association; Handbook of pharmaceutical excipients. https://www.abebooks.com/9781582120225/Handbook-Pharmaceutical-Excipients-4th-Edition-1582120226/plp

Safina G (2012) Application of surface plasmon resonance for the detection of carbohydrates, glycoconjugates, and measurement of the carbohydrate-specific interactions: a comparison with conventional analytical techniques. A critical review. Anal Chim Acta 712:9–29. https://doi.org/10.1016/j.aca.2011.11.016

Sahoo SK, Parveen S, Panda JJ (2007) The present and future of nanotechnology in human health care. Nanomedicine: nanotechnology. Biol Med 3:20–31. https://doi.org/10.1016/j.nano.2006.11.008

Sahoo D, Mandal A, Mitra T, Chakraborty K, Bardhan M, Ak D (2018) Nanosensing of pesticides by zinc oxide quantum dot: an optical and electrochemical approach for the detection of pesticides in water. J Agric Food Chem 66:414–423. https://doi.org/10.1021/acs.jafc.7b04188

Salam F, Uludag Y, Tothill IE (2013) Real-time and sensitive detection of Salmonella typhimurium using an automated quartz crystal microbalance (QCM) instrument with nanoparticles amplification. Talanta 115:761–767. https://doi.org/10.1016/j.talanta.2013.06.034

Schaller E, Bosset JO, Escher F (1998) 'Electronic noses' and their application to food. LWT Food Sci Technol 31:305–316. https://doi.org/10.1006/fstl.1998.0376

Schleh C, Semmler-Behnke M, Lipka J, Wenk A, Hirn S, Schäffler M, Schmid G, Simon U, Kreyling WG (2012) Size and surface charge of gold nanoparticles determine absorption across intestinal barriers and accumulation in secondary target organs after oral administration. Nanotoxicology 6:36–46. https://doi.org/10.3109/17435390.2011.552811

Schlundt J (2002) New directions in foodborne disease prevention. Int J Food Microbiol 78:3–17. https://doi.org/10.1016/s0168-1605(02)00234-9

Sekhon BS (2014) Nanotechnology in agri-food production: an overview. Nanotechnol Sci Appl 7:31–53. https://doi.org/10.2147/nsa.s39406

Shin GH, Kim JT, Park HJ (2015) Recent developments in nanoformulations of lipophilic functional foods. Trends Food Sci Technol 46:144–157. https://doi.org/10.1016/j.tifs.2015.07.005

Si SH, Li X, Fung YS, Zhu DR (2001) Rapid detection of Salmonella enteritidis by piezoelectric immounosensor. Microchem J 68:21–27. https://doi.org/10.1016/s0026-265x(00)00167-3

Silva HD, Cerqueira MA, Vicente AA (2012) Nanoemulsions for food applications: development and characterization. Food Bioprocess Tech 5:854–867. https://doi.org/10.1007/s11947-013-1094-8

Singh NA (2016) Nanotechnology definitions, research, industry and property rights. In: Ranjan S, Dasgupta N, Lichtfouse E (eds) Nanoscience in Food and Agriculture 1, Sustainable agriculture reviews, vol 20. Springer, Cham, pp 43–64. https://doi.org/10.1007/978-3-319-39303-2

Skalickova S, Milosavljevic V, Cihalova K, Horky P, Richtera L, Adam V (2017) Selenium nanoparticles as a nutritional supplement. Nutrition 33:83–90. https://doi.org/10.1016/j.nut.2016.05.001

Skocaj M, Filipic M, Petkovic J, Novak S (2011) Titanium dioxide in our everyday life; is it safe? Radiol Oncol 45:227–247. https://doi.org/10.2478/v10019-011-0037-0

Sonaje K, Lin KJ, Tseng MT, Wey SP, Su FY, Chuang EY, Hsu CW, Chen CT, Sung HW (2011) Effects of chitosan-nanoparticle-mediated tight junction opening on the oral absorption of endotoxins. Biomaterials 32:8712–8721. https://doi.org/10.1016/j.biomaterials.2011.07.086

Sozer N, Kokini JL (2009) Nanotechnology and its applications in the food sector. Trends Biotechnol 27:82–89. https://doi.org/10.1016/j.tibtech.2008.10.010

Srivastava SK, Shalanbney A, Khalaila I, Gruner C, Rauschenbach B, Abdulhalim I (2014) SERS biosensor using metallic nano-sculptured thin films for the detection of endocrine disrupting compound biomarker vitellogenin. Small 10:3579–3587. https://doi.org/10.1002/smll.201303218

Srivastava AK, Dev A, Karmakar S (2017) Nanosensors and nanobiosensors in food and agriculture. Environ Chem Lett 16:161–182. https://doi.org/10.1007/s10311-017-0674-7

Sun Y, Fang L, Wan Y, Gu Z (2018) Pathogenic detection and phenotype using magnetic nanoparticle-urease nanosensor. Sensors Actuators B Chem 259:428–432. https://doi.org/10.1016/j.snb.2017.12.095

Taitt CR, Anderson GP, Ligler FS (2015) Evanescent wave fluorescence biosensors: advances of the last decade. Biosens Bioelectron 76:103–111. https://doi.org/10.1016/j.bios.2015.07.040

Tang VW, Goodenough DA (2003) Paracellular ion channel at the tight junction. Biophys J 84:1660–1673. https://doi.org/10.1016/s0006-3495(03)74975-3

Teow Y, Asharani PV, Hand MP, Valiyaveettil S (2011) Health impact and safety of engineered nanomaterials. Chem Commun 47:7025–7038. https://doi.org/10.1039/C0CC05271J

Vidic J, Grosclaude J, Persuy MA, Aioun J, Salesse R (2006) Quantitative assessment of olfactory receptors activity in immobilized nanosomes: a novel concept for bioelectronic nose. Lab Chip 6:1026–1032. https://doi.org/10.1039/b603189g

Viswanathan S, Radecki J (2008) Nanomaterials in electrochemical biosensors for food analysis- a review. Polish J Food Nutr Sci 58:157–164. https://www.researchgate.net/publication/277309495_Nanomaterials_in_electrochemical_biosensors_for_food_analysis-A_review
Wang Y, Zhang Q, Zhang CL, Li P (2012) Characterisation and cooperative antimicrobial properties of chitosan/nano-ZnO composite nanofibrous mambranes. Food Chem 132:419–427. https://doi.org/10.1016/j.foodchem.2011.11.015
Wani KA, Kothari R (2018) Agricultural nanotechnology: applications and challenges. Ann Plant Sci 7:2146–2148. https://doi.org/10.21746/aps.2018.7.3.9
Wesley SJ, Raja P, Raj AAS, Tiroutchelvamae D (2014) Review on nanotechnology applications in food packaging and safety. Int J Eng Res 3:645–651. https://doi.org/10.17950/ijer/v3s11/1105
Yakes BJ, Lipert RJ, Bannantine JP, Porter MD (2008) Detection of Mycobacterium avium subsp. Paratuberculosis by a sonicate immunoassay based on surface-enhanced Raman scattering. Clin Vaccine Immunol 15:227–234. https://doi.org/10.1128/cvi.00334-07
Yang LJ, Li YB (2005) Quantum dots as fluorescent labels for quantitative detection of Salmonella typhimurium in chicken carcass wash water. J Food Prot 68:1241–1245. https://doi.org/10.4315/0362-028x-68.6.1241
Yildirim N, Long F, Gao C, He M, Shi HC, Gu AZ (2012) Aptamer-based optical biosensor for rapid and sensitive detection of 17beta-estradiol in water samples. Environ Sci Technol 46:3288–3294. https://doi.org/10.1021/es203624w
Yoshida T, Yoshioka Y, Fujimura M, Yamashita K, Higashisaka K, Morishita Y, Kayamuro H, Nabeshi H, Nagano K, Abe Y, Kamada H, Tsunoda S, Itoh N, Yoshikawa T, Tsutsumi Y (2011) Promotion of allergic immune responses by intranasally-administered nanosilica particles in mice. Nanoscale Res Lett 6:1–6. https://doi.org/10.1186/1556-276x-6-195
Zhang Y, Chen Y, Jin G (2011) Serum tumor marker detection on PEGylated lipid membrane using biosensor based on total internal reflection imaging ellipsometry. Sens Actuators B Chem 159:121–125. https://doi.org/10.1016/j.snb.2011.06.059
Zhao R, Torley P, Halley PJ (2008) Emerging biodegradable materials: starch- and protein-based bio-composites. J Mater Sci 43:3058–3071. https://doi.org/10.1007/s10853-007-2434-8

Chapter 4
Micro/Nanoencapsulation of Active Food Compounds: Encapsulation, Characterization and Biological Fate of Encapsulated Systems

Semih Calamak

Abstract The micro/nanoencapsulation methods for active food compounds have attracted great interest and opened the door to innovative applications in the food and pharmaceutical sciences. In food science, active compounds have major problems associated with their bioavailability and biocompatibility. These limitations have been overcome through encapsulation approaches, which improve the sensory effect, biocompatibility and bioavailability. Also, the encapsulation of active food compounds enables a protected environment from external conditions. This chapter emphasizes the current know-how and approaches for the production of micro/nanoencapsulation systems for active food compounds and application in new generation foods along with their future progress. We elaborately discussed the importance of micro/nanoencapsulation, the application of complex coacervates, electrospun and electrosprayed micro/nanoparticles, lipid and biopolymeric-based systems with their advantages of encapsulation. Also, this chapter describes the characterization techniques and biological fate of the micro/nano encapsulated systems. In conclusion, the functionality of various micro/nano encapsulated systems is compressively discussed, and future developments are highlighted.

Keywords Microencapsulation · Nanoencapsulation · Active food compounds · Complex coacervates · Lipid based carriers · Biopolymeric micro/nano carriers · Nanoliposomes · Emulsion systems · Electrospun · Polysaccharide-protein complex

---

S. Calamak (✉)
Department of Basic Pharmaceutical Sciences, Faculty of Pharmacy, Hacettepe University, Ankara, Turkey
e-mail: semihcalamak@hacettepe.edu.tr

V. K. Maurya et al. (eds.), *Sustainable Agriculture Reviews 55*, Sustainable Agriculture Reviews 55, https://doi.org/10.1007/978-3-030-76813-3_4

Abbreviations

AG	Acacia gum
AMPS	Allyl methyl disulfide
DLS	Dynamic light scattering
FTIR	Fourier transform infrared spectroscopy
GRAS	Generally recognized as safe
MBAX	Maize bran arabinoxylans
MWAX	Waste water arabinoxylans
O/W	Oil in water emulsion
PEO	Poly (ethylene oxide)
PVA	Poly (vinyl alcohol)
SAXS	Small angle X-ray Scattering
SEM	Scanning electron microscopy
TEM	Transmission electron microscopy
XRD	X-ray Diffraction
β-lg	β-lactoglobulin

4.1 Introduction

Encapsulation of active compounds has attracted great interest in polymer chemistry and various research areas such as food, cosmetic, pharmaceutical and agriculture (Sarıgöl et al. 2017; Sarıgöl et al. 2018; Cota-Arriola et al. 2013). The encapsulation process comprises of entrapment of active compounds within a carrier material (polysaccharide, protein, lipid, biopolymer). The carried matrix is mostly called as shell, capsule, coating and membrane. The encapsulation of active compounds provides a protected environment from external conditions such as heat, light, shear and moisture (Augustin and Hemar 2009). In food science and pharmaceutical applications, the encapsulation method is also used for masking any unpleasant taste or odors of active compounds. Likewise, encapsulation is an efficient approach to control the delivery of the active compounds to the desired area with required concentration and optimal release kinetics (Tampau et al. 2018; Sarigol-Calamak and Hascicek 2018). Encapsulation methods are able to control release mechanisms and kinetics at the desired level and appropriate time with physiological triggers such as heat, light, pH, etc.

In food science, phenolic active compounds (high antioxidant activity) have a major problem with respect to their bioavailability. Also, essential oils have organoleptic problems such as poor water solubility, unpleasant odor and taste. However, such limitations have been overcome through encapsulation approaches, which improve the sensory effect, biocompatibility and bioavailability (Nedovic et al. 2011; Gupta et al. 2016).

The encapsulation carrier materials for active compounds must be biocompatible, food-grade and durable in food systems. The first step for the encapsulation process is the selection of a suitable carrier matrix. The most commonly used group of materials consists of carbohydrate polymers (cellulose, starch and their derivatives). Plant extracts and exudates include galactomannans, gum, soybean polysaccharides, and pectins. Chitosan, gellan, xanthan, and dextran belong to microbial and animal-derived polysaccharides. This is in addition to lipids and proteins. In the food industry, low-cost carrier materials such as corn starch, gelatin and alginate are mainly preferred (Kavitake et al. 2018; Assadpour and Jafari 2019; Gümüşderelioğlu et al. 2020).

4.1.1 Encapsulation of Active Food Compounds and Its Significance in Food Applications

Encapsulation is an approach that entraps an active compound such as drugs, probiotics, vitamins, antioxidants or living cells within a carrier matrix (carbohydrate, protein, lipids or polymers). Encapsulation enables increase biocompatibility and bioavailability, controlled release of active compounds. Also, it provides odorless and tasteless materials (De Matteis et al. 2019).

Encapsulation methods have attracted great interest in food science and applications for 60 years. An ideal encapsulation should shield the active compound against external conditions, including pH, temperature and ion concentration and enable controlled release of active compounds. In the literature, many techniques have been reported to produce micro/nano encapsulated particles. These methods have their own merits and demerits. For instance, in the emulsion approach, nano-sized particles are produced in the liquid phase that needs an optimum drying process to produce nanocapsules in powder form. Likewise, electrospraying and electrospinning methods are single-step and easy methods for the fabrication of micro and nanocapsules in powder structure. Also, the encapsulation materials intended for food incorporation should contain food-grade ingredients, i.e., materials that are commonly recognized as safe (GRAS) (Bhushani and Anandharamakrishnan 2014). Therefore, proteins, carbohydrates and natural biopolymers are widely used for encapsulation of active compounds due to their biocompatibility and bioavailability. Encapsulated particles are defined as microparticles as the size is between 0.2 and 5000μm, macroparticles when the scale is higher than 5000μm and nanoparticles under 1μm (Akhavan et al. 2018).

4.2 Encapsulation Techniques

Multifunctional micro/nano carries such as emulsion, microcapsules, polymer gels, core-shell capsules and self-assembly structures are mainly used as active compounds delivery systems to increase stability, solubility biocompatibility and bioavailability of encapsulated active compounds. The selection of the micro/nanoencapsulation method is managed by the physicochemical properties of active compounds (antioxidants, vitamins peptides) and the carrier matrix materials. Encapsulation methods of the active food compounds are classified as physico-chemical (coacervation and phase separation and emulsion) and physicomechanical (spray drying, electrospray and electrospinning) methods.

4.2.1 Micro/Nano Encapsulation in Protein-Polysaccharide Complex Coacervates

It has been reported that there are two forms of coacervation: simple and complex coacervations. In simple coacervation, a macromolecule solute phase is transferred to the coacervation phase by changing the condition parameters, including temperature, molecular weight, ionic strength, electrostatic interaction and pH (Fig. 4.1). On contrast, complex coacervation is formed by mixing two oppositely charged ions into two immiscible liquid phases (Kizilay et al. 2011). Polysaccharide-protein complexes are the leading carrier system for the encapsulation of active food compounds. Recently, there has been great attention on potential applications of polysaccharide-protein complexes such as food, cosmetics and pharmaceutical. The electrostatic interactions between oppositely charged polymers control the complex structure during the synthesis.

In complex coacervate systems, soluble protein and polysaccharide form aggregate structure through electrostatic interaction, non-covalent and H-bonding interactivity to minimize the free energy of the complex coacervate during their chemical

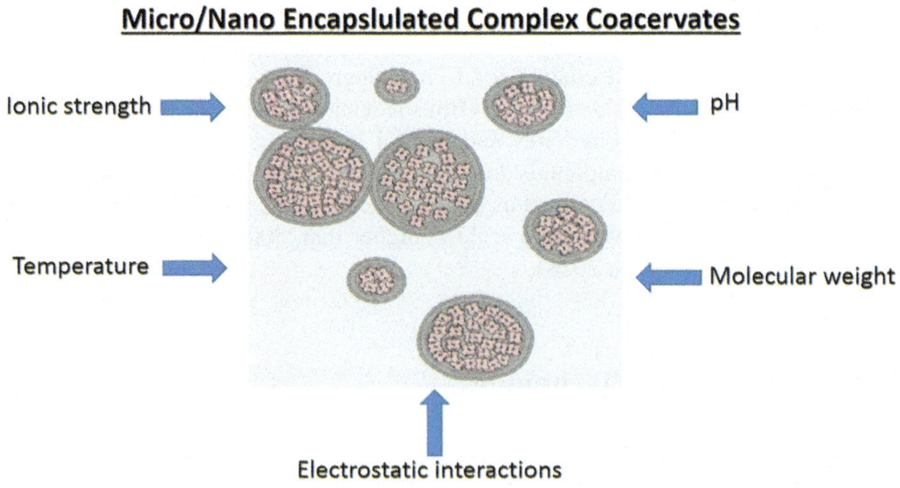

Fig. 4.1 Schematic representation of synthesis parameters which affect the formation of complexes coacervates

and structural properties ensure coacervation (Schmitt and Turgeon 2011). In nature, complex coacervation (polysaccharide-protein complex) can be seen in various living organizations that initiate biological functions. For instance, the sandcastle worm *Phragmatopoma californica* produce sandcastle glue naturally. This process originates from complex coacervation of various oppositely charged proteins and polysaccharides (Zhao et al. 2005; Cooper et al. 2005).

Total polymer concentration, protein and polysaccharide ratio, pH and molecular weight of the proteins and polysaccharides affect the formation of complex coacervation. In addition, the most important thermodynamic parameter is the Gibbs free energy of complex coacervation that increases with an increase in electrostatic enthalpy. Due to its excellent physicochemical properties, biocompatibility and bioavailability, there has been great attention in complex coacervatives for the usage of encapsulation applications. The synthesized complex coacervatives based systems mostly have diameters of nm to mm scale. In the literature, negatively charged polysaccharides and positively charged proteins are widely preferred to form complex coacervates. Schmitt et al. used acacia gum (AG) polysaccharide as a negatively charged molecule, which formed coacervate with β-lactoglobulin (β-lg) (positively charge) (Schmitt et al. 2001).

Polysaccharide-protein based complex coacervates are suitable for most of the active compounds. Their carrier system is able to interact with a great variety of active compounds via their functional groups. In addition, they can be considered as an optimum carrier system if a high-temperature process is required. Polysaccharide structure provides them stability under high temperatures. They are resistant to high temperature compare to lipid-based emulsion systems.

Proteins as carrier matrix have a strong binding capacity to several active compounds via hydrogen bonding and ionic interactions. The functional groups (carboxyl, amine and sulfate groups) of proteins enable physical and chemical surface modifications to designed novel micro/nano encapsulated materials. Likewise, polysaccharides are already widely used as food ingredients and physical, chemical and biochemical properties tailor the processes. Polysaccharides consist of monosaccharides linked by glycosides bonds. The hydrolysis of the polysaccharides results in their constituent oligosaccharides and monosaccharides. Polysaccharides have various functional groups and chemical organizations. A great variety of polysaccharide derivatives can be found in variable molecular weight and linear to branched structure. In nature, they are in amorphous structure and water-insoluble. Cellulose, chitosan, carrageenan, gum arabic, etc. are mainly utilized for complex coacervation of polysaccharides and proteins (Devi et al. 2017). Although coacervation is an expensive method of encapsulation, it can be used for encapsulation of unstable but high-value bioactive substances such as polyphenols and essential oils (Fang and Bhandari 2010).

4.2.2 Spray Drying

Drying is one of the oldest and widely used methods for the protection of foods. By drying methods, the moisture content of the food is reduced and the development of microorganisms and chemical reactions are slowed down (Assadpour and Jafari 2019). Thus, the shelf life of the food extends. Spray drying method was used for the production of milk powder and detergent in 1920s. Spray drying is commonly utilized in food, pharmaceutical, cosmetic, agricultural and chemical industries. This method is fast, cheap, automatize and reproducible method for encapsulating active compounds for food applications. Micro/nano size and encapsulation efficacy depend on several parameters, including solution viscosity, atomizer type, flow rate and inlet/outlet temperature. Suitable materials for the spray drying method should show good drying properties, emulsification and film formation and have low viscosity in concentrated solutions (Chen 2009).

The first step of this process is based on dissolving the active compound and polymer in a suitable solution. After that, the polymer/active compound mixture is put in the atomized heating chamber. This chamber removes the solvent and dried particles are formed. To achieve microparticle production, spray drying uses atomizers and nozzles, which are assisted by pressure. The production of nanosized particles by using conventional spray drying is not possible. To form nanosized particles, a new generation spray drying methods have been developed in these days. The new generation spray drying methods utilize efficient particle collector and a vibrating mesh for ultrafine droplet generation. After nanoparticle production, dried particles are gathered by an electrostatic particle collector. Due to the production process of the spray drying contains heating, this method is not suitable for thermosensitive active compounds. Some carbohydrates such as starch are not suitable because of gelation properties. On the other hand, cyclodextrins and hydroxypropyl cellulose are suitable for spray drying approach at high temperatures (Maurya et al. 2020a).

In food systems, water-soluble dispersions are widely utilized. However, most of the food ingredients are water-insoluble. To cope with this obstacle, the modification of functional groups such as hydroxyl groups of cellulose, chitosan, cyclodextrin lead enhanced water solubility and increased the potential usage of the food carrier matrix (Fathi et al. 2014). Depending on the starting solution and system parameters of spray-drying process result in microparticles, which have a particle size of 1–1000μm. It has been reported that whey protein and casein have attractive coating properties. They have been successfully produced into microparticles integrating anhydrous milk fat, conjugated linoleic acid, avocado oil and probiotic microorganisms (Bae and Lee 2008; Jimenez et al. 2004). The starches such as glucose, lactose, corn syrup and maltodextrin are often incorporated as a secondary carrier matrix to promote drying properties during the spray drying process. They also reduce oxygen permeability of the carrier system and increase the oxidative stability of the encapsulated active compounds (Kagami et al. 2003).

4.2.3 Electrospray and Electrospinning

Electrospray and electrospinning methods are widely used to provide biocompatible, biodegradable and food-grade encapsulations of active compounds (Calamak et al. 2015a, b; Çalamak et al. 2014; Ulubayram et al. 2015). These methods utilize electrostatic forces to generate micro/nanofiber and micro/nanoparticles (Fig. 4.2a, b). Both methods work on the same working principle. The polymer concentration and morphology of the final product determine the method. When the solution concentration is high, elongation occurs at the tip of the nozzle (Taylor cone is stable) and nanofibers are formed on the collector. If the polymer concentration is low, the polymer jet destabilized and micro/nanoparticles are produced (Bhushani and Anandharamakrishnan 2014). In the electrospray approach, the polymer solution or liquid, which contains active compounds is atomized by electrical forces. The solvent evaporates during the flight of the micro/nanoparticles through the collector. Electrospray method can fabricate nanosized particles compare to spray drying (Pérez-Masiá et al. 2015).

In recent years, new generation methods have been developed in electrospraying and electrospinning technologies. These methods are coaxial electrospinning or emulsion electrospinning (Fig. 4.2c). Coaxial electrospinning and electrospraying methods enable ultrafine core-shell micro/nanofibers and particles. In this approach, inner capillary nozzle contains an active compound and the shell material comes from the outer capillary nozzle. These new methods enable single-step

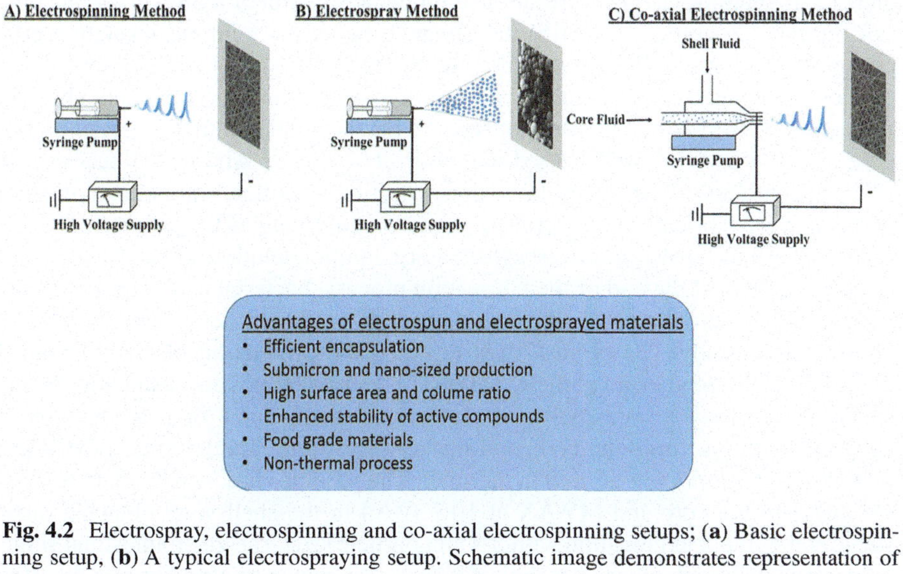

Fig. 4.2 Electrospray, electrospinning and co-axial electrospinning setups; (**a**) Basic electrospinning setup, (**b**) A typical electrospraying setup. Schematic image demonstrates representation of electrospraying process, (**c**) A typical new generation co-axial electrospinning setup. Schematic image shows representation of co-electrospinning process

encapsulation of multiple active compounds with different carrier matrix compared to conventional single nozzle electrospinning.

Electrospinning and electrospray methods provide functional and structural advantages for the encapsulation of active compounds (Mavis et al. 2009). The final particle size can be adjusted by changing system parameters, including polymer concentration, viscosity and dielectric constant. Also, particle size can be controlled by system parameters such as distance between tip (nozzle) and collector, electric field, flow rate and collector material. In addition, the ambient conditions of the system, such as humidity, temperature and chamber air flow affect the particle size.

In the literature, electrospinning and electrospraying methods are well studied as tissue scaffold, drug delivery system and bioelectronics (Maurya et al. 2020a). However, its usage in the field of food science is not well studied. It has been reported that collagen, gelatin, whey protein isolate and whey protein concentrate are widely used as protein sources (Neo et al. 2013; Okutan et al. 2014). Electrospray and electrospinning methods are very suitable for protein encapsulation because these techniques do not require heat that can denature the protein structure. Lopez et al. showed that whey protein concentrate based micro (1724 ± 524 nm) and sub-micron (83.1 ± 11.5 nm) particles could be produced by electrospray method. In this study, they achieved to encapsulate antioxidant β-carotene. The results showed that the difference in pH of the whey protein solution resulted in significant particle size change. Micro-sized particles were obtained at pH 6.4 (López-Rubio and Lagaron 2012).

Aside from these food active compounds, the food scientists focus on encapsulation methods which enable the stability and viability of probiotic bacteria and bacteriocins for food processing and storage. Many reports have shown that electrospray and electrospinning methods are suitable for encapsulation of living probiotic cells. For instance, Zaeim et al. (2018) investigated the acacia gum encapsulation efficiency by using an electrospray method to protect probiotic cells. To optimize production parameters acacia gum concentration, surfactant addition and physical properties of feed solution were adjusted. It has been shown that increasing gum concentration up to 40 wt% caused to a viscosity increase. At 35 wt.% acacia gum solution containing 1 wt.% Tween-80 concentration ultra-fine, smooth and uniform particles were fabricated by electrospray reinforced drying of the autoclave. In this method thermal sterilization increased the acacia gum solution viscosity and electrospray ability. At the end of the fabrication process, bacterial cell viability results indicated that more than 96% of probiotic cells were alive (Zaeim et al. 2018).

In another study, Paz et al. (2018) reported the production of electrosprayed core-shell arabinoxylan gel particles for insulin and probiotics encapsulation. In this study, electrosprayed core-shell particles consisted of maize bran arabinoxylans (MBAX) with insulin in the core, and maize waste water arabinoxylans (MWAX) with probiotic *(Bifidobacterium)* in the shell. The particles produced with MBAX at 6% (w/v) in the core and MWAX at 10% (w/v) in the shell were obtained more stable and without aggregation with 2.9 mm particle size. The gastrointestinal simulation and insulin release studies indicated that core-shell particles were not digested in stomach and small intestine and core-shell system was released 76% of carried insulin in the colon (Paz-Samaniego et al. 2018).

Likewise, researchers have been working on the biocompatible composite materials for food applications. Synthetic polymers such as poly (ethylene oxide) (PEO), poly (vinyl alcohol) (PVA) enhance the physical and mechanical properties of the composite carrier materials. Liu et al. (2018) designed a composite film via electrospray method, which consisted of PVA and chitosan. The results indicated that the addition of PVA (75:25:PVA: chitosan) increased elongation at break, oxygen permeability and water barrier properties (Liu et al. 2018).

Electrospinning method does not allow many proteins and carbohydrates to be electrospun alone and needs synthetic polymers and plasticizer to form electrospun jet. In contrast, electrospray does not require any polymer blend or plasticizer. In the literature, it has been reported that the addition of PVA and PEO into electrospinning solution improves electrospinability and fiber formation (Abdel-Mohsen et al. 2019; Son et al. 2020). For instance, the egg albumen protein and low molecular weight collagen do not form fiber development. However, in such a case combining PEO or cellulose acetate with egg albumen provides fiber structure (Wongsasulak et al. 2010; Wongsasulak et al. 2007). The properties of encapsulation material can show a synergetic effect and increase the bioavailability of the active compounds. For instance, electrospun zein fibers enhanced oxidative and light stability of β-carotene was found (Fernandez et al. 2009). In addition, curcumin encapsulated in zein nanofiber (310 nm) enhanced free radical scavenging activity and sustained release properties (Brahatheeswaran et al. 2012).

Nanoparticles provide interesting features compared to microparticles. They have higher bioavailability, enhanced solubility of hydrophobic active compounds and higher surface area (Maurya and Aggarwal 2017). Nanoencapsulated structures can be produced by two different approaches. These are lipid- based vehicles and biopolymer based nanoparticles.

4.2.4 Lipid-Based Micro/Nano Encapsulated Systems for Protection and Delivery of Active Food Compounds

Lipid-based nanoencapsulation approaches are well-studied in the literature and they are widely used for pharmaceutical and food applications. Previous encapsulation approaches were comprised of carbohydrate-protein and biopolymers, which are not good candidates for industrial scale-up due to chemical and thermal processes. Besides, lipid-based nano-carrier matrix can easily be scaled up for industry for food and pharmaceutical applications and enables efficient encapsulation with lower systemic toxicity (Tamjidi et al. 2013).

Most of the active compounds that are used in food applications such as aromas, preservatives, nutraceuticals and vitamins are hydrophobic (Maurya et al. 2020b). Therefore, lipid-based carriers offer higher bioavailability and intestinal absorption of active compounds. Therefore, lipid-based nano-carriers are known as powerful and flexible delivery agents (Tamjidi et al. 2013). Up to date, several lipid based nano-carriers have been developed. We can classify them into two groups. These are liposomes and emulsions.

4.2.4.1 Liposomes

Liposome term is defined as a spherical amphiphilic lipid carrier, which is consists of an internal aqueous cavity. The production of liposomes includes amphiphilic lipid and aqueous phase interactions. These interactions are led the formation of bilayer structures like cell membrane. The presence of both lipid and aqueous phases provide the encapsulation and delivery of active compounds. The phospholipids comprise of a hydrophobic head and a hydrophilic tail (Fig. 4.3). During the

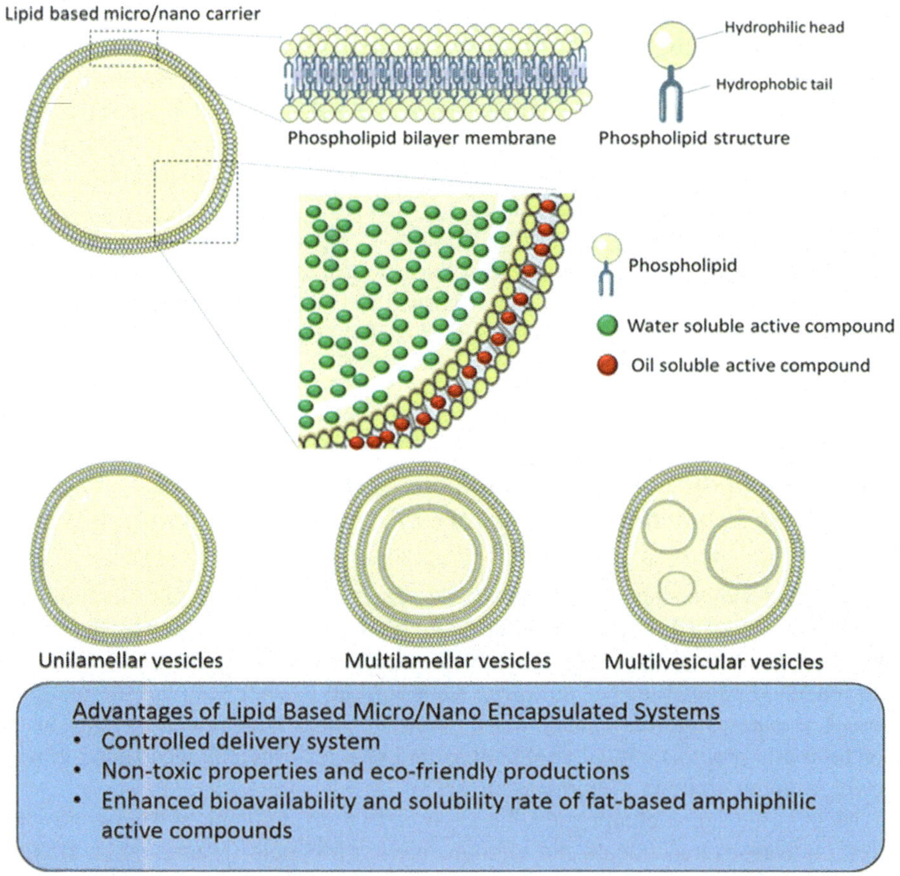

Fig. 4.3 Lipid based micro/nano carrier systems

liposome synthesis, the polar head aligned in the location of the aqueous phase. Liposomes have the ability to mimic cell membrane model due to its bilayer structure and this behavior of liposomes makes them a great candidate for drug formulation and controlled release (Fig. 4.3).

The type of phospholipids, which is mostly used as wall material for liposomes affects the liposome properties. To date, various liposome production methods have been developed in the literature (Lin and Malmstadt 2019; Trucillo et al. 2020). Conventional methods can be listed as thin-film dispersion (Bangham), ethanol/ether injection, probe ultrasonication, bath ultrasonication, reverse phase evaporation, freeze-dried rehydration vesicles, detergent depletion and membrane extrusion methods. Even if these methods offer rapid production and high stability, they require considerable sonication to achieve minimum size limit and longtime processes. To cope with production disadvantages of liposomes such as longtime process and size limits, high-throughput novel methods have been designed by researchers. Novel approaches can be classified as heating method, freeze drying of double emulsions, high-pressure homogenization, microfluidization, supercritical fluid injection and decompression, dual asymmetric centrifugation and dense gas techniques. New generation microfluidic-based methods do not require hazardous solvent and chemicals and may be a proper approach for the preparation of food grade liposomes (Liu et al. 2018; Calamak and Ulubayram 2019; Inci et al. 2018).

Entire production approaches for liposomes include three basic steps; (i) preparation of organic and aqueous phases with active compounds, (ii) drying down lipids from an organic solvent and (iii) purifying the final yield. In food applications, liposomes are typically used as carrier matrix for antioxidants, natural colors, aromas, vitamins and protein delivery (Akhavan et al. 2018). Yang et al. (2013) designed a complex nanoliposome system encapsulating both a hydrophilic drug vitamin C and hydrophobic drug medium-chain fatty acids by double emulsion method with dynamic high pressure microfluidization. The complex nanoliposomes showed high encapsulation efficiency of vitamin C (62.25 ± 3.43%) and relatively high entrapment efficiency of medium-chain fatty acids (44.26 ± 3.34)% with nano-size average diameter (110.4 ± 7.28) nm and excellent storage stability at 4 °C for 60 days (Yang et al. 2013). Shin et al. prepared chitosan-coated curcumin nanoliposomes via ethanol injection method. The entrapment efficiency of curcumin loaded nanoliposomes was 54.70%. The results showed that the encapsulated curcumin provided prolonged absorption in the gastrointestinal tract because of higher mucoadhesion (Shin et al. 2013). In another study, Velez et al. (2019) investigated the effect of lyophilization and rehydration medium on a liposome system for modified with linoleic acid. In this study, liposomes were produced by ethanol injection method employing soy phosphatidylcholine and linoleic acid. They have successfully produced efficient liposomal systems for bioactive compounds delivery in food applications (Vélez et al. 2019). Along with the beneficial attributes, nanoliposomes still have limitations, such as less stability and high cost of food-grade raw materials for nanoliposome.

4.2.4.2 Emulsions

Emulsion systems are mostly water and oil systems, where one of the two immiscible liquids is dispersed in small droplets in the other. The emulsions are classified in different ways depending on the relative dissemination of the oil and water phases in each other (McClements 2010). Emulsions in which oil droplets are dispersed in the water phase; called oil in water emulsions (O/W). The water-in-oil emulsions (W/O) are the ones where water droplets are dispersed in the oil phase. Emulsion systems are classified in three basic categories as macroemulsions (0.5–100 mm) microemulsions (10–100μm) and nanoemulsions (100–1000 nm) according to their particle size. It has been reported that macroemulsions are not thermodynamically stable. Besides, microemulsions are known as thermodynamically stable. However, nanoemulsions are merely kinetically stable (Gu et al. 2005; Doi et al., 2019). The growing interest in the exertion of nanoemulsions has increased significantly over the last decade. The most important advantage of nano-emulsions is the encapsulation of lipophilic functional compounds such as vitamins, flavors, colorants, antioxidants and preservatives (Maurya and Aggarwal 2019b). Lipophilic compounds are generally mixed with the oil phase prior to emulsion production so that when nanoemulsion is produced, these compounds are entrapped in the oil phase. The major components of the food-grade nanoemulsions can be classified as oil, water and surfactant. The optimized mixture of these components determines the properties and stability of the nanoemulsions. Nanoemulsions have high level of lipid moiety along with the scale-up potential with toxicological safety.

Nanoemulsions production techniques are closely related to thermodynamic and physicochemical properties of nanoemulsion systems. These spontaneous systems are produced either by high-energy emulsification and low-energy emulsification. The synthesis approaches for nanoemulsions can be divided as hot homogenization technique, cold homogenization technique, high pressure homogenization, solvent emulsification–evaporation method, solvent emulsification-diffusion technique, microemulsion technique, melting dispersion method, ultrasonication technique, solvent injection and double emulsion technique. Today, many food ingredients exist in the form of nanoemulsions such as sauces, soups, desserts and beverages (Maurya and Aggarwal 2019a; Jafari et al. 2015).

4.2.5 Biopolymeric Based Micro/Nano Encapsulated Systems

Natural biopolymers have attracted great interest in the design of biopolymeric based micro/nano carriers. Among them, hydrogel-based encapsulation methods are widely preferred systems due to their excellent structural and functional properties such as the huge volume of water absorption capacity and the ability for hydrophilic and lipophilic active compound encapsulation (Bourbon et al. 2016; Najafi-Soulari et al. 2016). With their high water absorbance capacity, they can protect the encapsulated active compounds from extreme conditions such as biochemical degradation and gastrointestinal tract. In a study, thermal gelation of lactoferrin and glycomacropeptide demonstrated good stability at pH 5 and pH 8 with high temperature and salt concentration (Bourbon et al. 2018). In another study Bourbon et al. (2016) designed lactoferrin and glycomacropeptide based curcumin (lipophilic) and caffeine (hydrophilic) loaded nano-sized hydrogel system. The results showed that lactoferrin and glycomacropeptide milk proteins encapsulated more than 90% of curcumin and caffeine with 112–126 nm particle size. The hydrogel-based nanoparticles showed controlled release of both active agent corresponding on pH (Bourbon, Cerqueira, and Vicente 2016). In another study, Wang et al. (2019) investigated encapsulation and controlled release of allyl methyl disulfide (AMDS), which is a lipophilic compound in garlic. It has flavoring, anticancer, antioxidant, and antimicrobial properties. They produced alginate microparticles by injecting a mixture of AMDS-loaded lipid droplets and sodium alginate into a calcium ion solution. Encapsulation of AMDS-loaded lipid droplets in microgels delayed flavor release appreciably (three-fold longer) (Wang, Doi, and McClements 2019). Gomez et al. (2019) developed biopolymeric based carrier materials to increase the storage of the active food compound. For this purpose, they used zein and gelatin as a carrier matrix to encapsulate two model active food compound i.e., epigallocatechin gallate as a model hydrophilic compound and α-linolenic acid as a model hydrophobic molecule. The results showed that encapsulation efficiency was dependent on the chemical structure between the bioactive and shell materials (Gómez-Mascaraque et al. 2019).

4.3 Characterization Techniques of Micro/Nano Encapsulated Systems

Several techniques could be implemented to characterize micro/nanoencapsulated systems. The average size of the microparticles has been generally characterized by Dynamic Light Scattering (DLS) method. DLS technique is based on measuring the intensity and change of light scattered from microparticles in the dilute solution. The change in the intensity of the scattered light depends on the movement and size of the particle and viscosity of medium and the temperature. DLS method is used to obtain hydrodynamic size, diffusion coefficient, distribution index and particle size distribution (Tosi et al. 2020; Dai et al. 2019). Phase-contrast microscopy is used to investigate morphological and structural changes in micro/nanoencapsulated materials. Besides, two and three-dimensional images of micro/nanoencapsulated materials can be visualized by confocal scanning laser microscopy (Mekhloufi et al. 2005; Lamprecht et al. 2000). The structure of micro/nanoencapsulated materials has been investigated by X-ray scattering (SAXS), Fourier transform infrared spectroscopy (FTIR), X-ray Diffraction (XRD) methods and Raman spectroscopy. FTIR and Raman spectroscopy methods include structurally relevant information with the vibrational bands of the materials as well as amorphous and crystalline structure of the proteins and biopolymers (Weinbreck et al. 2004; Chourpa et al. 2006). These methods also provide extent interactions between the carrier matrix and active compounds. The surface properties and morphology of the micro/nano encapsulated materials such as shape and size have been widely studied by Scanning electron microscopy (SEM), Transmission electron microscopy (TEM) and Cryogenic-TEM (Wei et al. 2017; Baxa 2018; Robson et al. 2018).

4.4 Biological Fate of Micro/Nano Encapsulated Active Compounds

In vitro and *in vivo* models are currently used to determine the biological fate of the micro/nanoencapsulated systems (Mao et al. 2019). Although *in vivo* animal studies are widely used, the collected data are often questioned due to variations in eating habits and physiological conditions of the digestion system between humans and animals (mice, rat, rabbit etc.). Currently, human studies are difficult due to ethical and social considerations. Therefore, *in vitro* systems are increasingly utilized as an alternative to human and *in-vivo* studies. *In-vitro* models can be classified into two sections; static and dynamic models (Bryszewska et al. 2019). The most widely used *in-vitro* models are static models. In these models, conventional laboratory equipment (a shaking and rotary bath) are used to mimic conditions of the stomach and small intestine. Also, these systems require gastro intestinal fluids to simulate digestion behaviors. Although static models are dominantly used for digestion model, none of the static models can mimic the dynamic conditions of the human body (Leyva-López et al. 2019). Compared to static models, dynamic models can mimic the conditions of the human gastrointestinal systems such as pH, enzyme secretion, fluid dynamics and microbial fermentation. The digestion system comprises of three stages: oral processing, gastric digestion and intestinal digestion (Fig. 4.4). The ionic strength, pH and enzyme content of saliva can affect the formation of the active compound encapsulated micro/nanoparticles (Table 4.1).

Enzymes such as pepsin, gastric lipase, protease and pancreatic lipase may affect the degradation of encapsulated materials and adsorption of the encapsulated active compounds. Especially for nanoliposomes and nanoemulsion system, differences in pH and concentration of ionic salts can affect the wall membrane and electrostatic interaction of the lipid based systems (McClements and Li 2010). Besides, digestion and exposure time also play a crucial role for digestion of encapsulated materials. Also, the thickness of the wall material and surface modifications are another two key factors that can significantly affect the degradation behaviors of micro/nanoencapsulation materials (Yu and Lv 2019).

Early studies on the biological fate of mico/nanoencapsulated active compounds were focused on insulin release as a model peptide. It has been reported that free insulin hydrolyzed rapidly after ingestion (Claessens et al. 2008). After encapsulation of insulin with mucin and polyethylene glycol, insulin resisted rapid hydrolysis

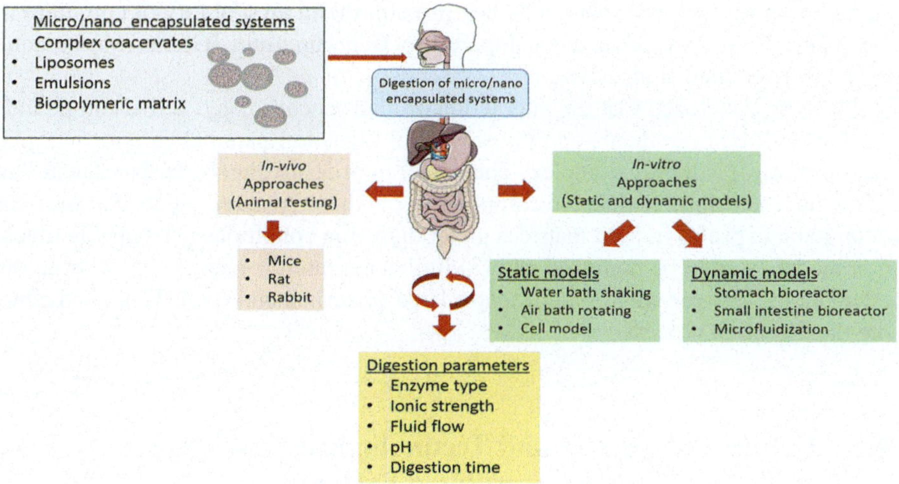

Fig. 4.4 Schematic image of biological fate of mico/nano encapsulated active compounds (Liu et al. 2019)

Table 4.1 Functions and ambient conditions of gastro intestinal system

Digestion system	Functions	Ambient conditions
Oral cavit	Chewing for minimizing the food particles	Enzyme: Amylase, lingual Lipase Saliva flow rate: 0.042–1.83 mL/min (unstimulated), 0.77–4.15 mL/min (stimulated) pH: 5–7
Stomach	Degradation, and chemical Hydrolysis of food particles	Enzymes: Pepsin, gastric Lipase Gastric juice secretion: 1–3 L/day pH: 1–3
Small intestine	Enzymatic catalysis of Macromolecules to Micromolecules and absorption of Nutrients	Enzymes: Pancreatic lipase, Protease, amylase Pancreatic juice secretion: ~ 1.5 L/day pH: 6–7.5
Large intestine and colon	Microbial fermentation and adsorption water	Microbiota:~10^{14} belonging To >1000 different species

and it gained stability in the gastrointestinal system (Iwanaga et al. 1997). Currently, researchers focus on the bioavailability of lipophilic active compounds after *in vitro* digestion. Curcumin is a member of polyphenol compounds and it has water solubility and bioavailability problems (Mutlu et al. 2018). It has been reported that after surface coating with chitosan and whey protein, the bioavailability of curcumin in small intestines was enhanced compared to free curcumin (Gómez-Mascaraque et al. 2017; Cuomo et al. 2018).

It can be concluded that the interaction of microencapsulated active compounds with other food ingredients and physiological digestion parameters (enzyme, pH, fluid flow etc.) is highly complex. Therefore, in order to clarify the biological fate of the microencapsulated active compounds; (1) there is an urgent need to monitor micro/nanocapsules in food matrices under digestion conditions (2) dynamic digestion models should be preferred and (3) further research is required to clear up the interactions between micro/nanoencapsulated materials and food compounds during the digestion process.

4.5 Future Perspective and Technological Challenges for Micro/Nano Encapsulated Systems

Micro/nanoencapsulation of active compound in food applications exhibit better functionality than conventional protection methods in terms of improved biocompatibility and bioavailability. A great variety of methods have been studied for the encapsulation of active compounds in food applications. However, a few of them i.e., spray drying and lipid- based approaches are widely applied in industrial food applications. Even though every approach has disadvantages with its unique characteristics, which make it challenging, they should be studied elaborately to overcome their limitations and enhance their level from laboratory bench scale to food industry scale. Nanoscale encapsulated materials are a promising approach that increases biocompatibility and bioavailability of active compounds and prolong retention time. To the best of our knowledge, the most suitable nano-sized carrier materials for food engineering are carbohydrate-polymer complexes and lipid-based emulsion systems. Besides, spray drying is the most preferred method. It is possible to make large-scale production with spray drying, which is widely available in the food industry. The successful encapsulation of active compounds mainly depends on the selection of carrier materials and encapsulation techniques. Polysaccharides and proteins offer an advantageous formulation for the micro-size encapsulation of active compounds by using spray drying and emulsion techniques. On contrary, electrospinning and electrospraying methods provide micro/nano sized high encapsulation efficiency, controlled release profile and increased thermal, oxidative and light stability. The digestion of micro/nanoencapsualtion materials and active compounds depends on other food ingredients, physicochemical properties of encapsulation materials, food intake time and gastrointestinal conditions such as age, sex and health status. To date, most micro/nanoencapsulation systems which have been developed, comprising of one active compound. On contrary, new generation food systems are much more complex and consisting of active compound mixtures. Therefore, further research on micro/nano encapsulation systems should focus on complex micro/nanocarriers for food science.

References

Abdel-Mohsen A, Pavliňák D, Čileková M, Lepcio P, Abdel-Rahman R, Jančář J (2019) Electrospinning of hyaluronan/polyvinyl alcohol in presence of in-situ silver nanoparticles: Preparation and characterization. Int J Biol Macromol 139:730–739. https://doi.org/10.1016/j.ijbiomac.2019.07.205

Akhavan S, Assadpour E, Katouzian E, Jafari SM (2018) Lipid nano scale cargos for the protection and delivery of food bioactive ingredients and nutraceuticals. Trends Food Sci Technol. 74:132–146. https://doi.org/10.1016/j.tifs.2018.02.001

Assadpour E, Jafari SM (2019) Advances in spray-drying encapsulation of food bioactive ingredients: from microcapsules to nanocapsules. Annu Rev. Food Sci Technol 10:103–131. https://doi.org/10.1146/annurev-food-032818-121,641

Augustin MA, Hemar Y (2009) Nano-and micro-structured assemblies for encapsulation of food ingredients. Chem. Soc. Rev. 38(4):902–912. https://doi.org/10.1039/B801739P

Bae E, Lee S (2008) Microencapsulation of avocado oil by spray drying using whey protein and maltodextrin. J Microencapsulation 25(8):549–560. https://doi.org/10.1080/02652040802075682

Baxa U (2018) Imaging of liposomes by transmission electron microscopy. In: Characterization of nanoparticles intended for drug delivery. Springer, pp 73–88. https://doi.org/10.1007/978-1-4939-7352-1_8

Bhushani JA, Anandharamakrishnan C (2014) Electrospinning and electrospraying techniques: Potential food based applications. Trends Food Sci Technol 38(1):21–33. https://doi.org/10.1016/j.tifs.2014.03.004

Bourbon AI, Cerqueira MA, Vicente AA (2016) Encapsulation and controlled release of bioactive compounds in lactoferrin-glycomacropeptide nanohydrogels: Curcumin and caffeine as model compounds. J Food Eng 180:110–119. https://doi.org/10.1016/j.jfoodeng.2016.02.016

Bourbon AI, Pinheiro AC, Cerqueira AA, Vicente AA (2018) In vitro digestion of lactoferrin-glycomacropeptide nanohydrogels incorporating bioactive compounds: Effect of a chitosan coating. Food Hydrocoll 84:267–275. https://doi.org/10.1016/j.foodhyd.2018.06.015

Brahatheeswaran D, Mathew A, Aswathy RG, Nagaoka Y, Venugopal K, Yoshida Y, Maekawa T, Sakthikumar D (2012) Hybrid fluorescent curcumin loaded zein electrospun nanofibrous scaffold for biomedical applications. Biomed Mater 7(4):045001. https://doi.org/10.1088/1748-6041/7/4/045001

Bryszewska MA, Tomás-Cobos T, Gallego E, Villalba M, Rivera SDLT, Gianotti A (2019) In vitro bioaccessibility and bioavailability of iron from breads fortified with microencapsulated iron. LWT 99:431–437. https://doi.org/10.1016/j.lwt.2018.09.071

Calamak S, Ulubayram K (2019) Controlled synthesis of multi-branched gold nanodendrites by dynamic microfluidic flow system. J Mater Sci 54(10):7541–7552. https://doi.org/10.1007/s10853-019-03403-0

Çalamak S, Erdoğdu C, Özalp M, Ulubayram K (2014) Silk fibroin based antibacterial bionanotextiles as wound dressing materials. Mater Sci Eng C 43:11–20. https://doi.org/10.1016/j.msec.2014.07.001

Calamak S, Aksoy EA, Erdogdu C, Sagıroglu M, Ulubayram K (2015a) Silver nanoparticle containing silk fibroin bionanotextiles. J Nanopart Res 17(2):87. https://doi.org/10.1007/s11051-015-2895-7

Calamak S, Aksoy EA, Ertas N, Erdogdu C, Sagıroglu M, Ulubayram K (2015b) Ag/silk fibroin nanofibers: Effect of fibroin morphology on Ag + release and antibacterial activity. Eur Polym J 67:99–112. https://doi.org/10.1016/j.eurpolymj.2015.03.068

Chen L (2009) Protein micro/nanoparticles for controlled nutraceutical delivery in functional foods. Designing Functional Foods. Elsevier, pp. 572–600. https://doi.org/10.1533/9781845696603.3.572

Chourpa I, Ducel V, Richard J, Dubois P, Boury F (2006) Conformational modifications of α gliadin and globulin proteins upon complex coacervates formation with gum arabic as studied

by Raman microspectroscopy. Biomacromolecules 7(9):2616–2623. https://doi.org/10.1021/bm060131d
Claessens M, Saris WH, van Baak MA (2008) Glucagon and insulin responses after ingestion of different amounts of intact and hydrolysed proteins. Br J Nutr 100(1):61–69. https://doi.org/10.1017/S0007114507886314
Cooper C, Dubin P, Kayitmazer P, Turksen S (2005) Polyelectrolyte–protein complexes. Curr Opin Colloid Interf Sci 10(1–2):52–78. https://doi.org/10.1016/j.cocis.2005.05.007
Cota-Arriola O, Cortez-Rocha MO, Burgos-Hernández A, Ezquerra-Brauer JM, Plascencia-Jatomea M (2013) Controlled release matrices and micro/nanoparticles of chitosan with antimicrobial potential: development of new strategies for microbial control in agriculture. J Sci Food Agric 93(7):1525–1536. https://doi.org/10.1002/jsfa.6060
Cuomo F, Cofelice M, Venditti F, Ceglie A, Miguel M, Lindman B, Lopez F (2018) In-vitro digestion of curcumin loaded chitosan-coated liposomes. Colloids Surf B 168:29–34. https://doi.org/10.1016/j.colsurfb.2017.11.047
Dai L, Zhou H, Wei Y, Gao Y, McClements DJ (2019) Curcumin encapsulation in zein-rhamnolipid composite nanoparticles using a pH-driven method. Food Hydrocoll 93:342–350. https://doi.org/10.1016/j.foodhyd.2019.02.041
De Matteis V, Cannavale A, Martellotta F, Rinaldi R, Calcagnile P, Ferrari F, Ayr U, Fiorito F (2019) Nano-encapsulation of phase change materials: From design to thermal performance, simulations and toxicological assessment. Energy Build 188:1–11. https://doi.org/10.1016/j.enbuild.2019.02.004
Devi N, Sarmah M, Khatun B, Maji TK (2017) Encapsulation of active ingredients in polysaccharide–protein complex coacervates. Adv. Colloid Interf Sci 239:136–145. https://doi.org/10.1016/j.cis.2016.05.009
Doi T, Wang M, McClements DJ (2019) Impact of proteins and polysaccharides on flavor release from oil-in-water emulsions during simulated cooking. Food Res Int 125:108549. https://doi.org/10.1016/j.foodres.2019.108549
Fang Z, Bhandari B (2010) Encapsulation of polyphenols–a review. Trends Food Sci Tech 21(10):510–523. https://doi.org/10.1016/j.tifs.2010.08.003
Fathi M, Martin A, McClements DJ (2014) Nanoencapsulation of food ingredients using carbohydrate based delivery systems. Trends Food Sci Tech 39(1):18–39. https://doi.org/10.1016/j.tifs.2014.06.007
Fernandez A, Torres-Giner S, Lagaron JM (2009) Novel route to stabilization of bioactive antioxidants by encapsulation in electrospun fibers of zein prolamine. Food Hydrocoll 23(5):1427–1432. https://doi.org/10.1016/j.foodhyd.2008.10.011
Gómez-Mascaraque LG, Sipoli CC, de La-Torre LG, López-Rubio A (2017) Microencapsulation structures based on protein-coated liposomes obtained through electrospraying for the stabilization and improved bioaccessibility of curcumin. Food Chem 233:343–350. https://doi.org/10.1016/j.foodchem.2017.04.133
Gómez-Mascaraque LG, Tordera F, Fabra MJ, Martínez-Sanz M, Lopez-Rubio A (2019) Coaxial electrospraying of biopolymers as a strategy to improve protection of bioactive food ingredients. Innovative Food Sci Emerg Technol 51:2–11. https://doi.org/10.1016/j.ifset.2018.03.023
Gu YS, Decker EA, McClements DJ (2005) Influence of pH and carrageenan type on properties of β-lactoglobulin stabilized oil-in-water emulsions. Food Hydrocoll 19(1):83–91. https://doi.org/10.1016/j.foodhyd.2004.04.016
Gümüşderelioğlu M, Sunal E, Demirtaş TT, Kiremitçi AS (2020) Chitosan-based double-faced barrier membrane coated with functional nanostructures and loaded with BMP-6. J Mater Sci Mater Med 31(1):4. https://doi.org/10.1007/s10856-019-6331-x
Gupta S, Khan S, Muzafar M, Kushwaha M, Yadav AK, Gupta AP (2016) Encapsulation: entrapping essential oil/flavors/aromas in food. Encapsulations, Elsevier:229–268. https://doi.org/10.1016/B978-0-12-804,307-3.00006-5

Inci F, Ozen MO, Saylan Y, Miansari M, Cimen D, Dhara R, Chinnasamy T, Yuksekkaya M, Filippini C, Kumar DK (2018) A novel on-chip method for differential extraction of sperm in forensic cases. Adv Sci 5(9):1800121. https://doi.org/10.1002/advs.201800121

Iwanaga K, Ono S, Narioka K, Morimoto K, Kakemi M, Yamashita S, Nango M, Oku N (1997) Oral delivery of insulin by using surface coating liposomes: improvement of stability of insulin in GI tract. Int J Pharm 157(1):73–80. https://doi.org/10.1016/S0378-5173(97)00237-8

Jafari SM, Fathi M, Mandala I (2015) Emerging product formation. In: Food waste recovery. Elsevier, pp 293–317. https://doi.org/10.1016/B978-0-12-800,351-0.00013-4

Jimenez M, Garcia H, Beristain C (2004) Spray-drying microencapsulation and oxidative stability of conjugated linoleic acid. Eur Food Res Technol 219(6):588–592. https://doi.org/10.1007/s00217-004-0992-4

Kagami Y, Sugimura S, Fujishima N, Matsuda K, Kometani T, Matsumura Y (2003) Oxidative stability, structure, and physical characteristics of microcapsules formed by spray drying of fish oil with protein and dextrin wall materials. J Food Sci 68(7):2248–2255. https://doi.org/10.1111/j.1365-2621.2003.tb05755.x

Kavitake D, Kandasamy S, Devi PB, Shetty PH (2018) Recent developments on encapsulation of lactic acid bacteria as potential starter culture in fermented foods–A review. Food Biosci 21:34–44. https://doi.org/10.1016/j.fbio.2017.11.003

Kizilay E, Kayitmazer AB, Dubin PL (2011) Complexation and coacervation of polyelectrolytes with oppositely charged colloids. Adv Colloid Interface Sci 167(1–2):24–37. https://doi.org/10.1016/j.cis.2011.06.006

Lamprecht A, Schäfer U, Lehr CM (2000) Structural analysis of microparticles by confocal laser scanning microscopy. AAPS PharmSciTech 1(3):10–19. https://doi.org/10.1208/pt010317

Leyva-López R, Palma-Rodríguez HM, López-Torres A, Capataz-Tafur J, Bello-Pérez LA, Vargas-Torres A (2019) Use of enzymatically modified starch in the microencapsulation of ascorbic acid: Microcapsule characterization, release behavior and in vitro digestion. Food Hydrocoll 96:259–266. https://doi.org/10.1016/j.foodhyd.2019.04.056

Lin WZS, Malmstadt N (2019) Liposome production and concurrent loading of drug simulants by microfluidic hydrodynamic focusing. Eur Biophys J 48(6):549–558. https://doi.org/10.1007/s00249-019-01383-2

Liu W, Ye A, Han F, Han J (2019) Advances and challenges in liposome digestion: Surface interaction, biological fate, and GIT modeling. Adv Colloid Interface Sci 263:52–67. https://doi.org/10.1016/j.cis.2018.11.007

Liu Y, Wang S, Lan W (2018) Fabrication of antibacterial chitosan-PVA blended film using electrospray technique for food packaging applications. Int J Biol Macromol 107:848–854. https://doi.org/10.1016/j.ijbiomac.2017.09.044

López-Rubio A, Lagaron JM (2012) Whey protein capsules obtained through electrospraying for the encapsulation of bioactives. Innov Food Sci Emerg 13:200–206. https://doi.org/10.1016/j.ifset.2011.10.012

Mao AS, Özkale B, Shah NJ, Vining KH, Descombes T, Zhang L, Tringides CM, Wong SW, Shin JW, Scadden DT (2019) Programmable microencapsulation for enhanced mesenchymal stem cell persistence and immunomodulation. PNAS 116(31):15392–15,397. https://doi.org/10.1073/pnas.1819415116

Maurya VK, Aggarwal M (2017) enhancing bio-availability of vitamin d by nano-engineered based delivery systems-An overview. Int J Curr Microbiol App Sci 6(7): 340–353. doi: https://doi.org/10.20546/ijcmas.2017.607.040

Maurya VK, Aggarwal M (2019a) Fabrication of nano-structured lipid carrier for encapsulation of vitamin D3 for fortification of 'Lassi'; A milk based beverage. J Steroid Biochem Mol Bio 193:105429. https://doi.org/10.1016/j.jsbmb.2019.105429

Maurya VK, Aggarwal M (2019b) A phase inversion based nanoemulsion fabrication process to encapsulate vitamin D3 for food applications. J Steroid Biochem Mol Bio 190:88–98. https://doi.org/10.1016/j.jsbmb.2019.03.021

Maurya VK, Aggarwal M, Ranjan V, Gothandam K (2020a) Improving bioavailability of vitamin a in food by encapsulation: An update, Nanoscience in medicine, vol 1. Springer, pp 117–145. https://doi.org/10.1007/978-3-030-29,207-2_4

Maurya VK, Bashir K, Aggarwal M (2020b) Vitamin D microencapsulation and fortification: Trends and technologies. J Steroid Biochem Mol Bio 196:105489. https://doi.org/10.1016/j.jsbmb.2019.105489

Mavis B, Demirtaş TT, Gümüşderelioğlu M, Gündüz G, Çolak Ü (2009) Synthesis, characterization and osteoblastic activity of polycaprolactone nanofibers coated with biomimetic calcium phosphate. Acta Biomater 5(8):3098–3111. https://doi.org/10.1016/j.actbio.2009.04.037

McClements DJ (2010) Emulsion design to improve the delivery of functional lipophilic components. Annu Rev Food Sci Technol 1:241–269. https://doi.org/10.1146/annurev.food.080708.100722

McClements DJ, Li Y (2010) Review of in vitro digestion models for rapid screening of emulsion-based systems. Food Funct 1(1):32–59. https://doi.org/10.1039/C0FO00111B

Mekhloufi G, Sanchez C, Renard D, Guillemin S, Hardy J (2005) pH-induced structural transitions during complexation and coacervation of β-lactoglobulin and acacia gum. Langmuir 21(1):386–394. https://doi.org/10.1021/la0486786

Mutlu G, Calamak S, Ulubayram K, Guven E (2018) Curcumin-loaded electrospun PHBV nanofibers as potential wound-dressing material. J Drug Deliv Sci Tec 43:185–193. https://doi.org/10.1016/j.jddst.2017.09.017

Najafi-Soulari S, Shekarchizadeh H, Kadivar M (2016) Encapsulation optimization of lemon balm antioxidants in calcium alginate hydrogels. J Biomater Sci Polym Ed 27(16):1631–1644. https://doi.org/10.1080/09205063.2016.1226042

Nedovic V, Kalusevic A, Manojlovic V, Levic S, Bugarski B (2011) An overview of encapsulation technologies for food applications. Procedia Food Sci 1:1806–1815. https://doi.org/10.1016/j.profoo.2011.09.265

Neo YP, Ray S, Jin J, Gizdavic-Nikolaidis M, Nieuwoudt MK, Liu D, Quek SY (2013) Encapsulation of food grade antioxidant in natural biopolymer by electrospinning technique: A physicochemical study based on zein–gallic acid system. Food Chem. 136(2):1013–1021. https://doi.org/10.1016/j.foodchem.2012.09.010

Okutan N, Terzi P, Altay F (2014) Affecting parameters on electrospinning process and characterization of electrospun gelatin nanofibers. Food Hydrocoll 39:19–26. https://doi.org/10.1016/j.foodhyd.2013.12.022

Paz-Samaniego R, Rascón-Chu A, Brown-Bojorquez F, Carvajal-Millan E, Pedroza-Montero M, Silva-Campa E, Sotelo-Cruz N, López-Franco YL, Lizardi-Mendoza J (2018) Electrospray-assisted fabrication of core-shell arabinoxylan gel particles for insulin and probiotics entrapment. J Appl Polym Sci 135(26):46411. https://doi.org/10.1002/app.46411

Pérez-Masiá R, López-Nicolás R, Periago MJ, Ros G, Lagaron JM, López-Rubio A (2015) Encapsulation of folic acid in food hydrocolloids through nanospray drying and electrospraying for nutraceutical applications. Food Chem 168:124–133. https://doi.org/10.1016/j.foodchem.2014.07.051

Robson AL, Dastoor PC, Flynn J, Palmer W, Martin A, Smith DW, Woldu A, Hua S (2018) Advantages and limitations of current imaging techniques for characterizing liposome morphology. Front Pharmacol 9:80. https://doi.org/10.3389/fphar.2018.00080

Sarıgöl E, Pehlivan SB, Ekizoğlu M, Sağıroğlu M, Çalış S (2017) Design and evaluation of gamma-sterilized vancomycin hydrochloride-loaded poly (ε-caprolactone) microspheres for the treatment of biofilm-based medical device-related osteomyelitis. Pharm Dev Technol 22(6):706–714. https://doi.org/10.3109/10837450.2015.1102280

Sarıgöl E, Ekizoğlu M, Pehlivan SB, Bodur E, Sağıroğlu M, Çalış S (2018) A thermosensitive gel loaded with an enzyme and an antibiotic drug for the treatment of periprosthetic joint infection. J Drug Delivery Sci Technol 43:423–429. https://doi.org/10.1016/j.jddst.2017.11.004

Sarigol-Calamak E, Hascicek C (2018) Tissue scaffolds as a local drug delivery system for bone regeneration. Cutting-edge enabling technologies for regenerative medicine. Springer, pp 475–493. https://doi.org/10.1007/978-981-13-0950-2_25
Schmitt C, Turgeon SL (2011) Protein/polysaccharide complexes and coacervates in food systems. Adv Colloid Interface Sci 167(1–2):63–70. https://doi.org/10.1016/j.cis.2010.10.001
Schmitt C, Sanchez C, Lamprecht A, Renard D, Lehr CM, de Kruif CG, Hardy J (2001) Study of β-lactoglobulin/acacia gum complex coacervation by diffusing-wave spectroscopy and confocal scanning laser microscopy. Colloids Surf B 20(3):267–280. https://doi.org/10.1016/S0927-7765(00)00200-9
Shin GH, Chung SK, Kim JT, Joung HJ, Park HJ (2013) Preparation of chitosan-coated nanoliposomes for improving the mucoadhesive property of curcumin using the ethanol injection method. J Agric Food Chem 61(46):11119–11,126. https://doi.org/10.1021/jf4035404
Son SJ, Hong SK, Lim G (2020) Emulsion electrospinning of hydrophobic ptfe-peo composite nanofibrous membranes for simple oil/water separation. J Sens Technol 29(2):89–92. https://doi.org/10.5369/JSST.2020.29.2.89
Tamjidi F, Shahedi M, Varshosaz J, Nasirpour A (2013) Nanostructured lipid carriers (NLC): A potential delivery system for bioactive food molecules. Innovative Food Sci Emerg Technol 19:29–43. https://doi.org/10.1016/j.ifset.2013.03.002
Tampau A, González-Martínez C, Chiralt A (2018) Release kinetics and antimicrobial properties of carvacrol encapsulated in electrospun poly-(ε-caprolactone) nanofibres. Application in starch multilayer films. Food Hydrocoll 79:158–169. https://doi.org/10.1016/j.foodhyd.2017.12.021
Tosi MM, Ramos AP, Esposto BS, Jafari SM (2020) Dynamic light scattering (DLS) of nanoencapsulated food ingredients. Characterization of nanoencapsulated food ingredients. Elsevier, pp. 191–211. https://doi.org/10.1016/B978-0-12-815,667-4.00006-7
Trucillo P, Ferrari P, Campardelli R, Reverchon E, Perego P (2020) A supercritical assisted process for the production of amoxicillin loaded liposomes for anti-microbial applications. J Supercrit Fluids:104842. https://doi.org/10.1016/j.supflu.2020.104842
Ulubayram K, Calamak S, Shahbazi R, Eroglu I (2015) Nanofibers based antibacterial drug design, delivery and applications. Curr Pharm Des 21(15):1930–1943. https://doi.org/10.2174/1381612821666150302151804
Vélez MA, Perotti MC, Hynes ER, Gennaro AM (2019) Effect of lyophilization on food grade liposomes loaded with conjugated linoleic acid. J Food Eng 240:199–206. https://doi.org/10.1016/j.jfoodeng.2018.07.033
Wang M, Doi T, McClements DJ (2019) Encapsulation and controlled release of hydrophobic flavors using biopolymer-based microgel delivery systems: Sustained release of garlic flavor during simulated cooking. Food Res Int 119:6–14. https://doi.org/10.1016/j.foodres.2019.01.042
Wei X, Patil Y, Ohana P, Amitay Y, Shmeeda H, Gabizon A, Barenholz Y (2017) Characterization of pegylated liposomal mitomycin C lipid-based prodrug (Promitil) by high sensitivity differential scanning calorimetry and cryogenic transmission electron microscopy. Mol Pharmaceutics 14(12):4339–4345. https://doi.org/10.1021/acs.molpharmaceut.6b00865
Weinbreck F, Tromp R, De Kruif C (2004) Composition and structure of whey protein/gum arabic coacervates. Biomacromolecules 5(4):1437–1445. https://doi.org/10.1021/bm049970v
Wongsasulak S, Kit M, McClements DJ, Yoovidhya T, Weiss J (2007) The effect of solution properties on the morphology of ultrafine electrospun egg albumen–PEO composite fibers. Polymer 48(2):448–457. https://doi.org/10.1016/j.polymer.2006.11.025
Wongsasulak S, Patapeejumruswong M, Weiss J, Supaphol P, Yoovidhya T (2010) Electrospinning of food-grade nanofibers from cellulose acetate and egg albumen blends. J Food Eng 98(3):370–376. https://doi.org/10.1016/j.jfoodeng.2010.01.014
Yang S, Liu C, Liu W, Yu H, Zheng H, Zhou W, Hu Y (2013) Preparation and characterization of nanoliposomes entrapping medium-chain fatty acids and vitamin C by lyophilization. Int J Mol Sci 14(10):19763–19,773. https://doi.org/10.3390/ijms141019763

Yu Y, Lv Y (2019) Degradation kinetic of anthocyanins from rose (Rosa rugosa) as prepared by microencapsulation in freeze-drying and spray-drying. Int J Food Prop 22(1):2009–2021. https://doi.org/10.1080/10942912.2019.1701011

Zaeim D, Sarabi-Jamab M, Ghorani B, Kadkhodaee R, Tromp RH (2018) Electrospray-assisted drying of live probiotics in acacia gum microparticles matrix. Carbohydr Polym 183:183–191. https://doi.org/10.1016/j.carbpol.2017.12.001

Zhao H, Sun C, Stewart RJ, Waite JH (2005) Cement proteins of the tube-building polychaete Phragmatopoma californica. J Biol Chem 280(52):42938–42,944. https://doi.org/10.1074/jbc.M50845720

Chapter 5
Encapsulation of Herbal Extracts

Sadhna Mishra, Shalini Sahani, Arvind, and Vijayeta Pal

Abstract From antiquity to till now, humans preferred natural and easily consumable vegetables, herbs, shrubs, and essential oils which have been added to the different food, beverages, agriculture, and pharmaceutical industries. The phytoactive compounds present in the plant which flattering more attention-grabbing vicinity in prophylactic studies because of being health-promoting capabilities. Polyphenols are a major group of phytoactive constituents which includes flavonoids, anthocyanins, so on and besides, they are also measured as food ingredients and found unsurprisingly in approximately all vegetables, fruits, and nuts. These phytoactive compounds afford a lot of dietetic ideals at the side of curative and stabilizer actions. The health problems like kidney disease, appetite aches, intestinal problems, liver and gall bladder problems outstanding to the antimicrobial, antioxidant, and anti-carcinogenic can be cured by the bioactive compounds that frequently institute in herbs and shrubs. These bioactive or chemical compounds of herbs and shrubs boast many important functional groups such as oxygenated compounds like aromatics, alcohols, aldehydes, phenols, sesquiterpene alcohol, esters, lactones, oxides, ethers and they also bear monoterpenes, sesquiterpenes, and aromatics. All the bioactive/phytoactive compounds are extremely susceptible to the environmental and chemical factors which are responsible for the degradation and inactivation of the compound. The stability of the innate antioxidants such as flavonoids, polyphenols, and other phytoactive compounds is depending on the pres-

S. Mishra · Arvind (✉)
Department of Dairy Science and Food Technology, Institute of Agricultural Sciences, Banaras Hindu University, Varanasi, India
e-mail: sadhna.mishra@bhu.ac.com; arvind00000@gmail.com

S. Sahani
Department of Material Science and Engineering, Gachon University, Seongnam, South Korea
e-mail: shalinisahani42@gmail.com

V. Pal
School of Materials Science and Technology, Indian Institute of Technology, Banaras Hindu University, Varanasi, Uttar Pradesh, India

V. K. Maurya et al. (eds.), *Sustainable Agriculture Reviews 55*, Sustainable Agriculture Reviews 55, https://doi.org/10.1007/978-3-030-76813-3_5

ervation method. Hence, for the preservation of these bio or phytoactive compounds for their stability, encapsulation is the prospective strategy. In encapsulation, the inner phase is a phytoactive herbal compound, and the outer phase is of second core material phase, former lucratively tried for the deliverance of confident phytoactive compounds.

Keywords Encapsulation · Phytoactive · And bioactive compounds · Polyphenols · Flavonoids

5.1 Introduction

Comprehension and utilization of herbal extracts which are derived from foliage have occurred in an assortment of populations through creature progression and commencement. From the past decades, human beings were learning about the selection of plants in favor of foodstuff, to alleviate ailments and diseases (Ferreira and Pinto 2010). At an overall cost, various natural products derived from herbal resource have diverse organic properties which offer ailment for various diseases. Approximately all the medicinal plant extracts have properties like antioxidants, insecticidal, antibiotic, antifungal, anticancer, antiparasitic, hypoglycemic, and anti-hypertensive. The organic solvents are needed for herbal extraction which makes complicated formulation that is why human beings cannot take it directly. Bioactive compounds present in herbal extracts are very sensitive to the chemical and physical environmental factors so that to triumph over these hurdles, the research based on encapsulation technology has been focused on developing novel customs to preserve the plant extracts and their safe delivery with enhanced remedial worth. Over the last few years, there has been a mounting curiosity on the bioactive constituent of foodstuff while on the other hand industries like pharmaceutics are also looking for the integration of health-promoting compounds into various products formulations. The issues related to ingredients include their poor availability inside the body and their low solubility in aqueous solutions. Encapsulation is a very effective strategy to resolve all these problems of herbal-based bioactive components (Assadpour and Jafari, 2019). Almost bioactive compounds from the plant or herbal extracts might lose their activity before getting to the bloodstream due to enzymatic activity of the liver and pH of the stomach. Consequently, blood may not get the appropriate amount of the plant extracts. Hence, if the sufficient dose of the bioactive constituents (drug) will not be reached to the tainted area at a "minimum effective level," in that case possibly the drug will not be sufficient to illuminate a remedial consequence. Delivery of the encapsulated herbal extract can transmit an optimal quantity of the desired drug to their site of action evade all the obstructions such as the acidic pH of the stomach, liver metabolism, and an augmentation in the complete drug transmission due to their tiny size. On the other hand, the enhancement for the development of novel and functional food products with the fortification of nutraceuticals and bioactive compounds for health concerns (Ting et al. 2014; Maurya and Aggarwal 2017; Maurya et al.2019) because of the direct consumption of bioactive compounds in food matrices have many limitations. There are many limitations of medicinal plants by their impending to attain the spot of the remedial action. Encapsulated deliverance organizations can enhance drug stability and amplify the period of curative consequence; they also possess useful properties such as controlled drug release (Maurya and Aggarwal 2017; Maurya et al. 2019). All the drawbacks which occur with the bioactive compounds can be overcome by the food-grade delivery systems of nanoencapsulation. Lipid-based nanocarriers are the promising strategy among all the encapsulation delivery systems for the flourishing deliverance of the bioactive compounds which are present in the food product. Encapsulated food formulations may be particularly practical as delivery systems when direct utilization of the bioactive compound obstruct with human metabolism. Other advantages of encapsulation comprise controlled liberation, unscrambling incompatible constituents, camouflage disagreeable taste of bioactive (astringent flavor of polyphenolic substances), and improving ultimate product qualities (Stojanovic et al. 2012). Hence, this chapter contains more about herbal extract and different encapsulation techniques and their fate for the successful delivery of the desired bioactive compound.

5.2 Herbal Extracts and Bioactive Compounds

In the early nineteenth century, the chemical examination becomes accessible, which commence the withdrawal and amendments of herbal extract. For a long duration of time, due to lack of characterization, processing like extraction, identification of remedial constituents, and scientific proof herbal medication were not implemented for the novel food formulation. Though, nanoparticles, liposomes, matrix systems, microemulsion, solid lipid nanoparticles, and solid dispersion proffer the way for the fabricating the novel carriers based on modern phytopharmaceutical research dealt with the scientific requirements for herbal medicines as in modern medicine. For the remedial compounds such as curcumin, paclitaxel, and vitamin D (chemotherapeutic drugs) and many other compounds the nanotubes, nanoemulsion, micellar system, and colloidal nanogels have been developed (Maurya and Aggarwal 2019).

All the phytoactive or bioactive constituents of plants are coming under the category of secondary metabolites. Amongst all the secondary metabolites, some specific compounds are very effective for the remedial purpose on biological systems is considered as the bioactive or phytoactive compounds. Therefore, a straightforward explanation of bioactive compounds in plants is secondary plant metabolites extract toxicological or pharmacological consequences in human beings. The plant extracts with bioactivities are also related to compounds like phytosterols, carotenoids, fiber, sulfur-containing compounds, vitamins, and organic acid anions together with polyphenolic. Table 5.1 contains some of the common bioactive compounds present in plant extracts of different plant species and their extraction methods (Mosaddik et al. 2018).

5.3 Extraction Techniques

The diversity of extraction techniques is used for the past decades and is used for the extraction of the phytoactive constituents from the different plant sources. The common purposes of all the extraction techniques are as follows:

- For the selective extraction of targeted phytoactive constituents from multifarious plant sample
- For enhancing the selectivity of investigative methodology
- To amplify warmth of bioassay by mounting the attentiveness of embattled constituents
- To renovate the bioactive compounds into a more appropriate forum for recognition and partition
- To make available a strong and reproducible technique that is self-governing variation in the sample matrix (Smith 2003).

The different extraction techniques that have the potential to extract out most of the phytoactive or bioactive compounds are the conventional extraction methods including the soxhlet extraction method and maceration techniques whereas the techniques like supercritical fluid extraction (SFE), microwave-assisted extraction (MAE), pressurized liquid extraction (PLE), ultrasound-assisted extraction (UAE) and enzyme-assisted extraction (EAE) are called green techniques.

5.4 Encapsulation

Encapsulation is defined as a process of confining active compounds within a matrix or membrane in particulate form to achieve one or more desirable effects. From the standpoint of herbal products, it is possible to extend shelf-life, separate contrary compounds, controlled delivery, masking unpleasant taste of bioactive such as the bitter taste of polyphenolic compounds, and improving final product qualities by applying the encapsulation of herbal extracts (Stojanovic et al. 2012). Controlled-delivery of desired bioactive compounds enhances bioavailability by tailoring the discharge process or velocity of that particular encapsulated phytoactive compound in the gastrointestinal tract (Fig. 5.1) (Maurya and Agrawal 2017). In other words, we can say that encapsulation is a way to preserve the remedial and other advantageous properties of plant extracts inside a medium to accomplish the desirable and

Table 5.1 Reported application of different techniques for the extraction of bioactive compounds from different plant sources and their benefits

Herbal source	Extraction technique	Bioactive compound	Benefits and solvent/ enzyme used for extraction	Remedial Application	References
Prunella vulgaris L. plant	Ultrasonic-assisted extraction	Flavonoids		Against sore throat, accelerating wound healing and reducing fever	Zhang et al. (2011)
Forsythia suspensa plant	Ultrasonic-assisted extraction	Phillyrin		Anti-inflammatory, Vasorelaxant, antioxidant, and antiviral	Xia et al. (2011)
Spirulina platensis alga	Ultrasonic-assisted extraction	Beta-carotene	Application for food and pharmaceuticals	Protect against cancer, chronic diseases and diabetes	Dey and Rathod (2013)
Chilean papaya Seeds	Ultrasonic-assisted extraction	Isothiocyanates, phenolic acids,and flavanols	Rapid and enhanced extraction process	Antimicrobial and Antioxidant	Briones-Labarca et al. (2015)
Jabuticaba skin	Ultrasonic-assisted extraction	Anthocyanins	Better recovery and rapid extraction of compounds	Aesthetic and Food industries	Santos et al. (2012)
Green coffee Beans	Microwave-assisted extraction	Chlorogenic acid, caffeine, and polyphenols		Used as functional Foods	Upadhyay et al. (2012)
Rosemary leaves	Microwave-assisted extraction	Phenolic acids and flavonoids	Lower extraction time	Antioxidants for the food industry	Svarc-Gajic et al. (2013)
Grape skin from three varieties	Enzyme-assisted extraction	Anthocyanins	Pectinex B3-L,Vinozym EC, and G	Food additives providing health benefits	Oszmianski et al. (2011)

(continued)

Table 5.1 (continued)

Herbal source	Extraction technique	Bioactive compound	Benefits and solvent/ enzyme used for extraction	Remedial Application	References
Dunaliella tertiolecta and Cylindrotheca closterium microalga	Microwave-assisted extraction	Chlorophyll a and b and β-caroteneand fucoxanthin	Better yield than conventional extraction	Biotechnological applications, Food and health	Pasquet et al. (2011)
Pigeon pea leaves	Enzyme-assisted extraction	Flavones: Luteolin and apigenin	Pectinase, cellulose, and beta-glucosidase	Anti-inflammatory, antiallergic, antiproliferative	Chen et al. (2010)
Rice bran	Enzyme-assisted extraction	Enzymatic extract	Endoprotease mixture	Prevention of diseases including cancer, fatty liver, hypercalciuria, kidney stones, and so on	Wang et al. (2010)

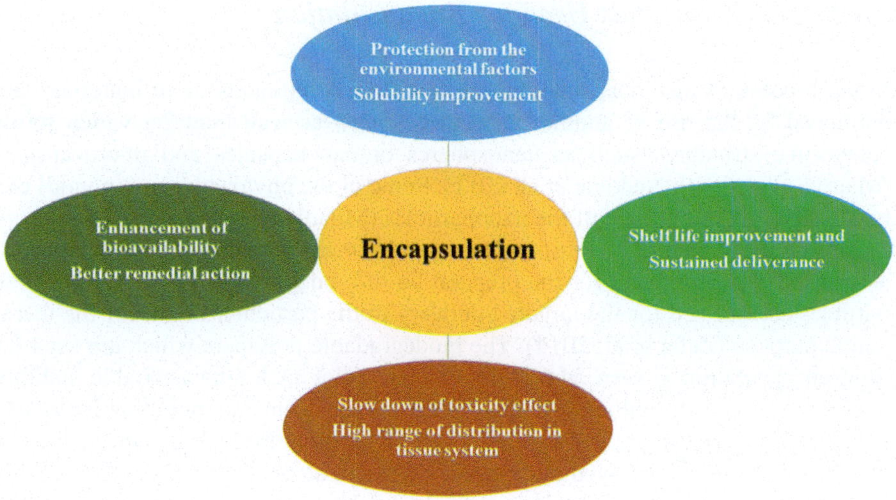

Fig. 5.1 Advantages of the use of encapsulation technology for encapsulation of herbal phytoactive compounds from plant extracts

most efficient actions. The main intention of encapsulation is to enhance the constancy of the desired extracted compounds throughout transportation and processing. It might be possible that the direct expenditure of the phyto or bioactive compounds obstruct with the human body so that a proper delivery system is mandatory. For example, polyphenols from the herbal source are generally devoured by making a tea or herbal mixture through the process of aqueous extraction. The different types of core materials which are used for encapsulation of bioactive compounds for food products are supposed to be of food-grade. Before a few decades, coacervation is one of the conventional process which attains interest and innovations to facilitate the commercialization of coacervated food products. Recently, in food division liposome attains increasing consideration because targeted delivery and high-quality stability still in water surrounding. Hydrogel made up of lipids are very complex systems and these are recently developed for the controlled deliverance of phytoactive constituents. Besides, the colloidal system of polymeric nanoparticles also works as carriers for the herbal extracts (Dordevic et al. 2015). Encapsulation possibly will be a very valuable scientific implement for the commercialization of value-added products or the differentiation of constructed products between competitors (Chan et al. 2010). Encapsulation of plant extracts by polymeric nanoparticles opens many opportunities in the fields of the health sector, medicine, cosmetics, and food industries. In other words, biological activity such as antidiabetic, antihypertensive, cosmetology, anticancer, the antibacterial activity of the herbal extracts can be enhanced by the different formulations based on polymeric nanoparticles (Armendariz-Barragan et al. 2016).

5.4.1 Wall Materials Used for Encapsulation

In the process of the encapsulation, the bioactive compounds (core materials) are entrapped by the use of another substance known as wall material which forms sphere-like structures such as nanospheres or nanocapsules and microcapsules (Maurya et al. 2019; Nedovic et al. 2011). Some of the phytoactive compounds can be absorbed on the surface of the nanoparticles (Miladi et al. 2016). Polymers from a natural source such as albumin, chitosan and some other synthetic polymers such as methacrylates are used for the preparation of biodegradable particles and these particles are utilized for the targeted delivery to the particular organ for the therapeutic purpose (Zafar et al. 2014). The biodegradable polymers which are used for drug encapsulation govern admirable characteristics including desirable stability and nontoxicity in the blood circulation. All the requirements including biological behavior like bioadhesion and increased cellular uptake, drug release profile may be prolonged, triggered, delayed and physicochemical attributes such as Particle size, zeta potential, and hydrophobicity can be obtained better by the nanoparticles which are made up of polymeric materials (Maurya et al. 2017). Commonly used biodegradable polymers used for the encapsulation of the active components are poly (lactic-co-glycolic acid), poly (glycolic acid) and Poly (lactic acid). The advantage of the use of biodegradable polymer is that based on polymer degradation kinetics, the release profile of the encapsulated compound inside the nanoparticles can be analyzed (Table 5.2). Many bioactive compounds comprise of progesterone, estradiol, dexamethasone, 9-nitrocamptothecin, insulin, tyrphostin, cisplatin, tamoxifen, haloperidol and paclitaxel with various remedial properties have effectively encapsulated by the use of various natural and synthetic polymers (Kumari et al. 2010). Usually, all the polymers are eco-friendly and biocompatible. The approaches like noninflammatory, very steady stability in bloodstream and non-toxicity have to be fulfilled by the use of Polymeric encapsulation. Furthermore, the polymeric nanoparticles also have some other advantages which are noticed (Armendáriz-Barragán et al. 2016) such as:

- Controlling profile of encapsulated drug release.
- Targeted deliverance to the particular tissue and organ.
- Protection of the bioactive compound from all the physical and chemical factors.
- Through nanoparticle elaboration the elimination of organic solvent is easy.

5.4.2 Criteria for the Selection of Wall Materials

The criteria for the selection of wall material for encapsulation include properties like the material should have good rheological properties, ability to scatter the bioactive compound and emulsion stabilization, non-reactive for active material, ability to release the core material completely in specific conditions, dissolve in non-toxic solvents. The wall materials like collagen and glycosaminoglycan are

Table 5.2 Different encapsulated products containing various bioactive compounds with better biological activity and their advantages

Encapsulated product	Wall material	Bioactive compound	Advantages	References
Microencapsulation of lutein, an extract from marigold flowers	Maltodextrin (polysaccharide base) and copovidone (polyvinyl pyrrolidone)	Lutein	Improve the bioavailability, antioxidant ability, and stability	Nalawade and Gajjar (2016)
The encapsulation of bitter melon by the use of spray-drying; antioxidant activity	Mixture of maltodextrin and arabic gum	Bitter melon	The infusion of bitter melon has been reported to improve antioxidant performance of about $\geq 87.9 \pm 2.6\%$	Tan et al. (2015)
Synthesis and characterization of polyphenols extracted from fresh strawberry fruits	Polymer chitosan	Polyphenols	Functional amino group is reported to enhance the loading of negatively charged polyphenols and improve bioavailability and sustained release	Pulicharla et al. (2016)
Encapsulation of lycopene from plant extract	Alginate gelatin	Lycopene	The stability against isomerization and release effect (diffusion coefficient) of lycopene was enhanced	Calvo et al. (2017)
Encapsulation of pantothenic acid	Liposome, alginate, oralginate-pectin mixture	Pantothenicacid	The efficiency and stability at acidic pH (4.0) improved	Ota et al.(2018)
Tragacanth gum for peppermint encapsulation	Natural polysaccharide tragacanth gum	Peppermint	The peppermint encapsulation showed better antimicrobial action over *C. albicans* than *S. aureus* and *E. coli*	Ghayempour et al. (2015)
Encapsulation of grape seed	Polylactide	Grape seed	The proanthocyanidins are reported to enhance sustained release and dental matrix stability	Yourdkhani et al. (2017)
Aloe vera extract encapsulation into natural polysaccharide tragacanth gum	Tragacanth gum	*Aloe vera*	*Aloe vera* extract reported as effective wound healer due to controlled release	Ghayempour et al. (2016)

used in combination due to a wide range of tissue-specific availability. A wall material must have been with good cell viability and low cytotoxicity (Dragostin et al. 2017).

5.5 Encapsulation Methodology

The bioactive compound that is suitable for consumption, as well as incorporation into any food product, the formulation for that, must be of food-grade. Encapsulation strategy is used for such bioactive compounds that have to be incorporated into any food product that should have good organoleptic properties. Encapsulation can elevate the physicochemical properties of the encapsulated compound and also protected to interact with other food components and also safe from degradation due to any other chemical and physical circumstances and controlled delivery of the remedial compound to specific environmental factors. The development of a variety of encapsulation techniques aims the broad-spectrum requirements of delivery systems (Dordevic et al. 2015). Encapsulation technologies for the encapsulation different bioactive molecule are classified into two main categories which are as follows:

(i) Chemistry-related processes (polymerization of monomers)
(ii) Physicochemical characteristic-based process (dispersal of preformed polymers).

Polymerization of monomers embraced processes such as interfacial polymerization, radical polymerization, mini emulsion, and microemulsion whereas in the dispersion of preformed polymer method include solvent diffusion, solvent evaporation, Nanoprecipitation, and dialysis (Armendariz-Barragan et al. 2016). The above techniques are used for the formation of different transporters such as microparticles, phytosomes, liposomes, and other nanoparticles (Miladi et al. 2013). Amongst all the abundant encapsulation methodologies, encapsulation by spray drying technology previously institutes and utilize for industrial purposes whereas on the other hand some new encapsulation technologies are evaluated including solid gel encapsulation, hydrogel formation, nanospheres, nanocapsules, liposomes, etc. gives better performance and have a great number of advantages for herbal extracts which is illustrated in Fig. 5.2 (Maurya et al. 2020). Hence, the herbal extracts or drugs from the plant source which are subjected to the nano formulation has a credible prospect for enhancing the desired action. The nature of the various active compounds and principles of the encapsulation techniques which are used for the encapsulation is the criteria which differentiate the encapsulation techniques from each other. The selection of the efficient encapsulation processes for in vivo or in vitro uses must be based on the formulation with proper characteristics (Armendariz-Barragan et al. 2016). Hydrophobicity of the active molecule is suitable characteristics for the selection of encapsulation (Mora-Huertas et al. 2010).

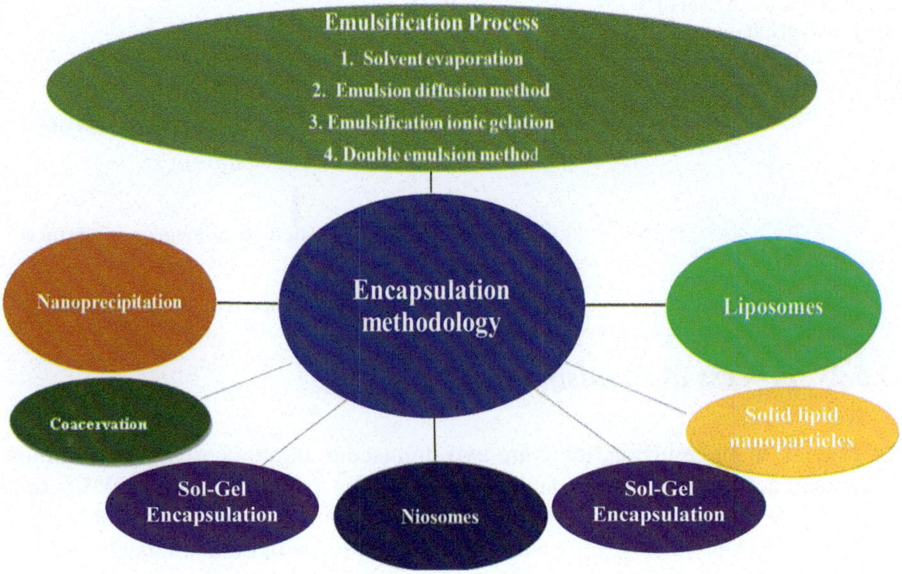

Fig. 5.2 Various encapsulation methodologies

5.5.1 Nanoprecipitation Technique

Fessi et al.(1989) developed the nanoprecipitation technique, also known as solvent displacement or interfacial deposition. It is an early developed encapsulation approach to encapsulate active ingredient. In the nanoprecipitation approach the two miscible phases are involved (Miladi et al. 2016). In the process of nanoprecipitation, the solvent phase can be formed by dissolving the film-forming substance, which may be a polymer, active ingredient, lipophilic surfactant. Besides, the non-solvent phase can be made from the film-forming substance non-solvent or a combination of non-solvents (Mora-Huertas et al. 2010). The particle formation in the process of the nanoprecipitation approach occurs throughout the three steps- nucleation, growth, and aggregation. The nanoprecipitation approach is roughly restricted to encapsulate the hydrophobic actives ingredients only (Fig. 5.3). Though, some modifications have been made in the nanoprecipitation method to encapsulate the hydrophilic active compounds. To encapsulate the hydrophilic active compounds the biodegradable polyesters, primarily polylactide-co-glicolide (PLGA), polylactide (PLA), and poly-e-caprolactone (PCL) are frequently used. Indeed, improved purity and reproducibility would occur by using synthetic polymers as compare to natural polymers (Mora-Huertas et al. 2010). The acetone is frequently used as a solvent polymer. Ethanol is also used to dissolve the active substance. Buffer solutions and polysorbate 80 are used as non-solvent and stabilizers. The mechanism on which the nanoprecipitation is based is the interfacial deposition of the polymer after the displacement of semi polar miscible solvent with water.

Fig. 5.3 Flow diagram of the nanoprecipitation approach

Organic phase
(Contains polymer with water soluble solvent)
↓
Drop wise addition by using syringe to the aqueous phase
(water with stabilizer)
↓
Put it on magnetic stirrer to form homogenous mixture
↓
Subjected it to the solvent evaporation to form Nanoparticle

5.5.2 Process of Emulsification

In general, in an emulsion, there are two immiscible liquid phases as a minimum, one phase act as a continuous, and the other acts as a dispersed phase (W/O emulsion or O/W emulsion). The emulsion can also be in a multiphase or double phase such as water/oil/water or oil/water/oil. Different types of emulsifiers can be used for the stabilization of the emulsion. In the emulsion, the encapsulation efficiency depends upon the size of the particles which depends on the nature and quantity of emulsifier and the technique of emulsification. The degradative and thermo oxidative protection of the bioactive compounds is carried out by embedding it into the continuous phase throughout the emulsification process. The physical appearance of the encapsulated active compounds depends on its allocation in the dispersed phase, the viscosity of the suspension, particle size, and process of the emulsification. The instruments like ultrasonicator, rotatory evaporator, and homogenizer are usually used to make nanoemulsion (Mosaddik et al. 2018).

5.5.3 Solvent Evaporation Process for Emulsification

The process of solvent evaporation is a very easy and most commonly used process. To form nanocapsules, an emulsion is formed by integrating the organic polymer solution in an aqueous phase. For the formation of the suspension, an organic polymer solution is mixed homogeneously with the bioactive oil in a non-solvent phase. During the process, the bioactive compounds are entrapped into the polymer are formed followed by the solvent evaporation. A researcher used a combination of solvent evaporation and double emulsion technique to form microcapsules (average diameter 1.38μm with 38% encapsulation efficiency) of grape seed extract in polylactide (Yourdkhani et al. 2017). The resulted microcapsules preserve the bioactivity of the extract. Encapsulation of the pink pepper extract in polylactic acid was made by the emulsification process followed by solvent evaporation. Pink pepper is a significant curative plant with properties like antitumor, antioxidant, and anti-inflammatory properties (Andrade et al. 2017).

5.5.4 Emulsion-Diffusion Method

This method of emulsion formation was developed by Quintanar-Guerrero and Fessi for the first time to form polylactide (PLA) nanoparticles (Quintanar-Guerrero et al. 1996). Though, this approach is mainly used to encapsulate the hydrophobic compounds but the lipophilic and hydrophilic bioactive compounds can also be encapsulated up to nano form. In this approach, the three liquid phases are prepared named as the organic phase, aqueous phase, and dilution phase (Miladi et al. 2014). The organic phase is partially miscible and has to saturate in water with polymer, active ingredient, oil, and an organic solvent, in which the lipophilic compounds are proposed to be nano encapsulated. The particle size can be affected by the working conditions rate of stirring during emulsification (RPM), diluting conditions (temperature and volume), polymer concentration, amount and ratio of the stabilizer. In this approach usually, the volume of the dilution phase is large, whereas the stabilizing agent with aqueous dispersion forms the aqueous phase. Polymers like Eudragit®, PCL, and PLA are frequently used in this approach (Mora-Huertas et al. 2010).

5.5.5 Emulsification-Ionic Gelation Method

The charged polymers like chitosan and alginate are used in the emulsification-ionic gelation method. These charged polymers are interacting with oppositely charged molecules to form particles and act as a cross-linking agent. Many lipophilic compounds were successfully encapsulated by using this technology like Turmeric oil is entrapped by emulsification in sodium alginate followed by gelification with chitosan and calcium chloride with subsequent solvent evaporation (Mosaddik et al. 2018).

5.5.6 Double Emulsion Method

Generally, the double emulsions are classified into two classes one is water-oil-water (w/o/w) and the other is oil-water-oil (o/w/o). The double emulsions are formed in two-steps and the droplets are dispersed in the emulsion. To obtain the primary emulsion (W1/O) the aqueous phase has to disperse into an organic solvent (non-miscible) for short-time and low-power sonication. After the formation of primary emulsion, it is dispersed in a second aqueous phase which contains

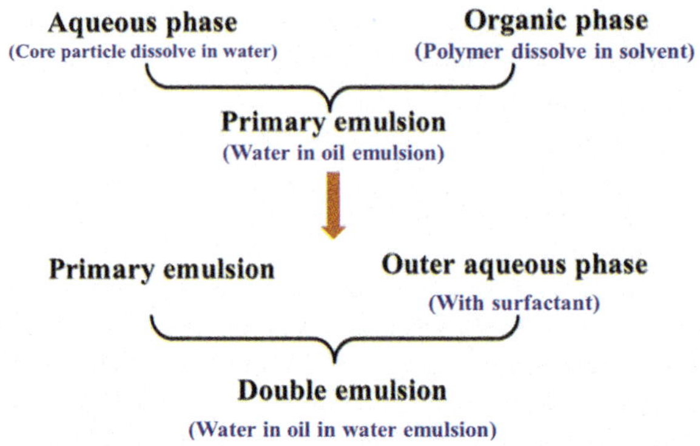

Fig. 5.4 Flow diagram of double emulsion formation

hydrophilic emulsifier and then subjected for homogenization or sonication. In the case of sonication, the second operation has to be carried out for a short time at low power to avoid the breaking of primary emulsion (Fig. 5.4). After the formation of multiple emulsions, the solvent evaporation (using rotatory evaporator) of the volatile organic phase occurs under low pressure and at ambient temperature which allows the amends in colloidal dispersion. The particle of double emulsion droplets contains one or more particles; sometimes droplets are large and contain many small particles inside it (Schuch et al. 2013). The process of the double emulsion is an appropriate technique to encapsulate hydrophilic bioactive compounds (Miladi et al. 2014). The stability and bioavailability of the particles can be significantly enhanced by altering the type and quantity of the stabilizer and wall material. The double emulsion technique coupled with the advantages including biodegradability, adaptability, and biocompatibility. The challenges including bulkiness, physical, and chemical degradation can be encountered by using multiple emulsion techniques. The complexity in the process, instability at the thermodynamic level, and heterogeneous size sensitivity of particles are some disadvantages of the double emulsion method. Both the hydrophilic and lipophilic types of bioactive compounds can be encapsulated by using a double emulsion approach (Mosaddik et al. 2018).

5.5.7 Liposomes

The liposome systems are defined as the systems made up of one or a few layers of phospholipid or other aqueous partitions. Phospholipids and cholesterol are the chiefly used constituents for liposomes formation. The spherical liposomes are categorized into unilamellar, oligolamellar, multilamellar, and multivesicular. Liposomes are broadly employed as carriers for hydrophobic and hydrophilic bioactive compounds (De Toni et al. 2012). The advantages of liposomes include the improvement of pharmacokinetics and biodistribution of the active compound and reduction of toxicity because they are nonimmunogenic, non-toxic, biocompatible, and biodegradable carriers of bioactive compounds (Drulis-Kawa and Dorotkiewicz-Jach 2010). The bioactive compounds of hydrophobic, hydrophilic, and amphiphilic nature can be encapsulated as liposomes (Yoshida et al. 2010). As it is well known that the herbal extracts are very prone to oxygen, temperature, and light degradation, which restrict their usage for remedial purposes. This approach of encapsulation is an attractive method to overcome the challenges that stumble upon the plant extracts such as low solubility in water which is associated with decreased bioavailability, stability problems due to volatility, oxygen, light, temperature, and toxicity (Detoni et al. 2012). As well, liposomes have enhanced tissue-specific targeting and also increase the biological activity of herbal extracts by modifying the physicochemical property of extracts.

5.5.8 Niosomes

These are the microscopic vesicle-like particles, the nonionic surfactants like span 60 or 80, and dialkyl polyglycerol ether and cholesterol are used to prepare niosomes, which are further hydrated in aqueous media. A small amount of anionic surfactant such as diacetyl phosphate is used with cholesterol to enhance stability (Makeshwar and Wasankar 2013). The components used to make niosome are nonionic surfactant, cholesterol, and charged molecules. Based on size the niosomes are divided into three classes (i) small unilamellar vesicles (0.025–0.05μm), (ii) multilamellar vesicles (>0.05μm), and (iii) large unilamellar vesicles (>0.10μm) (Moghassemi and Hadjizadeh 2014).

5.6 Future Forthcomings

The important impact of green chemistry is to change the industrialized and intellectual practices by the reduction in solvent and energy consumption. The enhancement of shelf life of any product aims to augment production and progression efficiency through the negligible changes in dietary and organic properties of foods. Hence, all the efforts are done for the development of environmentally sustainable production systems consecutively to extend safe and high-quality green products (Predrag et al. 2018). The antioxidant and free radical scavenging activity of the herbal extracts are very potent that can be made useful at the industrial level such as food and pharmaceutical industries (Sethiya et al. 2010). The main apprehension is the development of the most excellent delivery systems for the targeted deliverance of the drugs which are present in the herbal extract at the site of action, with an appropriate and prescribed amount of the drug that won't negotiate with the basic treatment (Yadav et al. 2011). Through the entire globe, remedial investigations based on natural products and the herbal extract is ongoing. The fundamental and medical investigations based on herbal formulation development are conceded out in several institutes (Namdari et al. 2017). In the upcoming duration, the concept of the nanoencapsulation attracts potential attention for infectious disease and cancer drug delivery to create considerable evaluations. Consequently, for the health benefits and the treatment of various chronic diseases the potential of herbal extracts is elevated by the nanoencapsulation. This category of integrative investigations in between the traditional herbal extract and contemporary drug delivery system called nanotechnology has instituted the desirability of the food and pharmaceutical industries that possibly will take benefits close to the upcoming time that will also have promotional effects on well-being's health.

5.7 Conclusion

In the area of nanoencapsulation technology, the investigations are still at the exploratory stage. A lot of hurdles in the examination, construction, and applications necessitate being solved. The utilization of nanoparticles devoid of any risk is still not possible because there is no unambiguous evidence to support the use of nanoparticles. Additionally, for the safe use of nano encapsulated products, it is necessary to stabilize mechanisms to overcome the toxic effects, removal of the accumulated product from the biological systems. There is a need to adapt the conventional methodologies which give more reliable results for the in vitro and in vivo evaluation of the encapsulated herbal active products. Besides all, it is very necessary to give more attention to investigate the suitable core substances for the development of an efficient formulation for the deliverance of the desired active compound. This could diminish the toxicity of drugs, improve their action, and also enhance the whole superiority of the agent so that the supplementary dose of the remedial component can be in attendance at the desired site of action including heart, brain, liver, stomach, kidney, and other organs. In spite having very excellent bioactivity the in vitro and in vivo actions, herbal bioactive compounds are not efficient due to the depressed molecular size and lipid solubility resulting pitiable bioavailability and absorption as lipid solubility and molecular size are the foremost restrictive reasons of the remedial molecules to cross the biological membrane. Phytoconstituents including tannins, polyphenols, flavonoids, and terpenoids are the standardized substituent of the herbal extracts which gives improved absorption and deliverance when they are administered by applying novel drug delivery system (nanoencapsulation) as it enables them to pass the biological membrane. Nanoparticles fulfill all the physical, chemical, and biological characteristics for the delivery of all the phytoactive components with different chemical properties. In the upcoming days, the areas including food, medicine, cosmetics, health, and pharmaceutics will possibly be an interesting field for research among others because of the employment of nanotechnology for the deliverance of the herbal extracts for safe utilization.

References

Armendariz-Barragan B, Zafar N, Badri W, Galindo-Rodriguez SA, Kabbaj D, Fessi H, Elaissari A (2016) Plant extracts: from encapsulation to application. Expert Opin Drug Deliv 13:1165–1175. https://doi.org/10.1080/17425247.2016.1182487

Assadpour E, Jafari SM (2019) An overview of lipid-based nanostructures for encapsulation of food ingredients. In lipid-based nanostructures for food encapsulation purposes. Academic, pp 1–34. https://doi.org/10.1016/B978-0-12-815673-5.00001-5

Briones-Labarca V, Plaza-Morales M, Giovagnoli-Vicuna C (2015) High hydrostatic pressure and ultrasound extractions of antioxidant compounds, sulforaphane and fatty acids from Chilean papaya (Vasconcelleapubescens) seeds: effects of extraction conditions and methods. LWT-Food Sci Technol 60:525–534. https://doi.org/10.1016/j.lwt.2014.07.057

Calvo TRA, Busch VM, Santagapita PR (2017) Stability and release of an encapsulated solvent-free lycopene extract in alginate-based beads. LWT-Food Sci Technol 77:406–412. https://doi.org/10.1016/j.lwt.2016.11.074

Chan ES, Yim ZH, Phan SH, Mansa RF, Ravindra P (2010) Encapsulation of herbal aqueous extract through absorption with ca-alginate hydrogel beads. Food Biopro Process 88:195–201. https://doi.org/10.1016/j.fbp.2009.09.005

Chen S, Xing XH, Huang JJ (2010) Enzyme-assisted extraction of flavonoids from Ginkgo biloba leaves: improvement effect of flavonoltransglycosylation catalyzed by *Penicillium decumbens*cellulase. Enzym Microb Technol 48:100–105. https://doi.org/10.1016/j.enzmictec.2010.09.017

De Toni M, Jonchiere R, Pullumbi P, Coudert FX, Fuchs AH (2012) How can a hydrophobic MOF be water-unstable? Insight into the hydration mechanism of IRMOFs. ChemPhysChem 13:3497–3503. https://doi.org/10.1002/cphc.201200455

Dey S, Rathod VK (2013) Ultrasound-assisted extraction of β-carotene from Spirulina platensis. UltrasonSonochem 20:271–276. https://doi.org/10.1016/j.ultsonch.2012.05.010

Dordevic V, Balanc B, Belscak-Cvitanovic A, Levic S, Trifkovic K, Kalusevic A, Nedovic V (2015) Trends in encapsulation technologies for delivery of food bioactive compounds. Food Eng Rev 7:452–490. https://doi.org/10.1007/s12393-014-9106-7

Dragostin I, Dragostin O, Pelin AM, Grigore C, Lacramioara Zamfir C (2017) The importance of polymers for encapsulation process and for enhanced cellular functions. J Macromol Sci A 54:489–493. https://doi.org/10.1080/10601325.2017.1320754

Drulis-Kawa Z, Dorotkiewicz-Jach A (2010) Liposomes as delivery systems for antibiotics. Int J Pharm 387:187–198. https://doi.org/10.1016/j.ijpharm.2009.11.033

Ferreira VF, Pinto AC (2010) A fitoterapia no mundoatual [Phytotherapy in the world today] quim Nova 33: 1829. doi:https://doi.org/10.1590/S0100-40422010000900001

Fessi HPFD, Puisieux F, Devissaguet JP, Ammoury N, Benita S (1989) Nanocapsule formation by interfacial polymer deposition following solvent displacement. Int J Pharm 55:R1–R4. https://doi.org/10.1016/0378-5173(89)90281-0

Ghayempour S, Montazer M, Rad MM (2015) Tragacanth gum as a natural polymeric wall for producing antimicrobial nanocapsules loaded with plant extract. Int J Biol Macromol 81:514–520. https://doi.org/10.1016/j.ijbiomac.2015.08.041

Ghayempour S, Montazer M, Rad MM (2016) Encapsulation of aloe Vera extract into natural Tragacanth gum as a novel green wound healing product. Int J Biol Macromol 93:344–349. https://doi.org/10.1016/j.ijbiomac.2016.08.076

Kumari A, Yadav SK, Yadav SC (2010) Biodegradable polymeric nanoparticles based drug delivery systems. Colloids Surf B Biointerfaces 75:1–18. https://doi.org/10.1016/j.colsurfb.2009.09.001

Maurya VK, Aggarwal M (2017) Enhancing bio-availability of vitamin D by Nano-engineered based delivery systems-an overview. Int J Curr Microbiol App Sci 6:340–353. https://doi.org/10.20546/ijcmas

Maurya VK, Aggarwal M (2019) Fabrication of nano-structured lipid carrier for encapsulation of vitamin D_3 for fortification of 'Lassi'; a milk based beverage. J Steroid Biochem Mol Biol 193:105429. https://doi.org/10.1016/j.jsbmb.2019.105429

Maurya VK, Aggarwal M, Ranjan V, Gothandam KM (2020) Improving bioavailability of vitamin a in food by encapsulation: an update. In: Nanoscience in Medicine, vol 1. Springer, Cham, pp 117–145. https://doi.org/10.1007/978-3-030-29207-2_4

Miladi H, Slama RB, Mili D, Zouari S, Bakhrouf A, Ammar E (2013) Essential oil of *Thymus vulgaris* L. and *Rosmarinus officinalis* L.: gas chromatography-mass spectrometry analysis, cytotoxicity and antioxidant properties and antibacterial activities against foodborne pathogens. J Nat Sci 5:729–739. https://doi.org/10.4236/ns.2013.56090

Miladi I, Alric C, Dufort S, Mowat P, Dutour A, Mandon C, Dutreix M (2014) The in vivo radiosensitizing effect of gold nanoparticles based MRI contrast agents. Small 10:1116–1124. https://doi.org/10.1002/smll.201302303

Miladi K, Sfar S, Fessi H, Elaissari A (2016) Nanoprecipitation process: from particle preparation to in vivo applications. In: Polymer nanoparticles for nanomedicines. Springer, Cham, pp 17–53. https://doi.org/10.1007/978-3-319-41421-8_2

Moghassemi S, Hadjizadeh A (2014) Nano-niosomes as nanoscale drug delivery systems: an illustrated review. J Control Release 185:22–36. https://doi.org/10.1016/j.jconrel.2014.04.015

Mora-Huertas CE, Fessi H, Elaissari A (2010) Polymer-based nanocapsules for drug delivery. Int J Pharm 385:113–142. https://doi.org/10.1016/j.ijpharm.2009.10.018

Mosaddik A, Ravinayagam V, Elaanthikkal S, Fessi H, Badri W, Elaissari A (2018) Development and use of polymeric nanoparticles for the encapsulation and administration of plant extracts. In: Natural products as source of molecules with therapeutic potential. Springer, Cham, pp 391–463. https://doi.org/10.1007/978-3-030-00545-0_11

Nalawade PB, Gajjar AK (2016) Microencapsulation of lutein extracted from marigold flowers (Tagetes erecta L.) using full factorial design. J Drug Deliv Sci Tech 33:75–87. https://doi.org/10.1016/j.jddst.2016.03.012

Namdari M, Eatemadi A, Soleimaninejad M, Hammed AT (2017) A brief review on the application of nanoparticle enclosed herbal medicine for the treatment of infective endocarditis. Biomed Pharmacother 87:321–331. https://doi.org/10.1016/j.biopha.2016.12.099

Nedovic V, Kalusevic A, Manojlovic V, Levic S, Bugarski B (2011) An overview of encapsulation technologies for food applications. Procedia Food Sci 1:1806–1815. https://doi.org/10.1016/j.profoo.2011.09.265

Oszmianski J, Wojdylo A, Kolniak J (2011) Effect of pectinase treatment on extraction of antioxidant phenols from pomace, for the production of puree-enriched cloudy apple juices. Food Chem 127:100–105. https://doi.org/10.1016/j.foodchem.2011.01.056

Ota A, Istenic K, Skrt M, Segatin N, Znidarsic N, Kogej K, Ulrih NP (2018) Encapsulation of pantothenic acid into liposomes and into alginate or alginate–pectin microparticles loaded with liposomes. JFood Eng 229:21–31. https://doi.org/10.1016/j.lwt.2016.11.074

Pasquet V, Cherouvrier JR, Farhat F (2011) Study on the microalgal pigments extraction process: performance of microwave assisted extraction. Process Biochem 46:59–67. https://doi.org/10.1016/j.procbio.2010.07.009

Pulicharla R, Marques C, Das RK, Rouissi T, Brar SK (2016) Encapsulation and release studies of strawberry polyphenols in biodegradable chitosan nanoformulation. Int J Biol Macromol 88:171–178. https://doi.org/10.1016/j.ijbiomac.2016.03.036

Quintanar-Guerrero D, Fessi H, Allémann E, Doelker E (1996) Influence of stabilizing agents and preparative variables on the formation of poly (D, L-lactic acid) nanoparticles by an emulsification-diffusion technique. Int J Pharm 143:133–141. https://doi.org/10.1016/S0378-5173(96)04697-2

Santos DT, Veggi PC, Meireles MA (2012) Optimization and economic evaluation of pressurized liquid extraction of phenolic compounds from jabuticaba skins. J Food Eng 108:444–452. https://doi.org/10.1016/j.jfoodeng.2011.08.022

Schuch NJ, Garcia VC, Vívolo SRGF, Martini LA (2013) Relationship between vitamin D receptor gene polymorphisms and the components of metabolic syndrome. Nutr J 12:96. https://doi.org/10.1186/1475-2891-12-96

Sethiya NK, Trivedi A, Patel MB, Mishra SH (2010) Comparative pharmacognostical investigation on four ethanobotanicals traditionally used as Shankhpushpi in India. J Adv Pharm 1:388–395. https://doi.org/10.4103/0110-5558.76437

Stojanovic R, Belscak-Cvitanovic A, Manojlovic V, Komes D, Nedovic V, Bugarski B (2012) Encapsulation of thyme (Thymus serpyllum L.) aqueous extract in calcium alginate beads. J Sci Food Agric 92:685–696. https://doi.org/10.1002/jsfa.4632

Svarc-Gajic J, Stojanovic Z, Carretero AS (2013) Development of a microwave-assisted extraction for the analysis of phenolic compounds from *Rosmarinus officinalis*. J Food Eng 119:525–532. https://doi.org/10.1016/j.jfoodeng.2013.06.030

Tan SP, Kha TC, Parks SE (2015) Effects of the spray-drying temperatures on the physiochemical properties of an encapsulated bitter melon aqueous extract powder. Powder Tech 281:65–75. https://doi.org/10.1016/j.powtec.2015.04.074

Ting Y, Jiang Y, Ho CT, Huang Q (2014) Common delivery systems for enhancing in vivo bioavailability and biological efficacy of nutraceuticals. J Funct Foods 7:112–128. https://doi.org/10.1016/j.jff.2013.12.010

Upadhyay R, Ramalakshmi K, Rao JML (2012) Microwave-assisted extraction of chlorogenic acids from green coffee beans. Food Chem 130:184–188. https://doi.org/10.1016/j.foodchem.2011.06.057

Wang T, Jonsdottir R, Kristinsson HG (2010) Enzyme-enhanced extraction of antioxidant ingredients from red algae *Palmariapalmata*. LWT-Food Sci Technol 43:1387–1393. https://doi.org/10.1016/j.lwt.2010.05.010

Xia EQ, Ai XX, Zang SY, Guan TT, Xu XR, Li HB (2011) Ultrasound-assisted extraction of phillyrin from Forsythia suspensa. Ultrasonics Sonochem 18(2):549–552

Yoshida T, Fujita Y, Sayama H, Kidokoro S, Maruyama K, Mizoi J, Yamaguchi-Shinozaki K (2010) AREB1, AREB2, and ABF3 are master transcription factors that cooperatively regulate ABRE-dependent ABA signaling involved in drought stress tolerance and require ABA for full activation. Plant J 61:672–685. https://doi.org/10.1111/j.1365-313X.2009.04092.x

Yourdkhani M, Leme-Kraus AA, Aydin B, Bedran-Russo AK, White SR (2017) Encapsulation of grape seed extract in polylactide microcapsules for sustained bioactivity and time-dependent release in dental material applications. Dent Mater 33:630–636. https://doi.org/10.1016/j.dental.2017.03.009

Zafar N, Fessi H, Elaissari A (2014) Cyclodextrin containing biodegradable particles: from preparation to drug delivery applications. Int J Pharm 461:351–366. https://doi.org/10.1016/j.ijpharm.2013.12.004

Zhang G, He L, Hu M (2011) Optimized ultrasonic-assisted extraction of flavonoids from *Prunella vulgaris* L. and evaluation ofantioxidant activities in vitro. Innovative Food Sci Emerg Technol 12:18–25. https://doi.org/10.1016/j.ifset.2010.12.003

Chapter 6
Improving Bioavailability of Nutrients Through Nanotechnology

Shalja Verma and Anand Kumar Pandey

Abstract Improving the nutritional value of food can enhance the quality of living and life expectancy. The increasing percentage of diseased and unhealthy population demands the improvement of food quality by adding nutrients having pharmaceutical property to prevent commonly developed diet-associated diseases. Nutraceutical treasure containing vitamins, antioxidants, stanols, sterols, poly unsaturated fatty acids, carotenoids, minerals, fibres, and biologically substantial peptides possess exceptional ability to treat highly prevalent diseases like osteoporosis, cancer, cardiovascular diseases, obesity, diabetes, and arthritis. Although the value of these nutraceuticals is immense, but their low bioavailability, chemical instability, and undesired flavour pose a great challenge. The science of nanotechnology has recently been amalgamated with food science. Miniaturizing nutraceuticals to nanoscale for *in-vivo* delivery has shown highly promising outcomes and seems to be an advantageous approach in this concern.

Here, we review significant aspects related to the bioavailability of such nutrients and varied developments associated with the application of nanotechnology in food science, which can considerably contribute to its improvement. Different fabrication technologies and food-grade formulation have been discussed in detail. Lipid-based formulations, naturally occurring nanoparticles, and biopolymers display high effectivity with least toxicity when formulated in nano-delivery systems for bioactive nutraceuticals and have been illustrated here in detail. Further safety and toxicity related issues associated with such systems have been briefly described.

Keywords Bioavailability · Functional foods · Nanotechnology · Nutraceuticals · Nutrients

---

S. Verma
Department of Biochemical Engineering and Biotechnology, Indian Institute of Technology, New Delhi, India

A. K. Pandey (✉)
Department of Biotechnology Engineering, Institute of Engineering and Technology, Bundelkhand University, Jhansi, India

V. K. Maurya et al. (eds.), *Sustainable Agriculture Reviews 55*, Sustainable Agriculture Reviews 55, https://doi.org/10.1007/978-3-030-76813-3_6

6.1 Introduction

"Let food be thy medicine and medicine be thy food", although this quote came into existence 2.5 thousand years ago, but its exact meaning has been realized recently with the growing incidence of diseased cases due to improper dietary habits. Food not only fulfils the appetite and the requirements of the body but can also act as a medicine to combat a large number of diseases (Goswami and Ram 2017).

Nutraceuticals are nutrients present in food which, when consumed in an adequate amount, can perform treasured therapeutic activities. A variety of such nutrients are known and are being formulated to develop functional foods. Vitamin A, procured from carotenoids and retinoids present in food like milk, butter, egg, and liver, shows highly beneficial effects against cancers, protects eyes, recovers the immune system, promotes bone development, growth and reproduction. Vitamin D enhances the intestinal calcium absorption from food and calcium recycling ability of kidney thus play a vital role in the recovery of osteoporosis and rickets or osteomalacia. Minerals like Ca, Fe and K show therapeutic effect against osteoporosis, anaemia and high blood pressure (which leads to stroke) respectively. Polyunsaturated fatty acids like Omega 3 reduces bad cholesterol and thus lowers heart diseases. Antioxidants like flavonoids, polyphenols, tocopherols present in fruits, vegetables and cereals, contribute to reducing oxidative damage in cancers and heart diseases by maintaining the levels of reactive oxygen species. Fiber supports bowel health, cholesterol, body weight, and blood sugar and hence promotes longevity. Proteins like casein present in milk and its products have excellent biological significance as they improve muscle growth. Many other ingredients of our daily diet contribute to varying medicinal effects (Das et al. 2011; Chauhan et al. 2013; Chanda et al. 2019).

Recently, the growing awareness about the advantages of such nutraceuticals has increased their amalgamation in the diet to a greater extent. A variety of functional foods are being developed, which consists of an adequate amount of specific nutraceutical which can cure and prevent, particular disease thereby uplifting the living standard. Although the effects of these nutraceuticals are quite prominent but a big challenge in their way of effectiveness is their low bioavailability (Cencic and Chingwaru 2010).

Bioavailability refers to the concentration and rate of absorption of a compound which is attained to bring that compound into the systemic circulation. Majority of these nutraceuticals are not fully absorbed by the gastrointestinal (GI) tract and are often excreted out of the body and thus their effective concentration in blood is rarely achieved leading to less availability than required, in the close vicinity of the target organ, hence low pronounced medicinal effects are distinguished (McClements et al. 2015a).

To counteract this problem nanotechnology has played ultimate roles. Transforming these nutraceuticals into nanoparticles or loading them onto targeted nanosystems has shown incredible outcomes to deal with this challenge. Also, the changes in the properties at nanoscale enhance the stability and hence the shelf life of these compounds. Fabrication of many such nanosystems, capable to be used as food supplements, has been done to enhance the bioavailability of nutraceuticals. The increasing number of publications from 2000 to 2019 on the application of nano-delivery systems for nutraceutical bioavailability improvement provide strong evidence for the effectiveness of the nano-approaches in this concern (Fig. 6.1). Lipid nanoparticles have successfully made a stand as food-grade nanotechnologies, as their structure resembles the cellular membrane and can easily be taken up by the targeted cells. Different biopolymers have also been discovered to be modulated into nanoparticles for the preparation of edible nano-nutraceutical formulations (Punia et al. 2019; Jampilek et al. 2019).

Though the approach of the application of nanoparticles for the development of a delivery system is quite efficient but safety and toxicity issues related to their in-vivo application may pose a significant challenge and require distinct consideration. Accumulation of nanoparticles in-vivo or delayed breakdown and excretion results in potent toxic effects; thus food-grade biodegradable materials can be of great benefit in this regard (McClements and Xiao 2017).

Henceforth, the present chapter exemplifies, major aspects related to the limited bioavailability of nutraceutical in-vivo, nanotechnological systems capable to deal with this shortcoming, wide range of fabrication materials, and techniques employed for the development of such nano-delivery systems and their safety and toxicity related facts. Moreover, a variety of researches associated with the utilization of nanotechnology for the development of high bioavailability dietary supplements

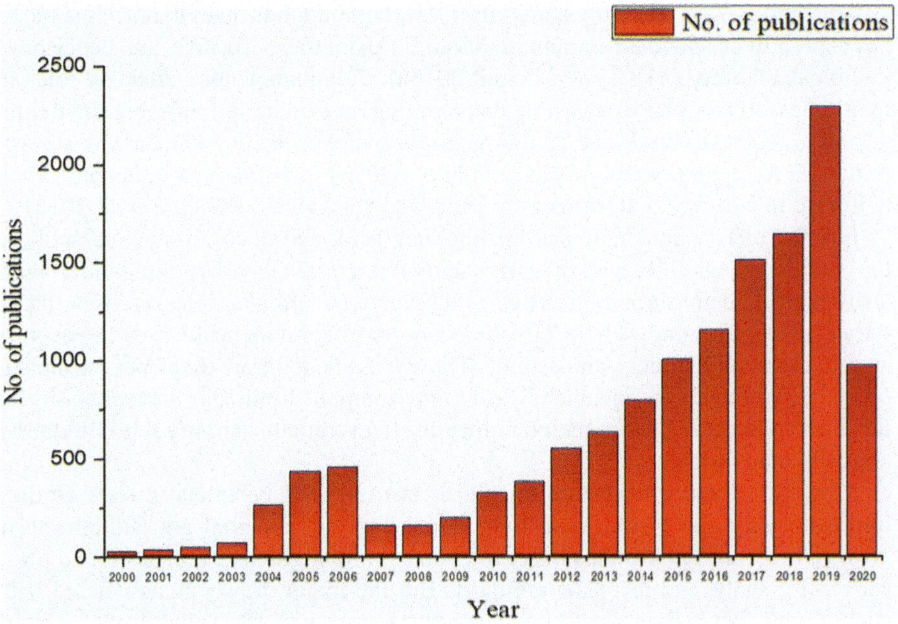

Fig. 6.1 Number of publications per year on application of nano-delivery systems for nutraceutical bioavailability improvement

and functional foods along with their emerging scope for large scale applications have been discussed in detail.

6.1.1 Definition

Food supply essential nutrients that deliver energy, act as units to encourage growth and repair, and control biochemical reactions necessary to support life. Under certain circumstances, due to imbalance in one or the other biochemical pathway, deficiency, or excess of some specific compound/s, infection from a foreign body or genetic mutations, the body suffers from disease (Cencic and Chingwaru 2010). Some nutrients present in food, along with supporting the normal function of the body, impart therapeutic effects and possess the ability to treat or prevent several diseases, thus are known as nutraceuticals (nutrients plus pharmaceutical). Functional foods are food forms which show exceptional health benefits beyond their conventional nutritive value due to the presence of these nutraceuticals (Adefegha 2018).

Bioavailability of a compound depends on its solubility and permeability across the epithelium, signifies the rate and extent of that compound at which it is available in systemic circulation so that it can be taken up and utilized by different parts of the body.

The nutraceuticals present in functional foods, as they have low solubility in the GI fluid and low permeability across the GI lining, find it difficult to reach the blood circulation in an adequate amount, required for them to be effective, and hence have low bioavailability (McClements et al. 2015a). Polyphenols play effective roles in treating cardiovascular diseases by encouraging vasodilation, inhibiting the oxidation of low-density lipids and agglutination of platelets but due to their low absorption in GI tract, these antioxidants could not prove their efficacy significantly when delivered in conventional forms as in fruits and vegetables (Khurana et al. 2013).

Further, eicosapentaenoic acid, α-linolenic acid, and docosahexaenoic acid are the major omega-3 forms of fatty acids which display hypolipidemic, anti-arrhythmic, and antithrombotic effects thus can treat cardiovascular diseases. These fatty acids are also known to be effective in promoting infant health, treating depressive and bipolar disorders, and asthma. Though the benefits are many but the insolubility of fatty acids in aqueous GI tract environment limits the bioavailability of these compounds and hence their therapeutic effects remain unnoticeable (Bradberry and Hilleman 2013).

Moreover, dietary fibers are known to have several beneficial effects as they improve binding at insulin receptors, faecal bulking, essential gut Bifidobacteria growth, levels of lipoproteins in serum, control blood glucose, reduces blood pressure and obesity, and increase immunity. But the major drawback associated with such fibrous diet is the reduction in absorption and hence bioavailability of various essential minerals, vitamins, and proteins which can not only lead to deficiency diseases but will also reduce protection against a variety of diseases including cancer, cataracts and cardiovascular disease (Kaczmarczyk et al. 2012). All these facts are evidential for the limited bioavailability of essential nutraceuticals and put forward an urgent need to develop approaches to work for the purpose.

Though many approaches have been considered to improve the bioavailability of these nutraceuticals like utilization of food additives, microorganism, enzymes and application of different cooking methods but nanotechnology based approaches, that deals with manipulation and modeling of matter at a scale of $1.0e^{-9}$ of a meter, have shown outstanding outcomes in numerous researches. The reduction of these therapeutic compounds to nanoscale affects their solubility and permeability profiles and enhance their concentration in circulation as well as at the binding target site to promote treatments. Thus, nanotechnology-based techniques improve the nutritional bioavailability and promote the development of highly effective natural therapies (Yu et al. 2018; Jampilek et al. 2019).

Before heading towards the wide variety of nanotechnology-based approaches it becomes necessary to have an apparent view of different aspects and conditions which act as limiting factors in concerns to nutraceutical bioavailability. Hence the following section further illustrates the effects of different factors on the bioavailability of nutraceuticals in detail and provides in-depth knowledge in this context.

6.1.2 Bioavailability of Nutraceuticals

Bioavailability of nutrients signifies their availability for biological systems to promote health. The food matrix with which the nutrients are consumed, the solubility of nutrients in GI fluid, interaction profile of nutrients with other components of food as well as of GI tract, degradation of nutrients in the GI environment having varying pH, metabolism and their permeability across epithelium are the determinant factors for bioavailability of nutrient (Maurya and Aggarwal 2017a, b, c). Nutraceuticals, nutrients which are naturally present in food having additional therapeutic effects, are usually disadvantaged due to their low bioavailability (Kumar and Smita 2017). This reduced bioavailability is due to various physiological and physicochemical characteristics, conveyed by the above-mentioned determinant factors, which maintains the amount of nutraceutical below the adequate level keeping the fullness of its potentials unnoticed. These characteristics are broadly classified as, bio-accessibility, absorption, and transformation in the GI tract (Nile et al. 2020).

Nutraceutical bio-accessibility depends on the physical form in which the nutraceutical is present before its absorption in the GI tract. This determines whether the nutraceutical will be absorbed by the body and the extent to which it will be absorbed. The quantity of nutraceutical liberated by the matrix of food, which gets solubilized in GI fluid and interacts with GI fluid components, making itself available for absorption denotes its bio-accessibility (Zou et al. 2015). The proportion of nutraceutical capable of getting dissolved in GI fluid instead of being present in a complex, crystalline or insoluble form, significantly governs the bio-accessibility of hydrophilic nutraceuticals whereas the portion of nutraceutical capable of getting solubilized in fat micelles present in GI fluid indicates the bio-accessibility of hydrophobic nutraceuticals (McClements et al. 2015a; Nile et al. 2020).

Nutraceutical absorption signifies the proportion that crosses the lining of mucus, goes through the epithelium cells and enters the systemic circulation. The intake can be restricted by deficient transport through mucus layer, endothelium bilayer, tight junction, active transporters, and/or efflux transporters (McClements et al. 2015b). The protective mucus layer over the endothelium limits the transport of abundant compounds which exceed the pore size of the sheet which is around 400 nm (Laura et al. 2012) Also, attractive hydrophobic and electrostatic interactions of nutraceutical with mucus layer components hinder its transport across the layer. Transportation across the hydrophobic phospholipid epithelium bilayer is significantly affected by the polarity of the nutraceutical. The nonpolar high partition coefficient molecules can travel through the bilayer more quickly and efficiently compared to the polar low partition coefficient molecules. Hydrophobicity or the logP value of molecule can provide the measure of transportability of a molecule across the hydrophobic bilayer and thus its absorption. Some nutrients with low hydrophobicity find it difficult to go across the phospholipid bilayer but can be transported via tight junctions which are present at the joints between the two epithelial cells. These are subtle channels which promote transport of small molecules nearly less than 0.7 nm (Crater and Carrier 2010). Active transporters are energy-consuming transporters which transfers some nutrients across the epithelial cells, which cannot pass the bilayer passively and affect absorption. Components like free form fatty acids, phytochemicals, and vitamins are usually transported by these active transporters. Another type of carriers are efflux transporters, they significantly affect the absorption of nutraceuticals but in a negative manner as they are responsible for transferring back the absorbed compound into the GI lumen. They limit the uptake into the blood circulation and hence reduces bioavailability (McClements et al. 2015b; Williamson et al. 2018).

Nutraceutical transformation is the conversion into an inactive form in the GI tract. Such transformations can be degradation by chemicals or metabolism. Chemical reactions can transform the nutraceuticals by hydrolysis, reduction or oxidation thus converts them into lowly absorbed forms. Metabolism inside the GI tract leads to the addition of hydrophobic groups to the nutraceuticals thus enhance their polarity which promotes their kidney resorption and urinary excretion. Metabolism of phase I induce oxidation, hydrolysis, or reduction but phase II involves action by enzymes like esterase, dehydrogenase, reductase, and CYP450 (Cytochrome P450 enzyme). Often the resulting molecules of phase I are subjected to phase II enzymes causing progressive changes in biological, molecular and physicochemical properties thus reducing the absorption and hence the bioavailability (McClements et al. 2015b; Williamson et al. 2018).

Therefore, bioavailability seems to be a major concern and its enhancement is highly desirous to exploit the sole potential of nutrients mainly nutraceuticals like quercetin, resveratrol, epicatechin, and other such bioactives, which have wide therapeutic effects on the body.

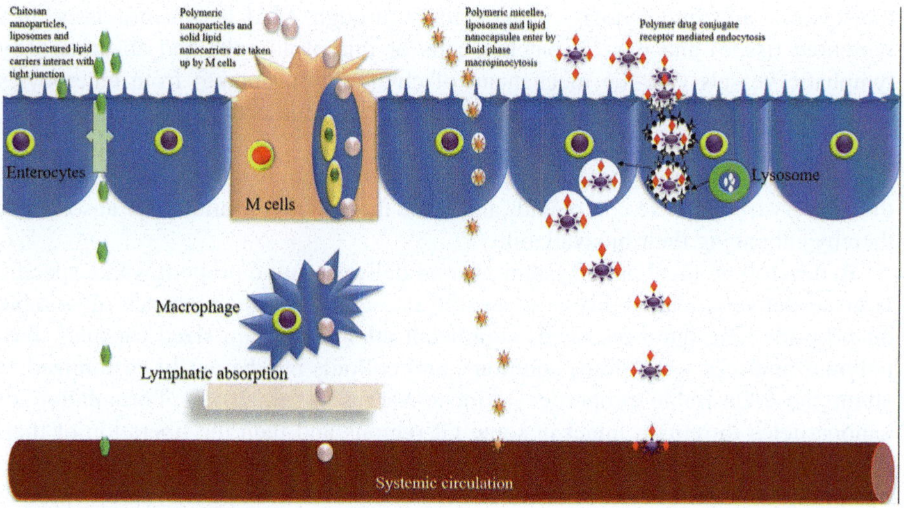

Fig. 6.2 Role of nanodelivery systems in enhancing the absorption across the cell of the gastrointestinal tract to increase the bioavailability

Numerous nanotechnology based approaches have immensely contributed to this purpose by modifying the relevant characteristics of nutraceuticals (Fig. 6.2). The characteristics that suffer significant changes when subjected to nanosize to convey increment in bioavailability are discussed in detail in the upcoming section.

6.2 Why Nanoparticles to Enhance Bioavailability?

Bringing down food materials in the size range of nanometre-scale increases the surface area to volume ratio and offer exceptional physiochemical properties. These properties are unique to nano conformations and rarely exist at the macroscale. Colour, diffusivity, strength, stability solubility, toxicity, thermodynamic, optical and magnetic properties are the major property types which get affected when materials are converted from macro to nanoscale and thus enhance the food sensory qualities like texture, taste, and colour along with its bioavailability (Srinivas et al. 2010). Researches have made it evident that the size of particles has a significant effect on their fate of getting absorbed by the cells. The efficient delivery of nutraceuticals or bioactive compounds to specific body sites is based on the size of their formulation as some cells allow efficient absorption of only submicron-sized particles, especially nano-sized instead of macro-scale particles. Also, most of the intake, entrapment, and digestion by the body cells occurs at the nanoscale, thus it is viable to opt nanosized delivery systems for delivering compounds of biological significance (Wang et al. 2014). Due to the very reasons, nano delivery systems enhance, favorable interaction with a mucus layer and tight junctions, receptor-based transcytosis and endocytosis, phagocytosis through MALT (mucosa-associated lymphoid tissue) and payer's patches cells or microfold cells and absorption by lymphatic vessels (via the mechanism of chylomicron uptake) from enterocytes concludingly improving the overall absorption of nutraceuticals (Srinivas et al. 2010; Wang et al. 2014; Maurya and Aggarwal 2017a, b, c; Martínez-Ballesta et al. 2018). Hence, processing of food by encapsulating them in nanoparticles improves the delivery of bioactive compounds and make them highly available for absorption, thereby enhancing their bioavailability.

To develop an ideal nano-system of food delivery, some properties like specific targeted delivery, availability at a specific rate and time, maintenance of suitable quantity for long-duration, needs significant attention. Nano sized capsules, biopolymer matrices, emulsions, solutions, and colloids can be easily customized to attain these desirable properties (Alpizar-Vargas et al. 2019). Formulation of nanoparticles to remain intact in some GI regions and then the liberation of their compositional nutraceutical at some other specific location is highly possible to maximize the biological effectiveness. Controlled release of ingredients and protection from harsh environment or undesirable interactions in the GI tract are further outstanding advantages communicated by nano-encapsulation (Rao and Naidu 2016). Many natural or synthetic polymer-based nano-encapsulating systems have been designed for efficient delivery which ultimately enhances bioavailability to a greater extent. Further, some nano-systems also contribute to the improvement of nutritional value and shelf-life. Different ways by which nano-encapsulation enhances the bioavailability of nutraceuticals are described in Fig. 6.3 and the technologies which are utilized for the development of such beneficial nanoencapsulation systems are illustrated in the following section.

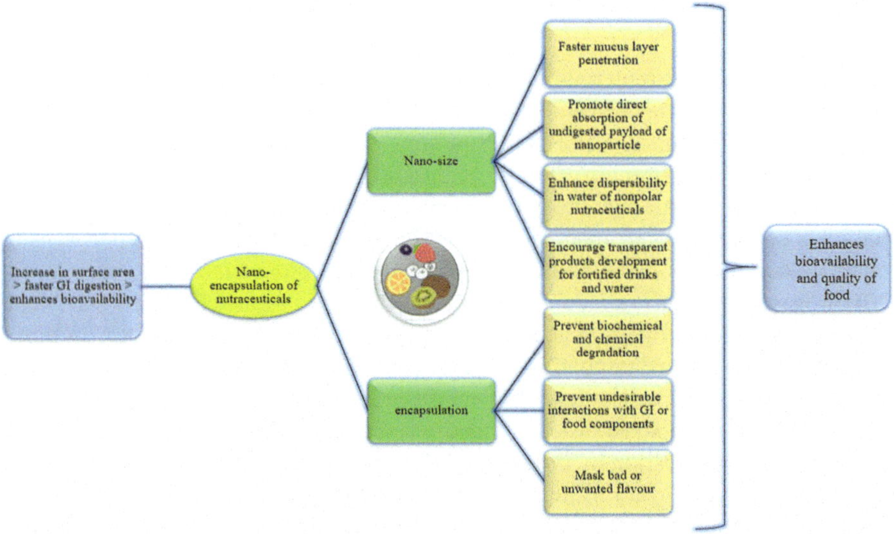

Fig. 6.3 Effect of nano-encapsulation of nutraceuticals on their bioavailability

6.3 Fabrication Technologies for Food-Grade Nanoparticles

A variety of encapsulation nanosystems have been developed for nutraceuticals which include nano-emulsions, microemulsions, biopolymer-based nanoparticles, lipid-based solid nanoparticles, lipid-based nano-structured carriers, and nanoliposomes (Maurya et al. 2020). Food grade materials like lipids, polysaccharides, proteins, surfactants, minerals, can be employed to formulate nanoparticles by a variety of methods (Pan and Zhong 2016). Though the majority of these methods of fabrication have been validated at the laboratory level and are not compatible with industrial production, but some of them seem to be highly promising for large scale too. Large scale production of nanoemulsions by employing process technologies can be done with great ease via high-pressure homogenizers, but an associated drawback of degradation after diffusion of a bioactive compound into the hydrophilic phase due to low relative oil phase viscosity limits its frequent application (Hamad et al. 2018).

Conventionally, nanoparticles fabrication approaches are classified into two groups: the bottom-up approach and the top-down approach. Bottom up fabrication approach compliment to an assemblage of smaller particles to larger particles of the desired size range by anti-solvent precipitation or micellization whereas top-down approach signifies breaking of larger particles of bulk phase into small particles by milling and homogenization (Pattekari et al. 2011). In the current scenario, the conventional classification has faded, and a new rating based on fabrication material, equipment, and techniques have come into the picture. This current classification consists of five classes, namely, natural nano-carriers, lipid-based formulations, biopolymer nanoparticles, nanoparticles using specialized equipment for production, and nanoparticles produced by different techniques (Fig. 6.4) (Assadpour and Jafari 2019).

Selection of technology of nano-encapsulation is mainly affected by the type of nutraceutical, desired particle size, physiochemical coating and core properties, safety, compatibility of the matrix of food associated, mechanism of release, cost of processing, method of delivery, performance, cost of the process, heftiness, viability at commercial scale and the requirement for labelling (Canizales et al. 2018). Thus, a specific class of fabrication approach which lies in the desirable range of parameters as mentioned above should be wisely selected for particular applications. In the upcoming sections, we will be dealing with some of the most acceptable food grade nanoformulation fabrication technologies in more detail.

6.3.1 Lipid-Based Nanoparticles Formulation Technologies

Lipid formulations due to their ease of production by technologies like microfluidization and homogenization which are already available in food industries seem to be highly promising in this context. In addition, the amalgamation of hydrophobic

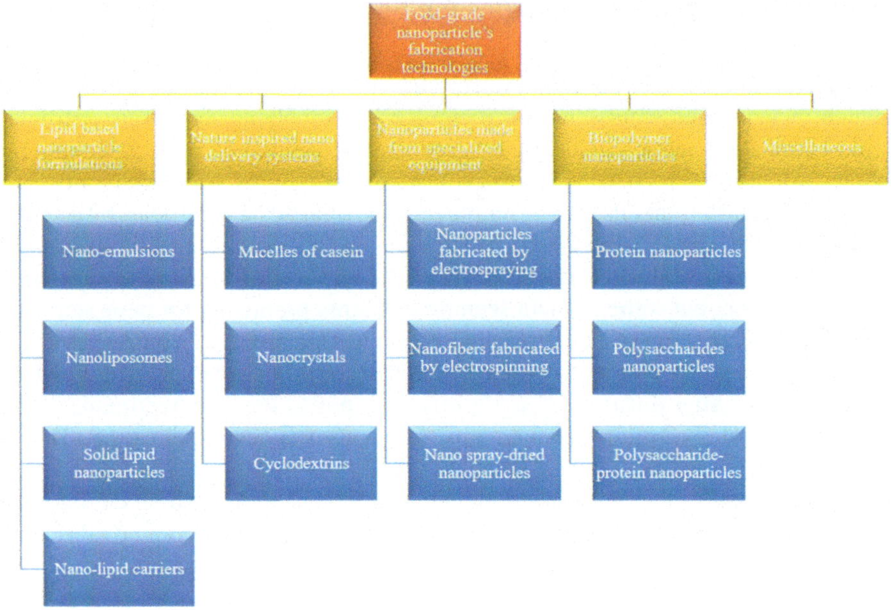

Fig. 6.4 Classification of food-grade nanoparticles based on fabrication technologies

food bioactive compounds like carotenoids, flavonoids, triglycerides, polyphenols, tocopherols, fat-soluble vitamins, colours, flavours and preservatives with beverages and aqueous foods require lipid-based encapsulation (Helal et al. 2019). Also, these lipids enhance the available quantity of micelles for solubilization and transport in the small intestine and thus promotes the bioactive compound absorption (Puri et al. 2009). Hence, due to the above-mentioned reasons fabrication of lipid-based nanoparticles, their characterization and their applications stand in high demand for exhaustive research. To date, various lipid-based nanoparticles types have been formulated by numerous researchers including nanoliposomes, nano-emulsions, solid-lipid nanoparticles and nano-lipid carriers (Fig. 6.5). Following are the illustrations of these types of nanoparticles:

6.3.1.1 Nano-emulsions

Nutraceutical compounds, due to their low solubility and absorption in GI tract suffers from low bioavailability. Lipid based nanoemulsions by altering the absorption, bioaccessibility, and stability of these compounds promote the increment in bioavailability (Salvia-Trujillo et al. 2016). These nanoemulsions are colloidal dispersions or heterogeneous mixture of two liquids which are immiscible, with one liquid dispersed into the other as small droplets. The two liquids are mainly oil and water,

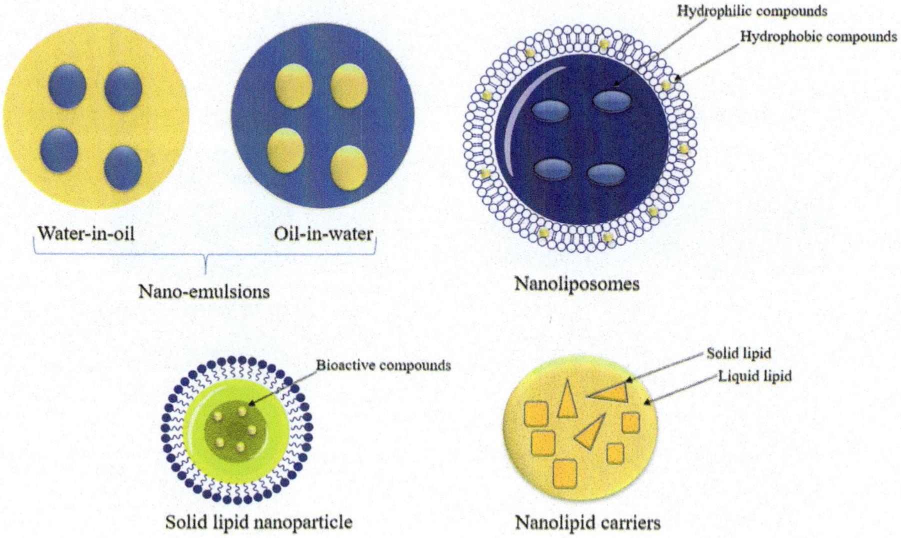

Fig. 6.5 Different types of lipid based nanoparticles frequently used for the oral delivery of nutrients

contributing to two major forms of emulsions, namely water in oil and oil in water emulsions (Fig. 6.6) (Donsì 2018; Maurya and Aggarwal 2019).

Nanoemulsion of oil in water contains oil droplets of less than 200 nm dispersed in aqueous medium or water where each droplet of oil is stabilized by aqueous or hydrophilic emulsifier coat. This type of nanoemulsions are usually employed for bioactive agents which are lipophilic. In the contrary, water in oil nanoemulsion is the dispersion of water droplets in oil where every water droplet is covered by an emulsifier which is hydrophobic, and this type is used for hydrophilic agents like polyphenols. The size of droplet and stability of emulsion depends on the water to oil ratio, type of oil, and its composition and co-solute or co-solvent used (Liu et al. 2019).

The formation of nanoemulsion can be done by either employing low energy consuming methods like spontaneous emulsification or phase inversion temperature or by high energy-consuming methods like sonication, homogenization at high pressure or microfluidization (Qian and McClements 2011; Kumar et al. 2019). Depending on the usage of nanoemulsions they can be developed into two forms, the liquid form or the powder form by employing freeze-drying or spray drying techniques. The major benefits conveyed by delivery systems based on nanoemulsions are high dispersibility in water, high transparency, good stability, high size control of droplet, high ease of manufacturing, and most importantly high bioavailability (Kumar et al. 2019).

Liu et al. in their study on the development of nanoemulsion systems for Astaxanthin which has low bioavailability, utilized oils having long triglyceride chains like olive, corn, and flaxseed oil. They evaluated the effectiveness of oil in

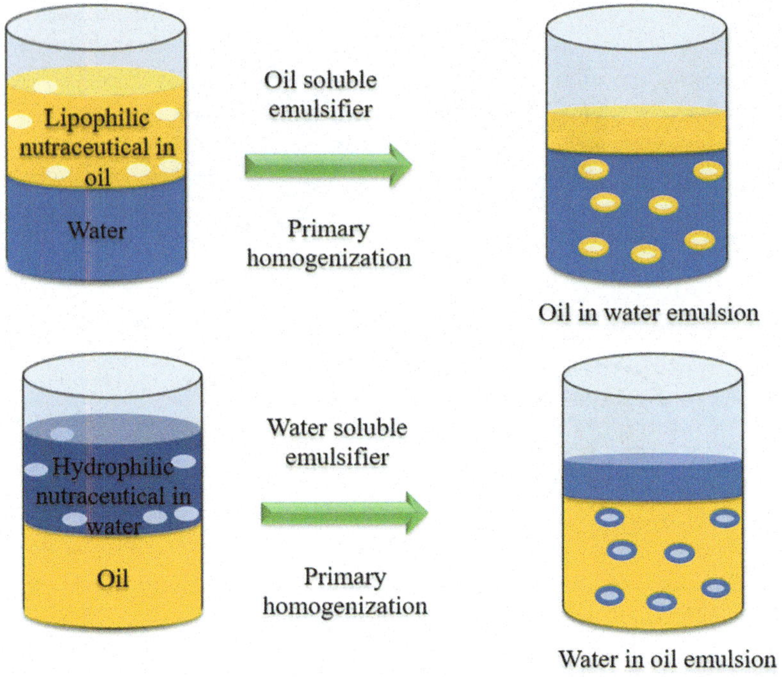

Fig. 6.6 Process of nano-emulsion fabrication

water nanoemulsions developed from the considered oils on the bioaccessibility of Astaxanthin (a keto-carotenoid) inside a simulated model of GI tract. Their results displayed significant improvement in the bioaccessibility of compound when in nanoemulsion form due to enhanced mixed micelles formation which increased the solubilization of the considered hydrophobic compound compared to control having no lipids (Liu et al. 2018). Sun et al. also employed olive oil and flaxseed oil for the preparation of the pterostilbene nanoemulsion delivery system to determine the carrier oil effectiveness on bioavailability. They concluded improved bioaccessibility in both types of formulations but nanoemulsion of olive oil displayed improved trans enterocyte transport than flax seed nanoemulsion. Further, the metabolic patterns during such transport were significantly different for different oil types, thus proving carrier oil selection a crucial task in nanoemulsion development. Fish oil due to its low solubility in water, bad odor and high ease of oxidation is not suitable for preparing healthy food formulations although it has many health benefits (Sun et al. 2015). Zhong et al. prepared a nanoemulsion formulation of fish oil to be added in yogurt for better solubility and increment of health benefits along with the reduction in syneresis and acidity (Zhong et al. 2018).

Though nanoemulsions have significantly worked for enhancing the bioavailability of nutraceuticals which is evident by the above-mentioned studies but the fact that they are thermodynamically unstable poses a great challenge in their developmental path. The use of different surfactants improves the stability of nanoemulsions but excessive use can lead to toxicity in the biological system (Lui et al. 2019). Thus, the use of natural surfactant in place of synthetic chemicals can be of great benefit in this concern. Further, proper optimization of the formulation will reduce the overuse of such chemicals and can result in safe and efficient formulations (Maurya and Aggarwal 2017a, b, c). Moreover, nanoliposomes as discussed in the upcoming section can be an effective solution to treat the problem concerned.

6.3.1.2 Nanoliposomes

The discovery of liposomes by Alec D Bangham dates back in the 1960s at Cambridge University. The need to develop stable nanoformulations having the capability to encapsulate both hydrophilic and lipophilic compounds lead to the discovery of these bilayer lipid vesicles (Bozzuto and Molinari 2015). They are made up of polar phospholipid bilayers that margin a hydrophilic core. The exceptional property of amphiphilic lipids to get self-assembled in aqueous solutions contributes to the formation of liposomes. These amphiphilic lipids form concentric structures which enclose the interior hydrophilic phase, that plays the role of the reservoir for bioactive hydrophilic compounds (Fig. 6.7). Along with this, a bilayer of lipids contributes as a hydrophobic compound reservoir as they provide an environment which is relatively lipophilic (Panahi et al. 2017; Puri et al. 2009). Thus, liposomes are highly versatile, as they can stably encapsulate both hydrophobic and hydrophilic compounds within a single system. The structural resemblance of bilayer liposomes with cell membranes provide them exceptional characteristic to act as models for the investigation of the cell to particle interactions. Encapsulation of bioactive nutraceuticals into liposomes also alter their temporal and spatial distribution inside the body (Keller 2001).

Liposomes at nanoscale ranging around 200 nm in diameter have similarities in physiochemical characteristics with that of the conventional liposomes but also contribute additional benefits of high bioavailability and physical stability when taken orally. Nanoliposomes can utilize inexpensive natural materials for their large-scale production like lecithins and can encapsulate and deliver both hydrophobic and hydrophilic compounds either simultaneously or individually (Khorasani et al. 2018). The ease of biodegradability and weak immunogenicity with limited toxicity

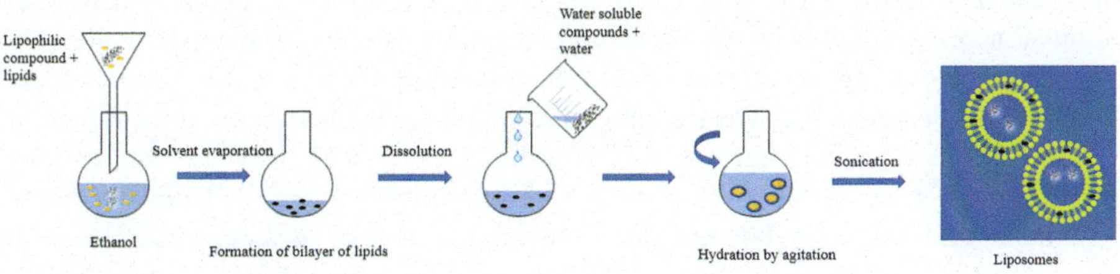

Fig. 6.7 Schematic diagram for process of nanoliposome fabrication

associated with nanoliposomes provide them a great advantage. Nanoliposomes can also be formulated for sustained release along with improving the bioavailability of sensitive and low bioavailability compounds to provide adequate amounts as and when required. High loading capacity of nanoliposomes indeed contributes to regulating long term release (Bozzuto and Molinari 2015).

Yang et al. in their study, developed nanoliposomes formulation, for the delivery of vitamin C and fatty acids of medium length, by lyophilization and stated that nanoliposomes can make improved bioavailability compared to liposomes which signifies advantage of nanotechnology in food supplement preparations (Yang et al. 2013). Mohammadi et al. developed Vitamin D3 nanoliposomal formulation with very high encapsulating efficiency of 93% for the fortification of beverage. Curcumin is a natural flavonoid, which has considerable pharmaceutical activities like antioxidant, antiviral, anti-inflammatory, antibacterial, anticancer, antifungal activities with no harmful effects. Despite of its high therapeutic qualities, its actual results remain unnoticed due to its low solubility in an aqueous medium, high instability, and very low bioavailability (Mohammadi et al. 2014). Gera et al., to overcome all these limitations developed a nanoliposome formulation of curcumin, having improved stability and solubility along with good physicochemical properties, thus proved high effectiveness of nanoliposomes to be employed for improving the bioavailability of lowly soluble compounds like curcumin (Gera et al. 2017).

Apart from several advantages, the need for highly specific, controlled, or targeted delivery and comparatively low efficiency of encapsulation in some conditions often limits the application of nanoliposomes. Also, sufficient removal of nanoliposomes by reticulo-endothelial system, in turn, poses a great challenge. Moreover, the utilization of organic chemicals for formulating nanoliposomes shows the potential for toxic side effects (Bozzuto and Molinari 2015). To deal with all these limitations new counterparts like solid lipid nanoparticles and nanolipid carriers were developed and are discussed in the following section.

6.3.1.3 Solid Lipid Nanoparticles and Nano-Lipid Carriers

Solid lipid nanoparticles and nano-lipid carriers were first identified in 1990 to overcome the limitations suffered by liposomal systems. Solid lipid nanoparticles are nanoscale carriers which are colloidal in nature and consist of a dispersion of physiological lipids in water or surfactant of aqueous nature (Naseri et al. 2015). These nanocarriers have been introduced in the last decade as new generation nanosized emulsions of lipids where the liquid form of lipid has been replaced by the solid form, thus providing an alternative to conventional lipid carriers (Gordillo-Galeano and Mora-Huertas 2018). The exceptional properties of solid lipid nanocarriers contribute following advantages to the incorporated material over the conventional nanocarriers: high stability, improved bioavailability, protection from the photo, chemical, and oxidative damage, due to its greater area of surface, small size, high biocompatibility and biodegradability and ease of drying, scale-up, and sterilization. Cumulatively these properties enhance the potential of these solid lipid nanocarriers for their application in improving the bioavailability of nutraceuticals (Katouzian et al. 2017). On the other hand, several drawbacks like poor loading capacity, chances of expulsion associated with incorporated compounds, the high water content of dispersion, and high particle aggregation susceptibility, limits the application of these solid lipid nanoparticles to a great extent (Naseri et al. 2015).

Nanostructured lipid carriers are another variety of nanoparticles which were developed to combat the above-mentioned shortcomings of solid liquid nanoparticles. Their composition consists of a mixture of solid and liquid lipids with non-ideal crystalized structure thus avoids lipid crystallization and hence prevent expulsion of incorporated bioactive compounds (Tamjidi et al. 2013). These nanocarriers consist of a variety of spatial lipids (that offer large distances among the crystals which are unstructured) and chains of fatty acids, therefore contributes to increased carrying capacity. The three types of these nanocarriers, namely imperfect, multiple, and amorphous further specifically increases the loading capacity and reduce the expulsion of the encapsulated compound (Jaiswal et al. 2016).

Imperfect type nanocarriers are made up of mixtures containing solid and liquid lipids where solid lipid is present in abundance. This type shows a comparatively high loading capacity than solid lipid nanocarriers (Akhavan et al. 2018). Multiple types of nanostructured lipid carriers contain a higher amount of oily lipid, thus provide high solubility as the lipophilic encapsulated compound will solubilize more in oily lipid as compared to solid lipids (Jaiswal et al. 2016). Another type is the amorphous type where additional lipids like hydroxyl octacosanyl, isopropyl myristate or hydroxyl stearate are used to avoid solid lipid crystallization when cooled. Such prevention of crystallization prevents encapsulated compound expulsion and hence shows good carrying properties (Khosa et al. 2018). In addition to this, reduced drug leakage, ease of modulation of release profiles, customization of dispersions by adding more solid lipids are other associated advantages with nanostructured lipid carriers which can ensure the development of good delivery systems for nutraceuticals to increase their bioavailability (Akhavan et al. 2018).

Hesperetin, a citrus fruit flavonoid, is well known for its cholesterol lowering ability. It has great potential to be used for food fortification for the development of a variety of functional foods, but its bitter taste and poor solubility limits its application. Fathi et al. developed solid lipid nanoparticles and nano lipid carriers for the development of hesperetin formulation to be used in functional foods. They tested the formulation by using milk as a model and no significant difference between sensory analysis scores of control and fortified milk was noticed. Also, their formulation masked the bitter taste of the compound along with improving the solubility (Fathi et al. 2013).

Zardini et al. in their food fortification study prepared solid lipid nanoparticles and nanostructured lipid carriers encapsulating lycopene and tested its effectiveness using orange drink as a model. Their sensory analysis confirmed no significant difference in the taste of drink upon addition and also proved improved solubility of lycopene, thus ensuring enhanced bioavailability (Zardini et al. 2018).

However, the scope of nanolipid carriers is highly significant but the utilization of these carriers for food fortification is still limited (Haider et al. 2020). Hence, further research to exploit their sole potential for the development of functional foods highly demanded. Though, man-made formulations possess the high capability to deal with the purpose but nature also provide inspirations for some exceptional technologies which can be formulated with great ease and have least or no toxic effects, unlike the synthetically formulated nano-systems.

6.3.2 Nature Inspired Nanoparticle Delivery Systems

Nature is full of inspirational wealth. Even the concept of nanoparticles is not new but has been procured from nature. A variety of nanoparticle assemblies exist naturally and can be employed for improving the bioavailability of various nutraceuticals thus can contribute to food fortification. Some common naturally existing examples of such assemblies include casein assemblies present in milk for encapsulating and delivering milk nutrients, starch granules and cyclodextrins inclusions with food nutraceutical compounds and chains of amylose conjugated with flavor compounds in bread which release flavors when heated subsequently while bread preparation (Guichard 2002; Semo et al. 2007; Ahmad et al. 2020; Doan et al. 2020). These type of nanocarriers are of great interest in the present scenario as they occur naturally; thus, no or low processing and preparation is needed along with null associated toxic effects. Details regarding most common types of nanocarrier lying under this category are elaborated as follows:

6.3.2.1 Micelles of Casein

Casein milk protein family contributes for 80% fraction of milk proteins in bovine. This family comprises insoluble phosphoproteins that are capable of binding secreted phosphate and calcium present in mammalian milk. These proteins act as a molecular chaperone for each other as well as for other proteins, thus stabilize them and prevent their unfavorable aggregation. Hence, under favorable conditions, the peptides of casein exist in the stable amorphous agglomerate form known as casein micelle having a radius of around 50 to 500 nm (Esmaili et al. 2011). Beau in 1921 first used the term casein micelles for all milk proteins consisting of aggregates of whey and casein proteins (Beau 1921). But at recent times these casein micelles are known to contain inner part of $\alpha s1$, $\alpha s2$, and β peptides and an outer hairy layer of κ peptide of casein that provides steric stability due to its hydrophilic glycosylated part (namely glycomacropeptide) which interact with the aqueous environment. They are considered safe and possess high biocompatibility, bioresorbability and biodegradability (Semo et al. 2007).

They also display exceptional pH-dependent behavior and thus can respond according to the variable pH conditions of gastrointestinal (GI) tract. In addition, they can travel across the plasma membrane via active transport thus can feasibly be taken up by cells when given orally. Amphiphilic nature of casein micelles contributes affinity for both hydrophilic and hydrophobic compounds hence increase their usage as delivery systems. Also, on subjection to proteolytic enzymes of the GI tract, these micelles are broken down and can quickly release the incorporated compounds (Głąb and Boratyński 2017). All these significant properties of casein micelles make them an excellent candidate for their application as delivery systems in food fortification to enhance the bioavailability of nutraceuticals. Loewen et al. in their optimization study on vitamin loading in re-assembled casein micelles, loaded vitamin A and vitamin D_3 and analysed their stability over a duration of 21 days. Their results showed high loading efficiency of re-assembled micelles and balance of vitamin D_3 in their optimized formulation (Loewen et al. 2017). Mohan et al. studied the association of vitamin A with unmodified casein micelles for the fortification of skimmed milk and found significant vitamin A binding results for differentially processed milk samples (Mohan et al. 2013).

The utilization of casein micelles to encapsulate fat soluble vitamins for the fortification of milk and milk products has been well documented but polyphenol encapsulation into these micelles has been less studied and often result in modification of proteinaceous matrix. In a past, research efforts have been made to reduce such modifications by the development of crosslinked hydrogels of casein micelles by spray drying which displayed high protection against heat and aging conditions to polyphenols (Kartsova and Alekseeva 2008). Thus, further research to develop the scope for uniform utilization of casein micelles for a wide range of products is highly required.

6.3.2.2 Nanocrystals

Naturally occurring nanocrystals are nano sized crystalline forms of polysaccharides and lipids. Polysaccharides like cellulose, chitin, and starch, by virtue, are present in mixed forms containing both crystalline and amorphous forms (Mu et al. 2019; Gutiérrez 2017). When exposed to controlled conditions, the amorphous form shows a high tendency to get hydrolysed, leaving behind highly ordered intact crystals. These nano-sized crystalline regions constitute nanocrystals. Ranby in 1949 hydrolysed the cellulose fibres which were dispersed in water by acid and kept the foundation for chemical synthesis of nanocrystals by utilizing natural polysaccharide (Ranby 1949). The exceptional associated advantages like high biocompatibility, bioavailability, biodegradability, surface area, strength, ease of processing, economic feasibility, and nanoscale effects, prove these natural nanocrystals an effective candidate to be used in biological systems (Wu et al. 2018; Hu et al. 2014). Additional advantages of polysaccharide nano counterparts like the presence of functional groups, high rigidity, large aspect ratio, highly crystalline nature, and associated chirality provide them significant ability to interact and form complex, with the majority of bioactive compounds (Hu et al. 2014). Moreover, their food-grade nature with the least toxicity, in turn, contributes to their use in functional foods as delivery systems for improving the bioavailability of nutraceuticals. Nanocrystals conjugated with physically and chemically unstable bioactive compounds can be further stabilized by encapsulating them in liposomes or layering them with biopolymers and surfactants (Sheikhi et al. 2019). Ntoutoume et al. developed a highly potent cellulose nanocrystal delivery system for a well-known nutraceutical, curcumin, to improve its bioavailability (Ntoutoume et al. 2016). Xiao et al. in their study of acetylated starch nanocrystals reported high biocompatibility and bioavailability of starch nanocrystals thus proving them an effective delivery system to be used for delivery of bioactive compounds having low bioavailability (Xiao et al. 2016).

Fabrication of nanocrystals is commonly conducted by using either heat controlled or acid hydrolysis technique, but the application of strong acid like sulphuric acid under controlled conditions of temperature, time, agitation and concentration of acid often convey low thermal stability to the nanocrystals which limits their wide application. To deal with this consequence instead of sulphuric acid other mineral acids like phosphoric acid, hydrochloric acid, hydrobromic acid were employed and found to confer acceptable biocompatibility and improved thermal stability to the extracted nanocrystals. Besides this, eco-friendly approaches like hydrolysis by enzymes and sonication at high intensity also gave promising outcomes and are gaining excessive attention in this regard in recent times (Vanderfleet et al. 2018).

Hence, further research on the extraction of nanocrystals and their application in food fortification shows excellent scope for further study.

Another class of natural nature inspired nanoparticle systems, which have gained much importance is of cyclodextrins. These cyclodextrins are prepared by starch hydrolysis and are discussed in detail in the following section.

6.3.2.3 Cyclodextrins

Cyclodextrins are cyclic oligosaccharides made up of glucopyranose monomers. They are non-reducing in nature and are produced by starch enzymatic degradation. The three well known types of cyclodextrins are alpha, beta, and gamma cyclodextrins which possess six, seven, and eight glucopyranose units respectively (Fig. 6.8) (Carneiro et al. 2019). The inner conical cylindrical cavity is hydrophobic in nature whereas the outer surface is hydrophilic. These characteristics provide them the ability to form inclusions with hydrophobic compounds and hence are widely used in pharmaceutical industries as an excipient. Also, these cyclic structures can be modified chemically to build a variety of desired nanostructures (Gidwani and Vyas 2015). They can form complexes with various bioactive molecules and improve their stability, solubility, and bioavailability by providing large hydrophilic surface (Tiwari et al. 2010).

Various types of nanostructures can be formulated by these cyclodextrins by self-aggregation, polymerization, chemical modifications, or by conjugating them with other biocompatible polymers like PEG, chitosan, and alginate (Haimhoffer et al. 2019). Nano sponges and nanospheres are widely investigated nanoformulations of cyclodextrins which enhances permeability and solubility of bioactive molecules and promotes controlled release (Omar et al. 2020). Amphiphilic cyclodextrins are

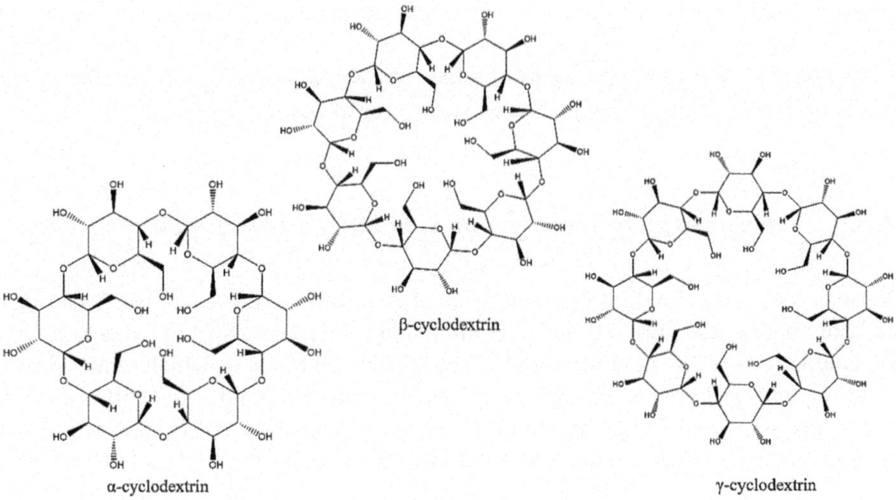

Fig. 6.8 Types of cyclodextrins used for the preparation of food grade nanoparticles

derivatives having hydrophobic chains grafted over the secondary and/or primary faces of cyclodextrin rings. They have the ability to self-assemble to form aggregates which are water-soluble like nanoparticles and micelles, or can also be fused into lipid membranes thereby improving cell targeting and permeability of bioactive compounds and hence improve their bioavailability. These spontaneously formed nanoparticles like nanospheres or nanocapsules also possess high loading capacity which is an additional advantage in this concern (Parrot-Lopez et al. 2010).

Cyclodextrin nanoparticles have recently gained much attention for their application in the development of functional foods. They can act as potent nutrient delivery systems by enhancing the characteristics of bioactive compounds having low bioavailability. In vivo studies have shown improvement in stability, solubility, and bioavailability of nutrients when given in complex form with cyclodextrins (Sharma and Baldi 2016). Nutraceuticals like curcumin, coenzyme Q10, and tocotrienol when combined with gamma-cyclodextrin form insoluble complexes. These complexes even being insoluble in nature, result in significant improvement in bioavailability. Recent findings reported that bioactive compounds or molecules dissociated from gamma cyclodextrins after encountering bile acids form micelles without being aggregated hence ensure increment in solubility and bioavailability (Uekaji and Terao 2019; Carneiro et al. 2019).

R-alpha-lipoic acid present in spinach, potatoes, and broccoli, have high antioxidant properties and act as a mitochondrial enzyme cofactor. But due to its instability at high temperature and pH, it suffers low intestinal absorption and hence low bioavailability. Ikuta et al. in their study on R-alpha-lipoic acid prepared gamma-cyclodextrin-R-alpha-lipoic acid complexes and evaluated their plasma concentration on oral administration. Their study resulted in a 2.5fold increase in R-alpha-lipoic acid concentration when given in cyclodextrin conjugated form compared to unconjugated form hence displaying a significant increase in bioavailability (Ikuta et al. 2016).

Hence, nature inspired nanoparticles have great potential to act as excellent food grade nano delivery systems for the enhancement of nutrient's bioavailability.

6.3.3 Nanoparticles Made from Specialized Equipment

Various types of techniques are used for the fabrication of nanoparticles. Some fabrication methods require specialized equipment to prepare a specific size and type of nanoparticles. The most commonly used fabrication methods which required specific equipment are electrospinning, electrospraying, and nanospray drying (Bhushani and Anandharamakrishnan 2014; Arpagaus et al. 2017). The variety of nanoparticles produced by these methods are as follows:

6.3.3.1 Nanofibers Fabricated by Electrospinning

Electrospun nanofibers are fabricated by electrospinning unit in which polymers, biopolymers, polymer blends, or bioactive compound impregnated polymer solutions are passed through a syringe needle shaped spinneret. High voltage is supplied to charge the solution particles thus generating a repulsive force. At a particular voltage, the surface tension of the solution becomes incapable to counter balance the generated repulsive force and hence the solution erupts out as a jet from the spinneret tip (Bhattarai et al. 2019). The solvent present in the erupting jet of the solution while travelling towards the low voltage grounded plate gets evaporated and thus results in fibre formation. The high production efficiency and low cost of this technique make it highly advantageous for industrial applications. The nanofibers fabricated possess high porosity and high ratio of surface area to the volume which are the most required characteristics to develop a nanocarrier to be used in the delivery of food nutrients having bioactive properties (Leidy and Ximena 2019).

6.3.3.2 Nanoparticles Fabricated by Electrospraying

The technique of electrospraying is an efficient fabrication method which works on the principle of enforcing a polymeric solution to form nanoparticles by applying high voltage (Fig. 6.9). In this fabrication method, the polymer solution filled syringe pump, is supplied with a high voltage supply, which acts as a functional electrode. Opposite to useful electrode, there is a collector made up of metal foil known as a ground electrode. The type of polymer solution used determines the rate of flow and the voltage to be applied for electrospraying. Similar to electrospinning the emerged liquid polymer solution due to surface tension forms tailored cone in the electric field. As the applied voltage increases the increment in electric field

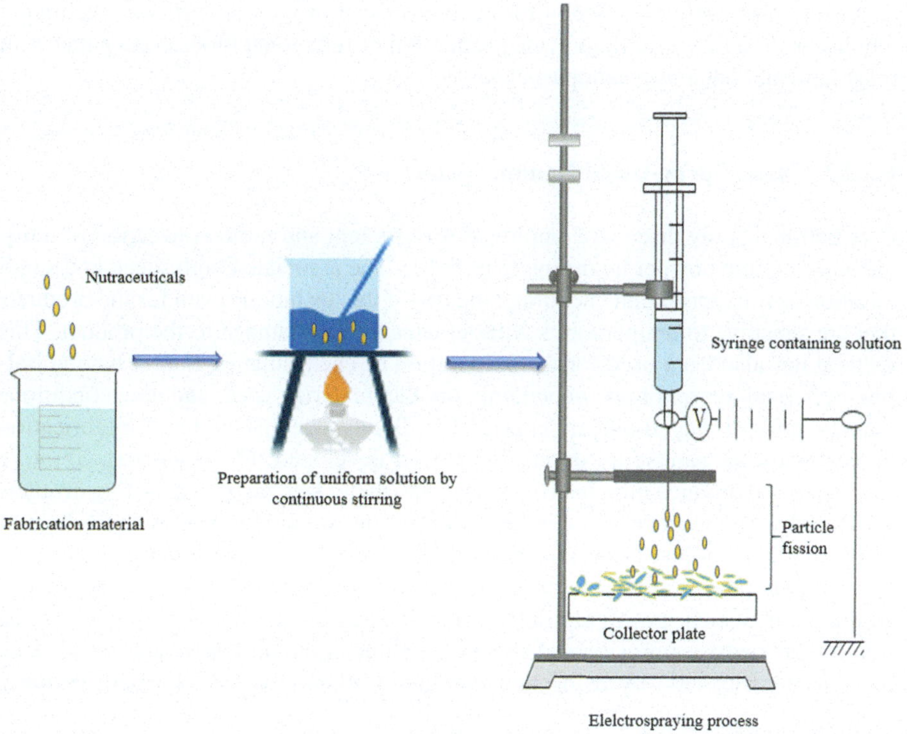

Fig. 6.9 Schematic representation of electrospraying technique for nanoparticle fabrication

breaks the cone and leads to the formation of droplets which are highly charged. The applied parameters of flow rate, electric field, and other suitable conditions determine the size of droplets hence by varying these parameters, the size of droplets can be customized from micro to nano range. Finally, solid nanoparticles are collected on collector after evaporation of the solvent (Sridhar and Ramakrishna 2013). These nanoparticles can be employed for a wide variety of applications like the development of nutraceutical delivery system, drug delivery system, and diagnostic and therapeutic techniques. Not only synthetic but natural polymers like carbohydrates or proteins can be utilized to fabricate nanoparticles by using this method. No reduction in the activity of polymer conjugated bioactive compounds was observed when fabricated to nanoparticles by electrospraying. The significant advantages associated with this method are its reproducibility, the high loading capacity of produced nanoparticles, and improved scalable synthesis (Boda et al. 2018; de Boer et al. 2019).

Several researchers have employed this technique for the fabrication of starch and chitosan nanoparticles for the delivery of bioactive compounds but still, limited research has been done for the implementation of this method for the development of functional food formulations (Boer et al. 2019). The high loading capacity of the prepared nanoparticles and the ease associated with this method seems to be highly promising and further research in this concern can provide an efficient technique which can be utilized for large scale production of functional foods conjugated with nutraceutical containing nanoparticles.

6.3.3.3 Nano Spray-Dried Nanoparticles

Conventional spray driers are employed for efficient and rapid conversion of a liquid solution into powder by drying (Fig. 6.10). The associated high speed and small duration of transformation encourage the use of this technique even for the products that are sensitive to temperatures without causing any damage to the product. This method has also been used for the preparation of encapsulating matrix having hollow spherical morphology depending on the material used and the conditions employed for drying (Bilancetti et al. 2010). To advance this method for fabrication of nanoparticles nanospray dryers have been developed which utilized vibrating mesh spray to produce minute droplets of nano meter size range. These tiny droplets are dried by drying gas flowing in laminar flow and are precipitated with the help of electrostatic precipitator in the form of dried nanoparticles. The stainless perforated, thin mesh is used to provide a narrow range of size distribution and high yield of formulation, which are highly desired advantages of nanospray technology. The size, shape, density, porosity, and chemical composition of the nanoparticles can be customized with ease by using this fabrication method (Li et al. 2010; Glaubitt et al. 2019).

This technology can be employed for transforming a variety of polymeric materials including natural polymers like carbohydrates and proteins to the ultrafine powder of desirable properties (Arpagaus et al. 2017). Various food-grade formulations of vitamins, proteins, antioxidants, and oils can be developed by this method

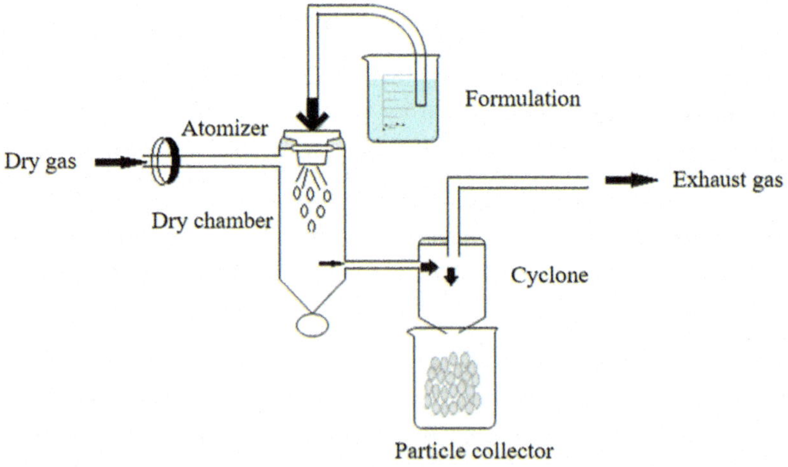

Fig. 6.10 Schematic representation of spray drying technique

to be employed to enhance the bioavailability of lipophilic nutraceuticals as these nanoparticle formulations provide high surface area to be encountered by the surrounding aqueous environment in GI tract (Jampilek et al. 2019). Xue et al. used nanospray drying technique for redispersion of colloidal solid lipid nanoparticles of curcumin to procure ultrafine nanoparticle powder which can in turn increase bioavailability of curcumin and also possess high GI stability (Xue et al. 2018).

Spray drying technique accounts for large part of marketed food nanoformulation based products as formulations developed by nano-spray drying can be customized to nanosize range contributing to the high efficiency of encapsulation and improved release rate along with high ease and low cost of production. The resulting powdered formulation prepared form this technique confers protection from light, oxidation and temperature. It makes the formulation highly stable and redispersible in an aqueous environment and also make it easy to handle and store. The low moisture content of powdered formulations also provides enhanced shelf life to food with which they are conjugated. Although, this technique is widely used, but the applicability of this technique for the development of nanoformulations suffers some limitations. Vibrating mesh technology which is common in nano-spray dryers, due to tiny pore size often gets clogged when a highly concentrated product or initial solution of large particle size is used. Even highly viscous solutions do not flow consistently across the mesh resulting in cessation of the process (Arpagaus et al. 2017). Regular cleaning of the apparatus like nebulizers and vibrating mesh is required to combat this limitation to some extent. Further utilization of low concentration solution can be an alternative but not a universal solution to deal with such limitation. Further, apparatus parameter optimization or development of versatile technology is required to enhance the applicability of this technique for all kinds of formulations (Jampilek et al. 2019).

Along with the fabrication technology, the material used to develop formulations also pose many limitations. The major concern with food grade formulation relates to the toxicity of material which can be dealt with some extent by utilizing biodegradable and biocompatible polymers as presented in the following section.

6.3.4 Biopolymer Nanoparticles

Generally recognised as safe (GRAS) materials are highly demanded for the development of functional food due to their low or null toxic effect and high biocompatibility. Biopolymers like proteins and carbohydrates are categorized as GRAS materials and have been potentially used to prepare food grade nanoparticle formulations (Joye and McClements 2014). Utilization of such nanoparticle formulations for protection, encapsulation and controlled release of nutraceuticals or other bioactive compounds (both hydrophobic and hydrophilic), have shown great benefits, as such formulations enhance their overall bioavailability and hence their effectiveness (Hudson and Margaritis 2014).

A variety of formulations has been developed by either using individual biopolymers or biopolymer combinations, without the use of harsh solvents or chemicals. Nanoparticles of different structures can be prepared by biopolymers and are classified as inclusions complexes, hydrogels, and polyelectrolyte complexes (Nitta and Numata 2013). Customization of particle size is highly possible, to modulate nanoparticle rheology, optics, stability, loading efficiency, retention, and rate of bioactive release. The interaction, degradation, transportation, and penetration of nanoparticle in the GI tract also suffer significant variations due to change in size (Lopes et al. 2016). Various types of biopolymer nanoparticles that can contribute to enhancing nutrient bioavailability in different functional food formulations have been identified and shows great potential for large scale employability. The major two categories of biopolymer nanoparticles, based on the material used that is, protein and carbohydrate nanoparticles, are briefly discussed below (Dima et al. 2020).

6.3.4.1 Protein Nanoparticles

Protein nanoparticles are highly customizable and can be employed for a wide variety of applications. Proteins can either be used in their conventional form or can be modified by physical, chemical or enzymatic means to vary their functional characteristics according to the requirement for nanoparticle formulation. Such nanoparticles can also be perfected for specific applications. The major advantages associated with protein nanoparticles are their high biodegradability and biocompatibility as they do not pose toxicity in the host, have no size limitations, do not accumulate in the body, and are not rapidly cleared out from the body (Verma et al. 2018). The majority of proteins are digestible and thus ensures eventual release of encapsulated compound in the GI tract. Some proteins protect the chemically unstable compound due to their antioxidant property. Also, protein nanoparticles can form conjugates with other carbohydrates and proteins and thus provide a broad scope to develop various types of nanoparticles (Martins et al. 2018). The proteins that can be used to fabricate nanoparticles are categorized as animal and plant proteins. Some leading animal proteins that can be used to formulate nanoparticles either individually or in combinations are albumins, casein, gelatin, fibroin, and whey protein. Several past studies have prepared combinations of gelatin or fibroin with albumin for the preparation of multifunctional nanoparticles. Plant-derived proteins which can be employed for this purpose are zein, gliadin, soy proteins, and pea legumin proteins (DeFrates et al. 2018).

Although many fabrication techniques have been used for nanoparticle formulation development like thermal gelation, desolvation, self-assembly, and precipitation but desolvation is the most frequently used one for protein nanoparticle formulation development due to its simple and versatile method and ability to prepare uniform sphere-shaped nanoparticles (Lohcharoenkal et al. 2014). It is a self-assembly method in which appropriate solvent is used to dissolve protein and after that, the prepared solution is subjected to an antisolvent which results in nanoparticle formation by protein precipitation (Pandey et al. 2017). For desolvation of hydrophilic proteins, water is used as solvent and alcohol act as anti-solvent but for hydrophobic ones, the solvent used is alcohol and water behave as antisolvent (Jahanban-Esfahlan et al. 2016). Globular proteins use a different fabrication method in which the protein is heated above its denaturation temperature under controlled conditions in the suitable solution of apt ionic strength and pH. This unfolds the protein molecules and exposes their non-polar buried groups which form links among each other due to hydrophobic forces and result in nanoparticles of spherical shape (Farooq et al. 2020). Fang et al. in their study employed bovine serum albumin, myoglobin, and lysozyme for the development of protein nanoparticles for delivery of hydrophobic compounds like quercetin, rutin, and kaempferol and concluded bovine serum albumin as a potential candidate to be used for the purpose due to better loading capacity, high control on release and highly significant protection of antioxidant property of bioactive compound (Fang et al. 2011). Penalva et al. developed a casein nanoparticle delivery system by nanospray drying technique for oral administration of resveratrol, an antioxidant commonly found in grapes. Their experimental result displayed high loading efficiency, protection of resveratrol from varying pH conditions of GI tract, high and constant plasma level for a duration of 8 h proving an increase in bioavailability (Peñalva et al. 2018).

In addition, protein nanoparticles can be customized by using recombinant proteins of desirable properties which can be exploited for varied purposes. Further research in this concern will increase the scope of this type of nanoparticles in a wide variety of formulations.

6.3.4.2 Polysaccharide Nanoparticles

Polysaccharides being cheap, biocompatible, easily available, biodegradable with low toxicity along with their exceptional property to act as pro and prebiotics can be highly potent candidates to develop food-grade nanoparticles for enhancing the nutritional bioavailability. Similar to proteins, they can be modified for different functional features by chemical, enzymatic and physical means (López-López et al. 2015). The gelation of polysaccharide leads to the formation of nanoparticles by three main mechanisms cold set, heat set, and ionotropic (Burey et al. 2008). Agar, alginate, carrageenan, cellulose, chitosan, dextran, gellan gum, inulin, pectin, pullulan, and starch are the potential polysaccharides which can be employed for the development of food grade nanoparticle formulations (Efthimiadou et al. 2015). Many cellulose derivatives have been used for oral delivery systems in pharmaceutical industries which prove them capable to be employed for the formulation of functional foods too (Arca et al. 2018). Chitosan forms biopolymer nanoparticles utilizing electrostatic interactions. It has the exceptional property to increase the absorption of the conjugated bioactive compound by increasing the time of contact of the absorption area with the bioactive. It is highly useful for hydrophilic compounds which form hydrogen or electrostatic bonds with chitosan (Priyadarshi and Rhim 2020). Starch is a highly efficient polysaccharide to be used for the purpose due to its native granular structure which can be modified by various means and its ability to get degraded in GI tract which may be beneficial for the preparation of formulations based on controlled release mechanisms. Starch has been well studied by past studies for specific delivery of probiotics to the colon (Zhu 2017). Moreover, starch hydrolysates have been reported to show positive results for the development of encapsulation systems for various polyphenols (Lin et al. 2011).

Various fabrication methods have been utilized for the development of nanoparticle formulations from polysaccharides based on their varying molecular and physicochemical properties. These properties like charge, molecular weight, conformations, hydrophobic nature, thickening, gelling, and surface activity contribute high versatility for the fabrication of nanoparticles. Most fabrication methods used for polysaccharide nanoparticles development are mild and do not employ organic solvents and chemicals hence are bio-friendly. Preparation of starch nanocrystals is possible either by hydrolysis of semi-crystalline form to remove the amorphous part or by gelatinization of starch under controlled conditions (Chen et al. 2016). Nanogels of polysaccharides can be prepared by polysaccharide self-assemblage in solutions via hydrophobic, covalent, electrostatic, or hydrogen bonding. These nanogels contain cross-linked three-dimensional networks which trap water in large amount (Neamtu et al. 2019). Hydrogels of polysaccharides are formed by cross-linking mineral ions with ionic polysaccharides like calcium alginate nanogels. Past researches proved that the ionic strength of the solvent and concentration of mineral ions plays a vital role in determining the size and polydispersity index of nanoparticles (Oliveira and Reis 2008).

6.3.4.3 Polysaccharide-Protein Nanoparticles

Combinations of biopolymers like protein-polysaccharide complexes can be utilized for the preparation of nanoparticles having an amalgamation of properties of both biopolymers. The most favourable fabrication methods that can be employed for preparing these complex nanoparticles are templating, injection, electrostatic complex formation, anti-solvent precipitation, and thermodynamic incompatibility (Jones et al. 2010). Tailoring of these nanoparticles can be done with ease by controlling the shape, size, composition, and charge by using optimized fabricating conditions. Biopolymer complex nanoparticles of protein and polysaccharide, are usually prepared by electrostatic complexation method (Jones and McClements 2010). A classical process includes mixing of ionic polysaccharide and protein at suitable pH, at which the two biopolymers have opposite charges which result in electrostatic interactions and complex formation. These complexes often have nanoscale range and can encapsulate bioactive agents (Peinado et al. 2010). Guadana et al. prepared protein-polysaccharide nanoparticles by hydrophobic ion pairing method of dextran sulphate and bovine serum albumin (Gaudana et al. 2011). Jones et al. prepared two types of beta-lactoglobulin-pectin nanoparticles by using different methods of fabrication. The first method includes the preparation of beta-lactoglobulin nanoparticle then forming a coat of pectin over them whereas the second method comprises heating together pectin and beta-lactoglobulin complex

(Jones et al. 2010). In another study by Al-obaidi et al. whey protein and chitosan nanoparticles were prepared for the development of an oral iron delivery system proving utilization of these complex nanoparticles for improving the GI absorption of iron (Al-Obaidi et al. 2016).

6.4 Safety and Toxicity of Nanostructures Applied in Food Systems

Nanotechnology has a wide range of applications in the food industry, and it can be employed to enhance the quality, nutritional benefits, safety, and cost of food products. Some nanomaterials are used to develop delivery systems for nutrients, which have low bioavailability in pure form and find it difficult to convey their health benefits. Also, in some cases, nanotechnology is applied to enhance the rheological, optical, and flow properties of food products (Yu et al. 2018). Moreover, some food products naturally contain nanomaterials like micelles of casein in milk or nano-sized cell organelles in some animal and plant cells and sometimes processing of food like grinding, homogenization or cooking result in the formation of some or the other types of nanoparticles (Semo et al. 2007). Though the presence of nano-sized materials in food is highly prevalent, but the safety or toxicity associated with their use demands great attention.

Many organic or inorganic nanoparticles have also been also used in food industry which pose varying effects on the health of consumers but to limit to the scope of this chapter the toxicity related to engineered organic food grade nanoparticles is discussed further. Mostly, the ability of ingested nanomaterial to cause harm to cells or organs of the human body determines the toxicity of nanoparticles. Such damage can occur both in the GI tract or in rest of the body after the absorption of nano species. Further nanoparticles may cause adverse effects on gut microbiota which can harm human health indirectly. In the case of organic nanoparticles, it is believed that they are least toxic but under specific situation, they too can pose dreaded effects (McClements and Xiao 2017). These nanoparticles may interfere with the GI tract functions as they have a large surface area and can adsorb and denature enzymes present in gastrointestinal fluid thus can reduce the digestion activity of the respective enzymes (Bergin and Witzmann 2013). Along with this high quantity of indigestible organic nanoparticles, in the GI tract may lead to a reduction in lipid, protein or starch digestion. Sometimes entry of nanoparticles into the body may trigger oxidative stress and inflammation in the GI tract due to immune responses (Gupta and Xie 2018). Though accumulation and aggregation of nanoparticles in different cells and tissues is a significant contributor of toxicity but the nanomaterials used in food or nanofoods are digestible in nature and pose the least toxicity in this concern. Also, due to low accumulation in the body, the carcinogenic or genotoxic effects are not significant in concerns to nanoparticles used in food (Ameta et al. 2020). Many studies have been conducted on animal or cell models to check the toxicity of food-grade particles but still, clinical trials on humans are yet to be undertaken (McClements and Xiao 2017).

Moreover, the processes used to formulate nanoparticles often employ harsh chemicals which can lead to high toxicity in-vivo. In nanoemulsions, the utilization of different types of ionic and non-ionic surfactants are the leading cause of toxicity. Along with this nanoliposomes formulation process also require use of organic solvents which needs wise selection as they can pose high toxic effects. In addition, some nanoparticles composed of indigestible proteins and carbohydrates may alter the absorption of other proteins, starch, and lipids and thus can cause potential harm (Farooq et al. 2020). Digestible lipids when encapsulated in nanolaminated fibres suffer delayed and slow digestion in the upper GI tract which leads to a higher amount of lipids to reach the colon where they get fermented and cause GI problems. Several nanoparticles which carry nutraceuticals having antibiotic properties and are not digested in the upper GI tract causes alterations in colonic microflora when they could reach the colon in large quantities hence cause toxic effects (Gupta and Xie 2018). Many such concerns related to safety and toxicity of food grade materials have been investigated, thus all these factors should be considered beforehand while formulating nanoformulation for dietary use.

6.5 Conclusion and Future Perspectives

The beneficial effects of a variety of nutrients often remain unnoticed due to their low bioavailability. Nano-sized delivery systems provided promising results to deal with this issue. Development of functional foods for improving the bioavailability of such nutrients by employing nano-delivery systems to protect, encapsulate, target, and release (in a controlled manner) the lowly bioavailable nutraceuticals, can be a great strategy to fully exploit their potential. Also, such nanosystems will contribute to reducing the nutrient and flavour loss and deterioration of texture, which usually occur during food processing. A variety of biocompatible and biodegradable materials have been discovered and developed to fabricate such delivery systems. Naturally occurring or functionally modified biomolecules have gained great interest in this concern as they pose least or no toxicity in biological systems. Numerous fabrication methods have been developed, which ensures the accuracy and precision of nanosized systems along with the least toxic side effects. Although much research has been conducted on such nanofoods containing products but their commercialization is yet to be done. But before the large-scale implementation of these nanotechnological approaches proper validation of health and safety-related factor is utmost necessary. Concludingly, application of nanotechnology in the food industry to enhance the nutrient bioavailability is a highly effective approach which shows great possibilities to improve the health status of the present population and thus extensive research in this concern is highly demanded.

References

Adefegha SA (2018) Functional foods and nutraceuticals as dietary intervention in chronic diseases; novel perspectives for health promotion and disease prevention. J Diet Suppl 15:977–1009. https://doi.org/10.1080/19390211.2017.1401573

Ahmad M, Gani A, Hassan I, Huang Q, Shabbir H (2020) Production and characterization of starch nanoparticles by mild alkali hydrolysis and ultra-sonication process. Sci Rep 10:1–11. https://doi.org/10.1038/s41598-020-60380-0

Akhavan S, Assadpour E, Katouzian I, Jafri SM (2018) Lipid nano scale cargos for the protection and delivery of food bioactive ingredients and nutraceuticals. Trends Food Sci Technol 74:132–146. https://doi.org/10.1016/j.tifs.2018.02.001

Al-Obaidi H, Patel N, Ghafarzada R (2016) Fabrication and characterisation of novel protein-polysaccharide biopolymer based nanoparticles for iron delivery. European Iron Club. Innsbruck, Austria 07–10 Apr 2016. https://ironmasterclass.eu/wp-content/uploads/2016/11/abstractbook-EIC-2016.pdf

Alpizar-Vargas L, Zúñiga-Montero C, Rodríguez-Murillo A et al (2019) Nutraceuticals: definition, applied nanoengineering in their production and applications. Int J Biosen Bioelectron 5:56–61. https://doi.org/10.15406/ijbsbe.2019.05.00154

Ameta SK, Rai AK, Hiran D, Ameta R, Ameta SC (2020) Use of nanomaterials in food science. Biogenic Nano-Particles Use Agro-ecosyst 21:457–488. https://doi.org/10.1007/978-981-15-2985-6_24

Arca HC, Mosquera-Giraldo LI, Bi V, Xu D, Taylor LS, Edgar KJ (2018) Pharmaceutical applications of cellulose ethers and cellulose ether esters. Biomacromolecules 19:2351–2376. https://doi.org/10.1021/acs.biomac.8b00517

Arpagaus C, John P, Collenberg A, Ruetti DP (2017) Nanocapsules formation by nano spray drying. In: Jafari SM (ed) Nanoencapsulation technologies for the food and nutraceutical industries. Academic, Cambridge, pp 346–401. https://doi.org/10.1016/B978-0-12-809436-5.00010-0

Assadpour E, Jafari SM (2019) A systematic review on nanoencapsulation of food bioactive ingredients and nutraceuticals by various nanocarriers. Critical Reviews in Food Sci Nutri 59:3129–3151. https://doi.org/10.1080/10408398.2018.1484687

Beau M (1921) Les matie` res albuminoı¨de du lait. Le Lait INRA Editions 1:19–26. https://hal.archives-ouvertes.fr/file/index/docid/894657/filename/hal-00894657.pdf

Bergin IL, Witzmann FA (2013) Nanoparticle toxicity by the gastrointestinal route: evidence and knowledge gaps. Int J Biomed Nanosci Nanotechnol 3:1–44. https://doi.org/10.1504/IJBNN.2013.054515

Bhattarai RS, Bachu RD, Boddu SHS, Bhaduri S (2019) Biomedical applications of electrospun nanofibers: drug and nanoparticle delivery. Pharmaceutics 11:1–30. https://doi.org/10.3390/pharmaceutics11010005

Bhushani JA, Anandharamakrishnan C (2014) Electrospinning and electrospraying techniques: potential food based applications. Trends Food Sci Tech 38:21–33. https://doi.org/10.1016/j.tifs.2014.03.004

Bilancetti L, Poncelet D, Loisel C, Mazzitelli S, Nastruzzi C (2010) A statistical approach to optimize the spray drying of starch particles: application to dry powder coating. AAPS Pharm Sci Tech 11:1257–1267. https://doi.org/10.1208/s12249-010-9492-y

Boda SK, Li X, Xie J (2018) Electrospraying an enabling technology for pharmaceutical and biomedical applications: a review. J Aerosol Sci 125:164–181. https://doi.org/10.1016/j.jaerosci.2018.04.002

Bozzuto G, Molinari A (2015) Liposomes as nanomedical devices. Int J Nanomedicine 10:975–999. https://doi.org/10.2147/IJN.S68861

Bradberry JC, Hilleman DE (2013) Overview of omega-3 fatty acid therapies. Pharmacy and Therapeutics 38:681–691

Burey P, Bhandari BR, Howes T, Gidley M (2008) Hydrocolloid gel particles: formation, characterization, and application. Crit Rev Food Sci Nutr 48:361–377. https://doi.org/10.1080/10408390701347801
Canizales JR, Rodríguez GRV, Avila JAD, Saldana AMP, Parrilla EA, Ochoa MAV, Aguilar GAG (2018) Encapsulation to protect different bioactives to be used as nutraceuticals and food ingredients. In: Mérillon JM, Ramawat K (eds) Bioactive molecules in food. Reference series in phytochemistry. Springer, Cham, pp 1–20. https://doi.org/10.1007/978-3-319-54528-8_84-1
Carneiro SB, Costa Duarte FÍ, Heimfarth L, Quintans JSS, Quintans LJ, da Veiga VF, Lima AAN (2019) Cyclodextrin-drug inclusion complexes: in vivo and in vitro approaches. Int J Mol Sci 20:1–23. https://doi.org/10.3390/ijms20030642
Cencic A, Chingwaru W (2010) The role of functional foods, nutraceuticals, and food supplements in intestinal health. Nutrients 2:611–625. https://doi.org/10.3390/nu2060611
Chanda S, Tiwari RK, Kumar A, Singh K (2019) Nutraceuticals inspiring the current therapy for lifestyle diseases. Adv Pharmacol pharmaceut Sci 2019:1–5. https://doi.org/10.1155/2019/6908716
Chauhan B, Kumar G, Kalam N, Ansari SH (2013) Current concepts and prospects of herbal nutraceutical: a review. J Adv Pharm Technol Res 4:4–8. https://doi.org/10.4103/2231-4040.107494
Chen L, Liu X, Wong K (2016) Novel nanoparticle materials for drug/food delivery-polysaccharides. Physical Sci Rev 2016:1–19. https://doi.org/10.1515/psr-2016-0053
Crater JS, Carrier RL (2010) Barrier properties of gastrointestinal mucus to nanoparticle transport. Macromol Biosci 10:1473–1483. https://doi.org/10.1002/mabi.201000137
Das L, Bhaumik E, Raychaudhuri U, Chakraborty R (2011) Role of nutraceuticals in human health. J Food Sci Technol 49:173–183. https://doi.org/10.1007/s13197-011-0269-4
de Boer FY, Imhof A, Velikov KP (2019) Encapsulation of colorants by natural polymers for food applications. Coloration Technol 135:183–194. https://doi.org/10.1111/cote.12393
DeFrates K, Markiewicz T, Gallo P, Rack A, Weyhmiller A, Jarmusik B, Hu X (2018) Protein polymer-based nanoparticles: fabrication and medical applications. Int J Mol Sci 19:1–20. https://doi.org/10.3390/ijms19061717
Dima C, Assadpour E, Dima S, Jafari SM (2020) Bioavailability of the nutraceuticals: role of the food matrix, processing conditions, the gastrointestinal tract, and nanodelivery systems. Compr Rev Food Sci Food Saf 19:954–994. https://doi.org/10.1111/1541-4337.12547
Doan VTH, Lee JH, Takahashi R, Nguyen PTM, Nguyen VAT, Pham HTT, Fujii S, Sakurai K (2020) Cyclodextrin-based nanoparticles encapsulating α-mangostin and their drug release behavior: potential carriers of α-mangostin for cancer therapy. Polym J 52:457–466. https://doi.org/10.1038/s41428-019-0296-y
Donsì F (2018) Applications of nanoemulsions in foods. In: Jafari SM, McClements DJ (eds) Nanoemulsions. Academic, Cambridge, pp 349–377. https://doi.org/10.1016/B978-0-12-811838-2.00011-4
Efthimiadou EK, Metaxa AF, Kordas G (2015) Modified polysaccharides for drug delivery. In: Ramawat K, Mérillon JM (eds) Polysaccharides. Springer, Cham, pp 1–26
Esmaili M, Ghaffari SM, Moosavi-Movahedi Z et al (2011) Beta casein-micelle as a nano vehicle for solubility enhancement of curcumin; food industry application. LWT-Food Sci Technol 44:2166–2172. https://doi.org/10.1016/j.lwt.2011.05.023
Fang R, Jing H, Chai Z, Zhao G, Stoll S, Ren F, Liu F, Leng X (2011) Design and characterization of protein-quercetin bioactive nanoparticles. J Nanobiotechnol 9:1–14. https://doi.org/10.1186/1477-3155-9-19
Farooq MA, Li L, Parveen A, Wang B (2020) Globular protein stabilized nanoparticles for delivery of disulfiram: fabrication, characterization, in vitro toxicity, and cellular uptake. RSC Adv 10:133–144. https://doi.org/10.1039/C9RA09468G
Fathi M, Varshosaz J, Mohebbi M, Shahidi F (2013) Hesperetin-loaded solid lipid nanoparticles and nanostructure lipid carriers for food fortification: preparation, characterization, and modeling. Food Bioprocess Technol 6:1464–1475. https://doi.org/10.1007/s11947-012-0845-2

Gaudana R, Khurana V, Parenky A, Mitra AK (2011) Encapsulation of protein-polysaccharide hip complex in polymeric nanoparticles. J Drug Deliv 2011:1–7. https://doi.org/10.1155/2011/458128

Gera M, Sharma N, Ghosh M, Huynh DL, Lee SJ, Min T, Kwon T, Jeong DK (2017) Nanoformulations of curcumin: an emerging paradigm for improved remedial application. Oncotarget 8:66680–66698. https://doi.org/10.18632/oncotarget.19164

Gidwani B, Vyas A (2015) A comprehensive review on cyclodextrin-based carriers for delivery of chemotherapeutic cytotoxic anticancer drugs. Biomed Res Int 2015:1–15. https://doi.org/10.1155/2015/198268

Głąb TK, Boratyński J (2017) Potential of casein as a carrier for biologically active agents. Top Curr Chem (Cham) 375:1–20. https://doi.org/10.1007/s41061-017-0158-z

Glaubitt K, Ricci M, Giovagnoli S (2019) Exploring the nano spray-drying technology as an innovative manufacturing method for solid lipid nanoparticle dry powders. AAPS Pharm Sci Tech 20:1–19. https://doi.org/10.1208/s12249-018-1203-0

Gordillo-Galeano A, Mora-Huertas CE (2018) Solid lipid nanoparticles and nanostructured lipid carriers: a review emphasizing on particle structure and drug release. Eur J Pharm Biopharm 133:285–308. https://doi.org/10.1016/j.ejpb.2018.10.017

Goswami HK, Ram HK (2017) Ancient food habits dictate that food can be medicine but medicine cannot be "food"!! Medicines (Basel) 4:1–23. https://doi.org/10.3390/medicines4040082

Guichard E (2002) Interactions between flavor compounds and food ingredients and their influence on flavor perception. Food Rev Int 18:49–70. https://doi.org/10.1081/FRI-120003417

Gupta R, Xie H (2018) Nanoparticles in daily life: applications, toxicity and regulations. J Environ Pathol Toxicol Oncol 37:209–230. https://doi.org/10.1615/JEnvironPatholToxicolOncol.2018026009

Gutiérrez TJ (2017) Chitosan applications for the food industry. In: Ahmed S, Ikram S (eds) Chitosan: derivatives, composites, and application. Wiley, New York, pp 183–232. https://doi.org/10.1002/9781119364849.ch8

Haider M, Abdin SM, Kamal L, Orive G (2020) Nanostructured lipid carriers for delivery of chemotherapeutics: a review. Pharmaceutics 12:1–26. https://doi.org/10.3390/pharmaceutics12030288

Haimhoffer A, Rusznyák A, Réti-Nagy K et al (2019) Cyclodextrins in drug delivery systems and their effects on biological barriers. Sci Pharm 87:1–21. https://doi.org/10.3390/scipharm87040033

Hamad AF, Han JH, Kim BC, Rather IA (2018) The intertwine of nanotechnology with the food industry. Saudi J Biol Sci 25:27–30. https://doi.org/10.1016/j.sjbs.2017.09.004

Helal NA, Eassa HA, Amer AM, Eltokhy MA, Edafiogho I, Nounou MI (2019) Nutraceuticals' novel formulations: the good, the bad, the unknown and patents involved. Recent Pat Drug Deliv Formul 13:105–156. https://doi.org/10.2174/1872211313666190503112040

Hu F, Fu S, Huang J, Anderson DP, Chang PR (2014) Structure and properties of polysaccharide nanocrystals. In: Huang J, Chang PR, Lin N, Dufresne A (eds) Polysaccharide-based nanocrystals. Wiley, New York, pp 15–62. https://doi.org/10.1002/9783527689378.ch2

Hudson D, Margaritis A (2014) Biopolymer nanoparticle production for controlled release of biopharmaceuticals. Crit Rev Biotechnol 34:161–179. https://doi.org/10.3109/07388551.2012.743503

Ikuta N, Okamoto H, Furune T et al (2016) Bioavailability of an R-α-Lipoic acid/γ-cyclodextrin complex in healthy volunteers. Int J Mol Sci 17:1–10. https://doi.org/10.3390/ijms17060949

Jahanban-Esfahlan A, Dastmalchi S, Davaran S (2016) A simple improved desolvation method for the rapid preparation of albumin nanoparticles. Int J Biol Macromol 91:703–709. https://doi.org/10.1016/j.ijbiomac.2016.05.032

Jaiswal P, Gidwani B, Vyas A (2016) Nanostructured lipid carriers and their current application in targeted drug delivery. Artif Cells Nanomed Biotechnol 44:27–40. https://doi.org/10.3109/21691401.2014.909822

Jampilek J, Kos J, Kralova K (2019) Potential of nanomaterial applications in dietary supplements and foods for special medical purposes. Nanomaterials (Basel) 9:1–42. https://doi.org/10.3390/nano9020296

Jones OG, McClements DJ (2010) Biopolymer nanoparticles from heat-treated electrostatic protein–polysaccharide complexes: factors affecting particle characteristics. J Food Sci 75:N36–N43. https://doi.org/10.1111/j.1750-3841.2009.01512.x

Jones OG, Decker EA, McClements DJ (2010) Comparison of protein–polysaccharide nanoparticle fabrication methods: impact of biopolymer complexation before or after particle formation. J Colloid Interface Sci 344:21–29. https://doi.org/10.1016/j.jcis.2009.12.017

Joye IJ, McClements DJ (2014) Biopolymer-based nanoparticles and microparticles: fabrication, characterization, and application. Curr Opin Colloid Interface Sci 19:417–427. https://doi.org/10.1016/j.cocis.2014.07.002

Kaczmarczyk MM, Miller MJ, Freund GG (2012) The health benefits of dietary fiber: beyond the usual suspects of type 2 diabetes mellitus, cardiovascular disease and colon cancer. Metabolism 61:1058–1066. https://doi.org/10.1016/j.metabol.2012.01.017

Kartsova LA, Alekseeva AV (2008) Effect of milk caseins on the concentration of polyphenolic compounds in tea. J Anal Chem 63:1107–1111. https://doi.org/10.1134/S1061934808110154

Katouzian I, Esfanjani AF, Jafari SM, Akhavan S (2017) Formulation and application of a new generation of lipid nano-carriers for the food bioactive ingredients. Trends Food Sci Technol 68:14–25. https://doi.org/10.1016/j.tifs.2017.07.017

Keller BC (2001) Liposomes in nutrition. Trends Food Sci Technol 12:25–31. https://doi.org/10.1016/S0924-2244(01)00044-9

Khorasani S, Danaei M, Mozafari MR (2018) Nanoliposome technology for the food and nutraceutical industries. Trends Food Sci Technol 79:106–115. https://doi.org/10.1016/j.tifs.2018.07.009

Khosa A, Reddi S, Saha RN (2018) Nanostructured lipid carriers for site-specific drug delivery. Biomed Pharmacother 103:598–613. https://doi.org/10.1016/j.biopha.2018.04.055

Khurana S, Venkataraman K, Hollingsworth A, Piche M, Tai TC (2013) Polyphenols: benefits to the cardiovascular system in health and in aging. Nutrients 5:3779–3827. https://doi.org/10.3390/nu5103777

Kumar B, Smita K (2017) Scope of nanotechnology in nutraceuticals. In: Oprea AE, Grumezescu AM (eds) Nanotechnology applications in food, vol 1. Academic, Cambridge, pp 43–63. https://doi.org/10.1016/B978-0-12-811942-6.00003-0

Kumar M, Bishnoi RS, Shukla AK, Jain CP (2019) Techniques for formulation of nanoemulsion drug delivery system: a review. Prev Nutr Food Sci 24:225–234. https://doi.org/10.3746/pnf.2019.24.3.225

Leidy R, Ximena QCM (2019) Use of electrospinning technique to produce nanofibres for food industries: a perspective from regulations to characterisations. Trends Food Sci Tech 85:92–106. https://doi.org/10.1016/j.tifs.2019.01.006

Li X, Anton N, Arpagaus C, Belleteix F, Vandamme TF (2010) Nanoparticles by spray drying using innovative new technology: the Büchinano spray dryer B-90. J Control Release 147:304–310. https://doi.org/10.1016/j.jconrel.2010.07.113

Lin N, Huang J, Chang ADP, Yu J (2011) Preparation, modification, and application of starch nanocrystals in nanomaterials: a review. Hindawi J Nanomater 2011:1–13. https://doi.org/10.1155/2011/573687

Liu X, Zhang R, McClements DJ, Li F, Liu H, Cao Y, Xiao H (2018) Nanoemulsion-based delivery systems for nutraceuticals: influence of long-chain triglyceride (LCT) type on in vitro digestion and astaxanthin bioaccessibility. Food Biophysics 13:412–421. https://doi.org/10.1007/s11483-018-9547-2

Liu Q, Huang H, Chen H, Lin J, Wang Q (2019) Food-grade nanoemulsions: preparation, stability and application in encapsulation of bioactive compounds. Molecules 24:1–37. https://doi.org/10.3390/molecules24234242

Loewen A, Chan B, Li-Chan ECY (2017) Optimization of vitamins a and D3 loading in re-assembled casein micelles and effect of loading on stability of vitamin D3 during storage. Food Chem 240:472–481. https://doi.org/10.1016/j.foodchem.2017.07.126

Lohcharoenkal W, Wang L, Chen YC, Rojanasakul Y (2014) Protein nanoparticles as drug delivery carriers for cancer therapy. Biomed Res Int 2014:1–12. https://doi.org/10.1155/2014/180549

Lopes M, Derenne A, Pereira C, Veiga F, Seica R, Sarmento B, Ribeiro A (2016) Impact of the in vitro gastrointestinal passage of biopolymer-based nanoparticles on insulin absorption. RSC Adv 6:20155–20165. https://doi.org/10.1039/C5RA26224K

López-López EA, Hernández-Gallegos MA, Cornejo-Mazón M, Hernández-Sánchez H (2015) Polysaccharide-based nanoparticles. In: Hernández-Sánchez H, Gutiérrez-López G (eds) Food nanoscience and nanotechnology, Food engineering series. Springer, Cham, pp 56–68. https://doi.org/10.1007/978-3-319-13596-0_1

Martínez-Ballesta M, Gil-Izquierdo Á, García-Viguera C (2018) Nanoparticles and controlled delivery for bioactive compounds: outlining challenges for new "smart-foods" for health. Foods 7:1–29. https://doi.org/10.3390/foods7050072

Martins JT, Bourbon AI, Pinheiro AC, Fasolin LH, Vicente AA (2018) Protein-based structures for food applications: from macro to nanoscale. Front Sustainable Food Syst 2:1–77. https://doi.org/10.3389/fsufs.2018.00077

Maurya VK, Aggarwal M (2017a) Factors influencing the absorption of vitamin D in GIT: an overview. J Food Sci Technol 54:3753–3765. https://doi.org/10.1007/s13197-017-2840-0

Maurya VK, Aggarwal M (2017b) Enhancing bio-availability of vitamin d by nano-engineered based delivery systems- an overview. Int J Curr Microbiol App Sci 6:340–353. https://doi.org/10.20546/ijcmas.2017.607.040

Maurya VK, Aggarwal M (2017c) Impact of aqueous/ethanolic goji berry (Lycium barbarum) fruit extract supplementation on vitamin D stability in yoghurt. Int J Curr Microbiol App Sci 6:2016–2029. https://doi.org/10.20546/ijcmas.2017.608.240

Maurya VK, Aggarwal M (2019) A phase inversion based nanoemulsion fabrication process to encapsulate vitamin D3 for food applications. J Steroid Biochem 190:88–98. https://doi.org/10.1016/j.jsbmb.2019.03.021

Maurya VK, Bashir K, Aggarwal M (2020) Vitamin D microencapsulation and fortification: trends and technologies. J Steroid Biochem Mol Biol 196:1–15. https://doi.org/10.1016/j.jsbmb.2019.105489

McClements DJ, Xiao H (2017) Is nano safe in foods? Establishing the factors impacting the gastrointestinal fate and toxicity of organic and inorganic food-grade nanoparticles. NPJ Sci Food 6:1–13. https://doi.org/10.1038/s41538-017-0005-1

McClements DJ, Li F, Xiao H (2015a) The nutraceutical bioavailability classification scheme: classifying nutraceuticals according to factors limiting their oral bioavailability. Annu Rev Food Sci Technol 6:299–327. https://doi.org/10.1146/annurev-food-032814-014043

McClements DJ, Zou L, Zhang R, Salvia-Trujillo L, Kumosani T, Xiao H (2015b) Enhancing nutraceutical performance using excipient foods: designing food structures and compositions to increase bioavailability. Compr Rev Food Sci Food Saf 14:824–847. https://doi.org/10.1111/1541-4337.12170

Mohammadi M, Ghanbarzadeh B, Hamishehkar H (2014) Formulation of nanoliposomal vitamin D3 for potential application in beverage fortification. Adv Pharm Bull 4:569–575. https://doi.org/10.5681/apb.2014.084

Mohan MS, Jurat-Fuentes JL, Harte F (2013) Binding of vitamin a by casein micelles in commercial skim milk. J Dairy Sci 96:790–798. https://doi.org/10.3168/jds.2012-5777

Mu R, Hong X, Ni Y, Li Y, Pang J, Wang Q, Xiao J, Zheng Y (2019) Recent trends and applications of cellulose nanocrystals in food industry. Trends Food Sci Tech 93:136–144. https://doi.org/10.1016/j.tifs.2019.09.013

Naseri N, Valizadeh H, Zakeri-Milani P (2015) Solid lipid nanoparticles and nanostructured lipid carriers: structure, preparation and application. Adv Pharm Bull 5:305–313. https://doi.org/10.15171/apb.2015.043

Neamtu I, Chiriac AP, Nita L, Diaconu A, Rusu AG (2019) Nanogels containing polysaccharides for bioapplications. In: Vasile C (ed) Micro and nano technologies, polymeric nanomaterials in nanotherapeutics. Elsevier, Amsterdam, pp 387–420. https://doi.org/10.1016/B978-0-12-813932-5.00011-X

Nile SH, Baskar V, Selvaraj D, Nile A, Xiao J, Kai G (2020) Nanotechnologies in food science: applications, recent trends, and future perspectives. Nano-Micro Lett 12:1–34. https://doi.org/10.1007/s40820-020-0383-9

Nitta SK, Numata K (2013) Biopolymer-based nanoparticles for drug/gene delivery and tissue engineering. Int J Mol Sci 14:1629–1654. https://doi.org/10.3390/ijms14011629

Ntoutoume GMAN, Granet R, Mbakidi JP et al (2016) Development of curcumin-cyclodextrin/cellulose nanocrystals complexes: new anticancer drug delivery systems. Bioorg Med Chem Lett 26:941–945. https://doi.org/10.1016/j.bmcl.2015.12.060

Oliveira JT, Reis RL (2008) Hydrogels from polysaccharide-based materials: fundamentals and applications in regenerative medicine. In: Reis RL, Neves NM, Mano JF et al (eds) Natural-based polymers for biomedical applications, Woodhead Publishing series in biomaterials. Woodhead Publishing, pp 485–514. https://doi.org/10.1533/9781845694814.4.485

Omar SM, Ibrahim F, Ismail A (2020) Formulation and evaluation of cyclodextrin-based nanosponges of griseofulvin as pediatric oral liquid dosage form for enhancing bioavailability and masking bitter taste. Saudi Pharm J 28:349–361. https://doi.org/10.1016/j.jsps.2020.01.016

Pan K, Zhong Q (2016) Organic nanoparticles in foods: fabrication, characterization, and utilization. Annu Rev Food Sci Technol 7:245–266. https://doi.org/10.1146/annurev-food-041715-033215

Panahi Y, Farshbaf M, Mohammadhosseini M, Mirahadi M, Khalilov R, Saghfi S, Akbarzadeh A (2017) Recent advances on liposomal nanoparticles: synthesis, characterization and biomedical applications. Artif Cells Nanomed Biotechnol 45:788–799. https://doi.org/10.1080/21691401.2017.1282496

Pandey AP, More MP, Karande KP, Chitalkar RV, Patil PO, Deshmukh PK (2017) Optimization of desolvation process for fabrication of lactoferrin nanoparticles using quality by design approach. Artif Cells Nanomed Biotechnol 45:1101–1114. https://doi.org/10.1080/21691401.2016.1202259

Parrot-Lopez H, Perret F, Bertino-Ghera B (2010) Amphiphilic cyclodextrins and their applications. Preparation of nanoparticles based on amphiphilic cyclodextrins for biomedical applications. Ann Pharm Fr 68:12–26. https://doi.org/10.1016/j.pharma.2009.12.002

Pattekari P, Zheng Z, Zhang X, Levchenko T, Torchilin V, Lvov Y (2011) Top-down and bottom-up approaches in production of aqueous nanocolloids of low solubility drug paclitaxel. Phys Chem Chem Phys 13:9014–9019. https://doi.org/10.1039/c0cp02549f

Peinado I, Lesmes U, Andrés A, McClements JD (2010) Fabrication and morphological characterization of biopolymer particles formed by electrostatic complexation of heat treated lactoferrin and anionic polysaccharides. Langmuir 26:9827–9834. https://doi.org/10.1021/la1001013

Peñalva R, Morales J, González-Navarro CJ, Larrañeta E, Quincoces G, Peñuelas I, Irache JM (2018) Increased oral bioavailability of resveratrol by its encapsulation in casein nanoparticles. Int J Mol Sci 19:1–17. https://doi.org/10.3390/ijms19092816

Priyadarshi R, Rhim JW (2020) Chitosan-based biodegradable functional films for food packaging applications. Innov Food Sci Emerg Technol 62:1–82. https://doi.org/10.1016/j.ifset.2020.102346

Punia S, Sandhu KS, Kaur M, Siroha AK (2019) Nanotechnology: a successful approach to improve nutraceutical bioavailability. In: Prasad R, Kumar V, Kumar M, Choudhary D (eds) Nanobiotechnology in bioformulations, Nanotechnology in the life sciences. Springer, Cham, pp 119–133. https://doi.org/10.1007/978-3-030-17061-5_5

Puri A, Loomis K, Smith B, Lee JH, Yavlovich A, Heldman E, Blumenthal R (2009) Lipid-based nanoparticles as pharmaceutical drug carriers: from concepts to clinic. Crit Rev Drug Carrier Syst 26:523–580. https://doi.org/10.1615/critrevtherdrugcarriersyst.v26.i6.10

Qian C, McClements DJ (2011) Formation of nanoemulsions stabilized by model food-grade emulsifiers using high-pressure homogenization: factors affecting particle size. Food Hydrocoll 25:1000–1008. https://doi.org/10.1016/j.foodhyd.2010.09.017

Ranby BG (1949) Aqueous colloidal solutions of cellulose micelles. Acta Chem Scand 3:649–650. https://doi.org/10.3891/acta.chem.scand.03-0649

Rao PJ, Naidu MM (2016) Nanoencapsulation of bioactive compounds for nutraceutical food. In: Ranjan S, Dasgupta N, Lichtfouse E (eds) Nanoscience in food and agriculture 2, Sustainable agriculture reviews, vol 21. Springer, Cham, pp 129–156. https://doi.org/10.17533/udea.vitae.v26n2a01

Salvia-Trujillo L, Martín-Belloso O, McClements DJ (2016) Excipient Nanoemulsions for improving Oral bioavailability of bioactives. Nanomaterials (Basel) 6:1–16. https://doi.org/10.3390/nano6010017

Semo E, Kesselman E, Danino D, Livney YD (2007) Casein micelle as a natural nano-capsular vehicle for nutraceuticals. Food Hydrocoll 21:936–942. https://doi.org/10.1016/j.foodhyd.2006.09.006

Sharma N, Baldi A (2016) Exploring versatile applications of cyclodextrins: an overview. Drug Deliv 23:729–747. https://doi.org/10.3109/10717544.2014.938839

Sheikhi A, Hayashi J, Eichenbaum J, Gutin M, Kuntjoro N, Khorsandi D, Khademhosseini A (2019) Recent advances in nanoengineering cellulose for cargo delivery. J Control Release 28:53–76. https://doi.org/10.1016/j.jconrel.2018.11.024

Sridhar R, Ramakrishna S (2013) Electrosprayed nanoparticles for drug delivery and pharmaceutical applications. Biomatter 3:1–12. https://doi.org/10.4161/biom.24281

Srinivas PR, Philbert M, Vu TQ et al (2010) Nanotechnology research: applications in nutritional sciences. J Nutr 140:119–124. https://doi.org/10.3945/jn.109.115048

Sun Y, Xia Z, Zheng J, Qiuab P, Zhang L, McClements DJ, Xiaoa H (2015) Nanoemulsion-based delivery systems for nutraceuticals: influence of carrier oil type on bioavailability of pterostilbene. J Functional Foods 13:61–70. https://doi.org/10.1016/j.jff.2014.12.030

Tamjidi F, Shahedi M, Varshosaz J, Nasirpour A (2013) Nanostructured lipid carriers (NLC): a potential delivery system for bioactive food molecules. Innov Food Sci Emerg Technol 19:29–43. https://doi.org/10.1016/j.ifset.2013.03.002

Tiwari G, Tiwari R, Rai AK (2010) Cyclodextrins in delivery systems: applications. J Pharm Bioallied Sci 2:72–79. https://doi.org/10.4103/0975-7406.67003

Uekaji Y, Terao K (2019) Bioavailability enhancement of hydrophobic nutraceuticals using γ-cyclodextrin. J Incl Phenom Macrocycl Chem 93:3–15. https://doi.org/10.1007/s10847-018-0856-3

Vanderfleet OM, Osorio DA, Cranston ED (2018) Optimization of cellulose nanocrystal length and surface charge density through phosphoric acid hydrolysis. Philos Trans A Math Phys Eng Sci 376:1–17. https://doi.org/10.1098/rsta.2017.0041

Verma D, Gulati N, Kaul S, Mukherjee S, Nagaich U (2018) Protein based nanostructures for drug delivery. J Pharm (Cairo) 2018:1–18. https://doi.org/10.1155/2018/9285854

Wang S, Su R, Nie S, Sun M, Zhang J, Wu D, Moustaid-Moussa N (2014) Application of nanotechnology in improving bioavailability and bioactivity of diet-derived phytochemicals. J Nutr Biochem 25:363–376. https://doi.org/10.1016/j.jnutbio.2013.10.002

Williamson G, Kay CD, Crozier A (2018) The bioavailability, transport, and bioactivity of dietary flavonoids: a review from a historical perspective. Compr Rev Food Sci Food Saf 17:1054–1112. https://doi.org/10.1111/1541-4337.12351

Wu C, Chen Z, Hu Y, Rao Z, Wu W, Yang Z (2018) Nanocrystals: the preparation, precise control and application toward the pharmaceutics and food industry. Curr Pharm Des 24:2425–2431. https://doi.org/10.2174/1381612824666180515124614

Xiao H, Yang T, Lin Q, Liu GQ, Yu F, Chen Y (2016) Acetylated starch nanocrystals: preparation and antitumor drug delivery study. Int J Biol Macromol 89:456–464. https://doi.org/10.1016/j.ijbiomac.2016.04.037

Xue J, Wang T, Hu Q, Zhou M, Luo Y (2018) Insight into natural biopolymer-emulsified solid lipid nanoparticles for encapsulation of curcumin: effect of loading methods. Food Hydrocoll 79:110–116. https://doi.org/10.1016/j.foodhyd.2017.12.018

Yu H, Park JY, Kwon CW, Hong SC, Park KM, Chang PS (2018) An overview of nanotechnology in food science: preparative methods, practical applications, and safety. J Chem 2018:1–10. https://doi.org/10.1155/2018/5427978

Zardini AA, Mohebbi M, Farhoosh R, Bolurian S (2018) Production and characterization of nano-structured lipid carriers and solid lipid nanoparticles containing lycopene for food fortification. J Food Sci Technol 55:287–298. https://doi.org/10.1007/s13197-017-2937-5

Zhong J, Yang R, Cao X, Liu X, Qin X (2018) Improved physicochemical properties of yogurt fortified with fish oil/γ-oryzanol by nanoemulsion technology. Molecules 23:1–11. https://doi.org/10.3390/molecules23010056

Zhu F (2017) Encapsulation and delivery of food ingredients using starch-based systems. Food Chem 229:542–552. https://doi.org/10.1016/j.foodchem.2017.02.101

Zou L, Liu W, Liu C, Xiao H, McClements DJ (2015) Utilizing food matrix effects to enhance nutraceutical bioavailability: increase of curcumin bioaccessibility using excipient emulsions. J Agric Food Chem 63:2052–2062. https://doi.org/10.1021/jf506149f

Chapter 7
Bacteriophage in Food Industry: NanoPhageBots

Avtar Sain and N. S. Jayaprakash

Abstract Food is the best medicine. However, healthy and safe food is a dire need as it keeps one healthy and prevents disease, thus more often than not obviates the use of medicine. Food spoilage by any means such as chemical additives, physical damage or biological contamination by bacteria and fungi leads to deterioration of food quality, taste, nutritional value, colour and texture. Nevertheless, bacteria are one of the main causative agents of food spoilage during storage as well as transportation due to which food poisoning is the biggest problem living being has ever encountered. Extensive use of the antibiotics has created an environment of distress and crisis, as the antibiotic resistant bacteria are on the rise. Use of the antibiotics in food and agro is one of the major causes of evolution of the multidrug resistant bacteria. When we look for the alternatives of the antibiotics in the scenario of MDR, bacteriophages prove themselves as potential candidates. Phages range from 50 nm to 250 nm in size placing them in a nanometre scale. Due to their size, shape, specificity and modus operandi, bacteriophage can be rightly called *bio robots* or *nanoPhagebots*. Application of specific bacteriophages and engineered phages at different stages of food production, transport, storage and pathogen detection has been proven to be highly efficient in combating food spoilage and subduing food borne illnesses caused by pathogenic bacteria. Moreover, encapsulation and formulation have been brought in the process for the efficient utility of the phage products. Several phages and phage products are available in the market for use as they have been certified as safe, whereas many are in the clinical phase trials stage. The current chapter focuses on the applications of bacteriophage and phage products in food sector, their health hazards, and safety regulations for their use in food industries.

Keywords Food · Pathogen · Drug resistance · Bacteriophage · Biofilms · Encapsulation · Preservation · Endolysin · Phage cocktail · Engineered phage

---

A. Sain · N. S. Jayaprakash (✉)
Centre for Bioseparation Technology, Vellore Institute of Technology, Vellore, Tamil Nadu, India
e-mail: nsjayaprakash@vit.ac.in

V. K. Maurya et al. (eds.), *Sustainable Agriculture Reviews 55*, Sustainable Agriculture Reviews 55, https://doi.org/10.1007/978-3-030-76813-3_7

Abbreviations

CFU	Colony forming unit
DNA	Deoxyribo nucleic acid
dsDNA	Double stranded Deoxyribo nucleic acid
dsRNA	Double stranded ribonucleic acid
ELISA	Enzyme linked immunesorbet assay
LAB	Lactic acid bacteria
MDR	Multidrug resistant
PCR	Polymerase chain reaction
PFU	Plaque forming unit
RNA	Ribonucleic acid
SPR	Surface plasmon resonance
ssDNA	Single stranded Deoxyribo nucleic acid
ssRNA	Single stranded ribonucleic acid
UV	Ultra-violate
XDR	Extensively drug resistant

7.1 Introduction

Since time immemorial, humans in various cultures across the world have strived to preserve their food using various methods of which pickling (Montaño et al. 2015), drying (Kumar et al. 2015), sugaring, salting (all of which targeted removing moisture) are a few (Hall 2010). Food preservation helps to combat several ways of nutrition deprivation such as those due to seasonal and geographical (which needs food to be transported) unavailability of food. It was not until the late nineteenth century that the underlying cause of food spoilage was discovered. Food spoilage occurs either by the virtue of microbial growth (Table 7.1) such as that of bacteria which thrive by feeding on the nutrients in food. This makes the food inedible for humans who not only consume the food deprived of nutrients or containing oxidized nutrients but also the bacteria itself which may have immediate life-threatening effects, known as food poisoning (Rawat 2015). Since the discovery of the culpable bacteria in food spoilage all the efforts were zeroed in on killing the microorganisms and creating an environment hostile for their growth. To fulfil this global need, scientists slowly pushed the boundaries of their contemporary research by discovering elegant methods of preservations such as air-tight storage, pasteurization, fermentation, canning, chemical additives, freezing, etc. each having its own limitations with respect to time of preservation (Varzakas and Tzia 2015). With the advancement in science and technology, preservation processes such as vacuum drying, irradiation, chemical preservatives and quick-freezing which increase the shelf-life of food have found applications in manufacturing packed food, frozen food and ready-to-eat food at food industries (Amit et al. 2017).

Table 7.1 A list of common food borne infectious bacteria, respective phages against them and their significance

Bacteria	Phage	Food	Significance	Year	References
Listeria monocytogenes	New isolates	Ready to eat food	Phage displayed oligo peptide magnetoelastic biosensor platforms for real time detection	2018	Chin et al. (2018)
Listeria monocytogenes	Mixture of phages	Honeydew melonslices	Reduced L. monocytogenes populations by 2.0–4.6 logcycles	2003	Leverentz et al. (2003)
Listeria monocytogenes	P100 (Myoviridae)	Food decontamination	Broad host range	2005	Carlton et al. (2005); Guenther et al. (2009)
S. aureus	Phage K	Raw milk and raw whey			Gill et al. (2006); O'Flaherty et al. (2005)
S. aureus	Cocktail of s88 and s35	Whole milk	Complete elimination of bacteria at MOI 100		Obeso et al. (2010); García et al. (2007)
Salmonella typhimurium and S. Enteritidis	Myoviridae phage-A	Broccoli and mustardseeds	Achieved 1.4 suppressions of Salmonella growth	2004	Pao et al. (2006)
S. Montevideo	Siphoviridae phage-B	Mustardseeds	1.5 log suppressions of Salmonella growth	2004	Pao et al. (2006)
S. Oranienburg	SSP5 (Myoviridae) and SSP6 (Siphoviridae)	Alfalfa seeds		2009	Kocharunchitt et al. (2009)
E. coli	DT1, DT5 and DT6	Milk	Inactivation of enteropathogenic and Shiga toxigenic *E. coli*	2013	Tomat et al. (2013)
E. coli O157:H7	Cocktail (ECP-100)	Broccoli, tomato	Reduced count 95 to 100%	2008	Abuladze et al. (2008)

Although the inventions had been successful in preserving food from rotting, most of them have proven to be lethal causing serious health hazards such as cancers. Food preservation which started for the benefit of human nutrition and survival in itself was being harmful which has warranted safe biological methods for the same. Bio-preservation is a term used to describe those methods that use certain biological entities to inhibit the growth of other organisms that cause food spoilage. Fermentation of food is one of the ancient methods of bio-preservation where certain bacteria and yeast (probiotics) when added in controlled conditions produce and release substances such as organic acids- lactic acid and acetic acid and alcohol-ethanol, which render the environment unsuitable for the growth of other microbes and also compete with the pathogenic organisms for nutrients in food (Franks 2011; Sain et al. 2018). The most common and renowned method to encounter bacterial growth in the field of health and medicine for more than half a century now, is the use of chemical molecules known as antibiotics. Antibiotic abuse has resulted in MDR strains and XDR of bacteria whose growth is impossible to be curbed by conventional antibiotics. Scientists across the globe have been striving to subdue antibiotic resistance and the discovery of bacteriophages served as a solace in establishing alternatives. Bacteriophage, phage or bacterial viruses are the most abundant biological units in biosphere with approximate numbers 10^{31} particles. Bacteriophages can dwell in all conditions, wherever their host is present, as they feed on bacteria specifically as obligate parasite and they out number their host by 10 times. There are enormous applications that bacteriophages have been isolated and studied for as depicted in Fig. 7.1, among which their use in food-preservation stands as a remarkable stride in combating food-spoilage and food-borne illness.

Any eukaryotic living system generally contains probiotics which helps in its living and the use of bacteriophages does not interfere with these probiotics while targeting the pathogenic bacteria by virtue of high specificity of bacteriophages. Furthermore, applications of bacteriophage are self-limiting i.e. they do not need successive dosage as they are capable of self-replication in proportion to the host

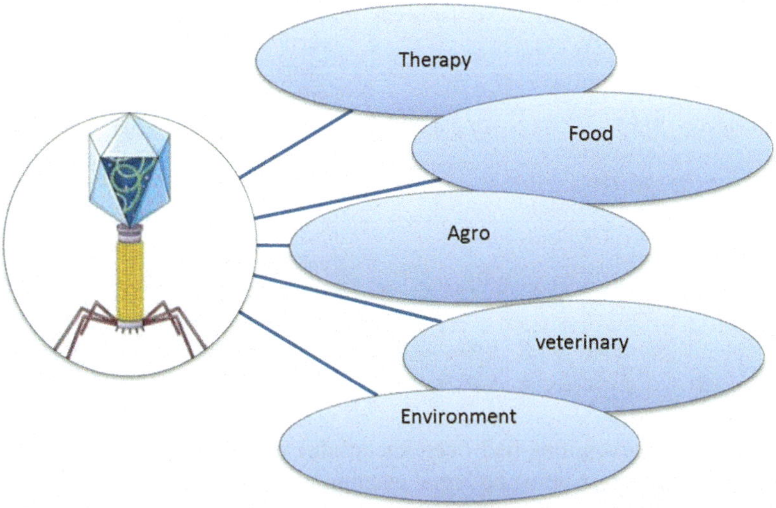

Fig. 7.1 Bacteriophage application: Phages can be applied in major fields such as therapy, food industry, agriculture science, veterinary field and environment as biocontrol agent against pathological bacteria

concentration and cease their growth with the clearance of bacteria. The co-evolution of bacteriophages along with bacteria also reassures that this anti-bacterial agent has very little chance of its host's resistance. Bacteriophages find wide range of applications in treating infections in humans and wound healing, treatment of tooth decay, control of biofilm, agriculture for bio-control of plant pathogens, molecular biology and protein related research as a laboratory technique- phage display (Morozova et al. 2018). Bacteriophage research in isolating and studying the potentiality of application has been making remarkable progress since a few decades to tame the growth of bacteria in various realms of existence. Moreover, Phage-based vaccination is one of the latter-day applications which supersedes conventional methods of vaccination delivery (Harada et al. 2018; Ul Haq et al. 2012). This chapter exclusively deals with the use of bacteriophages in food industry during manufacturing, packaging, storage, processing and transportation of food of all their other applications.

7.2 Basics of Phage Biology

7.2.1 Classification of Bacteriophage

Bacteriophage grouping or classification comes under the Bacterial and Archaeal Subcommittee (BAVS) within the International Committee on Taxonomy of Viruses (ICTV). The classification is based on the different characteristic properties possessed by a bacteriophage such as nucleic acid as genetic material (DNA or RNA), structure of capsid as shown in Fig. 7.2 (tailed, polyhedral, filamentous or pleomorphic), activity spectrum against various host, sequence similarity and pathogenicity (Chibani et al. 2019). Most known bacteriophages, approximately 96% belong to Caudovirales: an "Order of tail phage" consisting of three major families *Myoviridae, Podoviridae* and *Siphoviridae* containing phages of dsDNA as their genetic material (Ackermann 2011).

7.2.2 Life Cycle of the Bacteriophage

Figure 7.3 depicts the five phases of bacterial infection by phages. The first phase is the binding phase in which bacteriophage attaches itself to a surface receptor on a bacterium through one tail fiber. The attachment is facilitated by teichoic acid and lipoteichoic acid on gram positive bacteria and lipopolysaccharide on gram negative bacteria. The bacterial receptors for phage binding could be a protein on the surface of bacterium at any part of its structure. Tethering of one tail fiber restricts the movement of the phage and induces affinity of the rest of the tail fibers to bind to the receptor. This further orients the proteins of base plate leading to its three

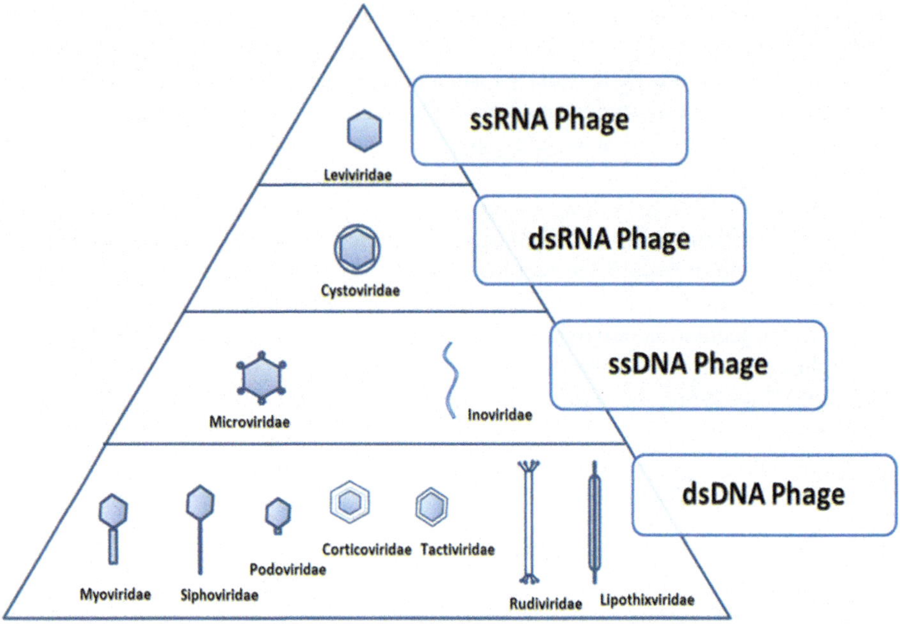

Fig. 7.2 Classification of phages based on the morphology and genetic material, ssDNA, dsDNA, ssRNA and dsRNA. Based on the tail morphology, phages have been classified as flexible noncontractile tail (Shiphoviridai), long nonflexible tail (Myoviridae and short tail (Podoviridae) (Harada et al. 2018)

dimensional conformation change which in turn induces the contraction of the sheath which pushes the phage further onto its host receptor (Harada et al. 2018).

The second stage, known as the penetration phase, is marked by the central spike protein of the base plate initiating a puncture on the host membrane which is followed by creation of an opening in the peptidoglycan layer by glycosidase enzyme. Certain bacteria contain a carbohydrate coating known as the glycocalyx which helps in its motility and adherence to surfaces creating aggregates also known as biofilms. Phages against such bacteria contain enzyme depolymerase which is an epoxypolysaccharide, a degrading enzyme, responsible for the degradation of glycocalyx (Wernicki et al. 2017). Penetration into the host cell is followed by the contraction of the capsid which pushes its genetic material into the host cytoplasm.

The third stage is the eclipse phase where the penetrated bacteriophage overpowers the metabolism of its host organism and begins to express proteins, necessary for replication, known as the early proteins. As the infection progresses, late proteins that form various parts of daughter phages are synthesized. This stage is followed by the assembly of the late proteins to form new daughter phages. The final stage is marked by the release of phages from its host. Tailed phages use the enzymes such as holin and lysin that help in puncturing holes and degrading the peptidoglycan layer respectively while the tailless phages contain lysis precipitating proteins that impair the maintenance machinery of the peptidoglycan layer (Fernandes and

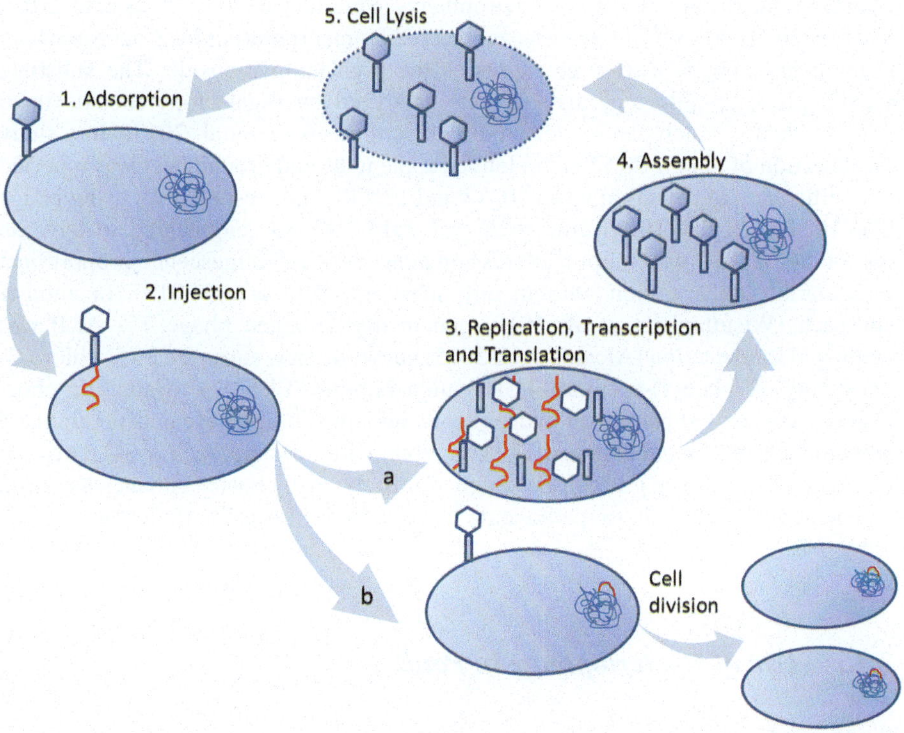

Fig. 7.3 Bacteriophage life cycle depiction: Phage can go under any of the two life cycles (**a**) Lytic cycle – the complete lytic cycle has been divided into 5 steps 1. adsorption 2. injection 3. replication 4. replication and 5. cell lysis, (**b**) lysogenic cycle

São-José 2018). The number of phages released per infected bacterium is known as the burst size which is the chief parameter for gauging the infection rate and ability of a particular phage (Ravi et al. 2017).

7.3 Application of Bacteriophage in Different Fields

7.3.1 Engineered Bacteriophages for Detection of Pathogenic Bacteria in Food

Bacterial pathogens in food can be detected using traditional techniques such as culture plating, PCR, ELISA and SPR but all these techniques have limitations related to cost, experience, skill, time and portability (Wei et al. 2019). Therefore, a sensitive, selective, cost effective, simple, novel and rapid detection technique needs to be developed. Bacteriophages have been engineered by using genetic engineering tools. These engineered phages have demonstrated great ability to detect pathogenic drug resistant bacteria in various environments (Smartt et al. 2012; Pires et al. 2016; Vinay et al. 2015). A T7 phage was engineered by incorporating *lac*Z operon which is upon infecting *E. coli* over expresses the β-galactopyranoside. The substrate 4-aminophenyl-β-galactopyranoside gets catalyzed by β-galactopyranoside in to p-aminophenol which can be detected by electrode (Wang et al. 2017). In a study the detection of *E. coli* O157:H7 in lettuce apple juice and ground beef was reported with efficiency of detection up to 10, 13 and 17 CFU/ mL respectively using phage phiV10. Phage phiV10 specific to *E. coli* O157:H7 was engineered to have an operon *luxCDABE* which upon expression generates bioluminescence proportional to bacterial concentration without any substrate (Kim et al. 2017). In another approach (Wisuthiphaet et al. 2019) genetically designed phage T7- ALP was employed for detection (Alcaine et al. 2015) but with a new substrate 2-(5′-chloro-2-phosphoryloxyphenyl)-6-chloro-4(3H)-quinazolinone (ELF-97) to alkaline phosphatase. This new substrate on hydrolysis by alkaline phosphatase gets precipitated and produces florescence. Phage T7-ALP along with new approach could detect up to 100 *E. coli* cells per gram of beverage. Similarly, many bacteriophages had been engineered for detection on pathogenic bacteria in food using different techniques Table 7.2.

7.3.2 Use of Bacteriophage in Poultry

Poultry is the most common non vegetarian food consumed worldwide, as poultry farming is the easiest and cheapest when compared to that of the other animals reared for meat. Chicken and egg consumption is very high in most developed nations with 80–95% of the population consuming chicken on a daily basis. Infections such as colibacillosis caused by *E. coli*, campylobacteriosis caused by *Campylobacter bacterium*, commonly *C. jejuni* and salmonellosis caused by *Salmonella* are very common poultry infections that pose substantial economic and health burden. These bacteria infect as many as 70–90% of the chickens in European countries and the United States (Goode et al. 2003). These bacteria show considerable resistance to antibiotics which has paved way for natural alternative i.e. bacteriophages (Wernicki et al. 2017). The most common bacteria in the digestive tract of poultry is *C. jejuni* which has not shown complete clearance by phage therapy but showed a significant reduction of about 2 log units. This could possibly be due to the bacteria developing resistance to phage as the faces contain both bacteria and phage. Preventive treatment with phages i.e. application before infection, in this case does not completely prevent the infection but cause a delay in colonization of the bacteria (Huff et al. 2002). *Clostridium perfringens* causes infection chiefly by the release of toxins. Phage treatments with whole phage, phage cocktail and phage endolysins have shown to be more effective than vaccines in decreasing the mortality rates (Miller et al. 2010).

Phage cocktail consisting of phages CNPSA1, CNPSA3 and CNPSA4 at a high single dosage of 10^{11} PFU/mL showed significant reduction in the infection caused

Table 7.2 detection of various pathogenic bacteria in different food items using engineered bacteriophage

Food	Pathogen	Phage	Technique	Significance	References
Egg	*Salmonella*	P22	Bioluminescence, Lux	Detection upto 10 CFU/ml	Chen and Griffiths (1996)
Water	*E. coli*	HK620, HK97	Luminescence, luxCDABE	Detection upto 10^4 bacteria/ mL in 1.5 h post infection	Franche et al. (2017)
Lettuce, sliced pork and milk	*Salmonella*	SPC32H-CDABE	Bioliminescencet, luxCDABE	Detection of at least 20 CFU/mL in 2 h	Kim et al. (2014)
Milk	*Salmonella*	E2 phage	Megnetoelastic	Detection limit of 5×10^3 cfu/ml	Lakshmanan et al. (2007)
Tomato	*Salmonella*	E2 phage	Megnetoelastic	Detected 6.1 and 7.8 logCFU/cm^2	Park et al. (2013)
Ground beef and milk	*Bacillusanthracis*	*B. Anthracis* phage Wβ	Bioluminescence, luxAB	Detection limit 80 to 8 CFU/mL in 7–16 h	Sharp et al. (2015)
Poulty	*Salmonella typhimurium*	P22	Bioluminescence, luxAB	Detection limit 5×10^2 to 1,65 $\times 10^5$ CFU/ mL	Thouand et al. (2008)
Water	*E.coli*	T4	Luminescent, LacZ, β-galactosidase gene	Detects <10 CFU/mL in 8 hour	Burnham et al. (2014)
Fresh spinach leaves	*Salmonella typhimurium*	E2 phage	Phage based megnetoelastic biosensor	Detects 100 CFU/25 g spinach	Wang et al. (2017)

by *Salmonella Enteritidis* as explained in the flow chart (Fig. 7.4) (Sklar and Joerger 2001; Fiorentin et al. 2005). *Salmonella Gallinarium* infected chicken showed a mortality rate of 5% when fed with bacteriophage as compared to 30% mortality rate in control population (Fiorentin et al. 2005). Bacteriophages are sometimes used in combination with probiotics for the treatment of infected chickens and resulted in tenfold decrease in bacterial concentration in different parts of chicken (Toro et al. 2005). Most of the studies have reported the reduction in infection (bacterial count) within the first week of phage administration and little effect of the same in the subsequent weeks when compared with untreated chickens. *Salmonella enterica* Serovar *Enteritidis* phage type 4 present in caeca of broiler chicken was found to be reduced in number upon treatment with its specific phage (Fiorentin et al. 2005). Bacteriophages administered through various route such as nasal, oral (through drinking water), intramuscular (Gigante and Atterbury 2019) and intracranial have significantly reduced *E. Coli* infections with 100% reduction in mortality

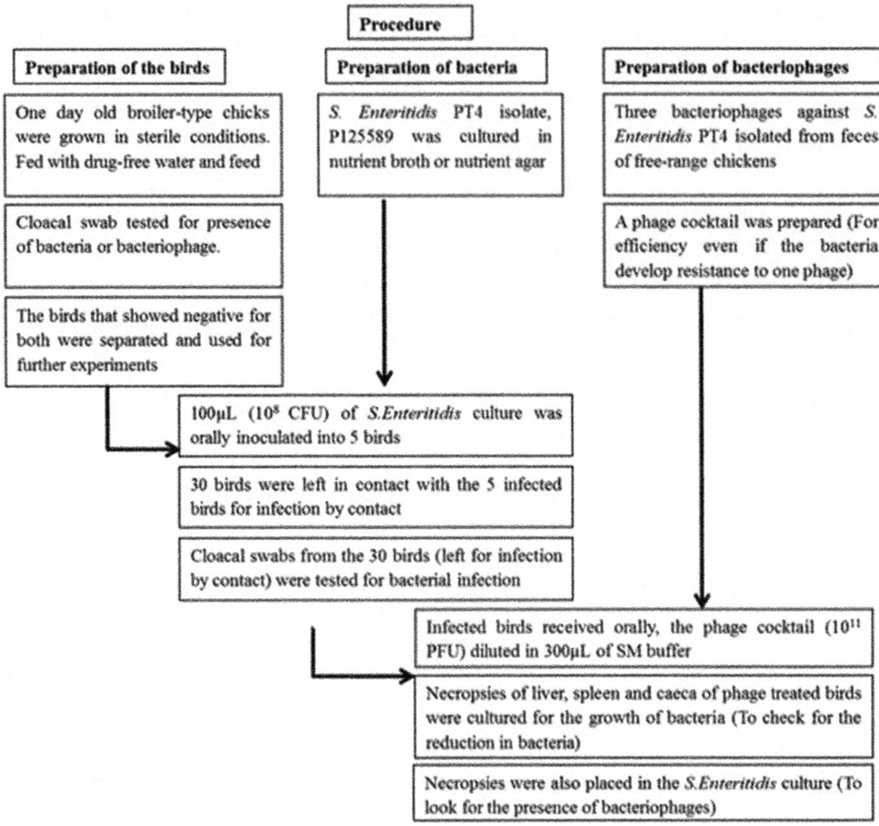

Fig. 7.4 The experimental process to determine the efficiency of bacteriophage cocktail against *S. Enteritidis*. During each of the steps mentioned in the flow chart, positive and negative controls were mandatorily maintained

rates in a few cases (Pouillot et al. 2012). However, application of phage preparations directly on to the site of infection has proved to be invariably more effective. Phage suspensions, in the form of aerosol, have also proved to be prophylactic to treat respiratory infections (Borie et al. 2008). A few other studies involving the use of cocktail of phages in combination with antibiotics have yielded positive outcomes in treating various types of infections (Tagliaferri et al. 2019).

Chorine water sprays, anti-bacterial sprays, UV light and heat have been commonly used to curb surface contamination of carcasses with some compromise having to be made with the quality of food or chemicals used. Phages used for decontamination of the surface of chicken skin proved to be efficient against *S. Enterica* Serovar *Enteritidis* and *C. jejuni* (Goode et al. 2003). Studies have also shown the bacteriophage's potential to decontaminate carcasses infected with *C. Jejuni* when used in combination with freezing (Atterbury et al. 2003). Bacteriophages against *Listeria monocytogenes* were effective in destroying surface bacteria on ready to eat poultry products and the food products showed to be free of bacterial contamination even after three weeks of treatment with phages in cold storage (Bigot et al. 2011). In the year 2006 FDA approved bacteriophage suspension 102-LMPTM against *L. monocytogenes* which has been effective against over 170 species of *Listeria* (Bren 2007). Optimizing concentration, route of delivery and age of the poultry is of cardinal importance for a particular phage preparation which would otherwise render the specific phages unavailing for use. Moreover, some phages may carry toxic genes or resistant genes which makes the phage unfit to use in biocontrol (Jamet et al. 2017). From the safety point of view, it is very important to characterize the full genome of any isolated phage (Sain and Jayaprakash 2020) before its use to have knowledge of encoded toxic proteins if any.

7.3.3 Use of Bacteriophage for Fish and Meat

Salmonella typhimurium, C. jejuni, Staphylococcus aureus, L. monocytogenes and *E. coli* O157:H7, are the most common bacteria present in meat and poultry. They are pathogenic and widely implicated in food spoilage. The various steps involved in processing and packaging of meat pave a major route of contamination. Bacteria have a very high chance of being spread to the entire lot from one part of the food by mere contact with the equipment either at the slaughter house or at the processing and packaging industry. Bacteriophages specific to the above mentioned organisms have been isolated and various methods of application have been explored to combat spoilage of meat. Bacteriophages can also be applied to the equipment used in the meat industry to forestall cross contamination. Treatment with ECP-100 of ground beef contaminated with 3400 CFU of *E. coli* O157:H7 reduced the bacteria by 95% at 10 °C in 24 h (Abuladze et al. 2008). A cocktail of three phages against *E. coli* O157:H7 when used on beef meat surface reduced the bacteria completely in seven cases out of nine. Even though there were bacteriophage-insensitive mutants, it did not seem to affect the preservation as these soon reverted and became sensitive to phage treatment (O'Flynn et al. 2004). Phages against *Salmonella typhimurium* and *Campylobacter jejuni* proved to be efficient on raw and cooked meat at 24 °C (Bigwood et al. 2008) and a phage preparation, FO1-E2 proved its efficiency on combating *Salmonella typhimurium* in sliced turkey/ turkey deli meat by more than 3 log units at 15 °C in 6 days (Guenther et al. 2012). Phage treatment against *Brochothrix thermosphacta* that causes spoilage of pork adipose tissue efficiently extended its storage period by 4 days (Greer and Dilts 2002). Contamination of pig carcasses with *Salmonella* was efficiently reduced by 99% when phage preparation PC1 was applied to post-slaughter pig skin which is most prone to contamination by *Salmonella typhimurium* U288 (Hooton et al. 2011).

Fish and other sea foods are generally contaminated by indigenous bacteria, present in marine environment, and exogenous bacteria that are introduced at the time of processing. Indigenous bacteria which include various species of *Vibrio* are not a major threat as far as spoilage is concerned as they are usually very low in number and can be completely obliterated by adequate cooking. The indigenous bacteria pose problems of spoilage only during transportation, processing and storage of sea food and lightly preserved fish products (LPFP). Exogenous bacteria include *Listeria monocytoogenes, Staphylococcus aureus, Clostridium perfringens, Salmonella, Shigella*, and *E. coli* which cause food spoilage even at low concentrations (Pilet and Leroi 2010). Simultaneous application of phage P100 and enterocin AS-48 against *L. monocytoogenes* in both raw and smoked salmon has shown a great reduction of the bacteria within 2 days of treatment (Baños et al. 2016). Listex P100 has also proven its efficiency on eradicating *L. monocytoogenes* contamination on the surface of fresh catfish fillets with reduction of 1 log units of bacteria in just half an hour of application and contamination free for about 10 days at 10 °C (Soni et al. 2010). *Shewanella putrefaciens* is the specific spoilage organism of chilled fish. Bacteriophage Spp001 extended *Paralichthys olivaceus* shelf life to about two weeks at 4 °C and proved more efficient than conventional potassium sorbate preservation (Li et al. 2014).

7.3.4 Use Bacteriophage for Fruits and Vegetables

A cocktail of three bacteriophages specific to *E. Coli* O15:H7 known as ECP-100 when sprayed on fresh cut lettuce and spinach showed bactericidal effect within the first half an hour of its application and resulted decline in pathogen population within 24 h (Sharma et al. 2009). The treatment proved to be more efficient with increase in dosage and temperature up to 37 °C (Abuladze et al. 2008). Another method of phage treatment of fresh cut green leafy vegetables is to immerse the produce in phage cocktail solution which is known to act slower compared to the spray technique but the product was pathogen free for one week when stored at 4 °C (Ferguson et al. 2013). The same phage cocktail against *E. coli*; ECP-100 when sprayed on tomatoes also reduced the bacterial concentration by 99% and also significantly reduced the pathogen on melons by spot treatment. Various other phage cocktails such as SCPLX-1 (four phages against *Salmonella enteritidis*) and LMP-102 9 (six phage cocktail) and LMP-103 (fourteen phage cocktail) against *Listeria monocytogens*) have also proved to be efficient in reducing bacterial growth on melons upon spot treatment (Sharma 2013). Although phage SCPLX-1 was not able to show any effect on sliced applies due to the low pH, both LMP-102 and LMP-103 were successful in their action (Leverentz et al. 2001). A bacteriophage cocktail ListShield™, has been approved by FDA for use on food products and has been successfully used on fresh cut leafy greens for their preservation (Boyacioglu et al. 2016).

A pore-forming bacteriocin known as nicin which is produced by lactic acid bacteria is the only approved bacteriocin in food preservation in various countries. Combination of bacteriophage cocktails have proved to be more effective in combating *L. monocytogens* than individual preparations. It is plausible that pores created on the bacterial cell membrane by Nisin would help in increased efficiency of phage in infecting the bacterium. The simultaneous application of phase and nisin would also result in the decreased development of bacterial mutants resistant against both the bacteriocin as well as the phage (Leverentz et al. 2003). Phages have also been tested for their efficiency in combating common scab caused by *Streptomycetes* in potatoes and bacterial spot in tomatoes caused by *Xanthomonas campestris* (McKenna et al. 2001; Obradovic et al. 2004).

7.3.5 Use of Bacteriophage in Dairy

For decades, bacteriophages were considered to be enemies of the dairy industry due to their implication in fermentation interference by infecting lactic acid bacteria (LAB) with detrimental effects both on quality of the product and also on the economic front. Intensive research on phages specific to the industry has unveiled various methods to circumvent the effect of phages on fermentation such as using mixed strains as starter cultures, highly concentrated frozen starter cultures, air-filtration and other sanitization techniques (Giraffa et al. 2017). Isolation and application of phage resistant starter strains (Madera et al. 2004), application of dynamic high pressure, phage inhibitory media, phage derived peptides that act against phages itself and phage-neutralizing antibody fragments are a few recently developed methods for inhibiting phage menace in dairy fermentation (Mc Grath et al. 2007).

Subsequent lysis of *Lactococcal* strains after fermentation to release intracellular peptidases are known to expedite cheese ripening and improve its flavor (O'Sullivan et al. 2000). This autolysis of bacteria varies with the strain type and environmental factors. Lysogenic/ temperate phages encode lytic genes and the prophage genes in the bacterial strains cause increase in their autolytic abilities (Fortier and Sekulovic 2013). Contamination by *Salmonella enteritidis* during manufacture, processing, storage and transport of cheddar cheese can be combated by SJ2 phage specific to the organism. The assumption was supported by a study that confirmed the absence of the organism even at the end of third month of storage after phage treatment (Modi et al. 2001). Listex P100, a phage preparation against *Lysteria monocytogenes,* (most common food spoilage bacterium) is an effective strategy in controlling the spoilage of cheese (Fernández et al. 2017). Milk is one of the most common sources of protein in most countries and is consumed daily. Phages against *Pseudomonas lactis* in raw milk have proved to be effective in the preservation of milk in cold storage. The phages are then inactivated by pasteurization (Tanaka et al. 2018). *Staphylococcus* and *Streptococcus* that cause mastitis in cattle and herd form the initial sources of milk contamination and phages (phiH5 and phiA72) against these microbes nips milk spoilage at the bud (Gutiérrez et al. 2019).

7.3.6 *Bacteriophage in Food Processing*

7.3.6.1 Bacteriophage in Food Packaging

The demand for safe, organic and natural products has grown over the time as the awareness for health and nutrition grew. Appropriate food packaging solves most of the problems associated with food spoilage and increase the shelf life of the product. Active packaging of the food items has been introduced to have enhanced shelf life, to maintain the quality of the product as well as the safety of the consumers. This mode of packaging called active, intelligent or smart packaging involves innovative ways which use the oxygen scavenging systems, CO_2 generating systems, ethanol generating systems and moisture controlling systems. Apart from these, some of the commonly used methods are listed in the Table 7.3 along with their limitations.

Bacteriophages have been proved as a promising alternate bio-control agent. In a recent study, bacteriophage was incorporated into an absorbent food pad and tested for the efficacy in food packing. According to this report, mixture of six salmonella phages were absorbed in a food pad which was used for packaging chilled meat. Study showed the significant reduction of bacterial load up to 0.87 log cycles in treated food items (Gouvêa et al. 2016). Bacteriophages could be administered in number of ways such as immobilizing on various surfaces, impregnating to paper and encapsulation in alginate beads and use in food packaging. Seed sprouts, cantaloupe and ready to eat food were stored for days in these materials to successfully prevent *E. coli* and *Listeria monocytogenes* (Lone et al. 2016). Polyethylene oxide (PEO) a food packaging material was studied for the adsorption and slow release of the phage particle while in contact with food. It was found that the thickness of the PEO fibre is directly proportional to the release rate of phage to a significant extent (Korehei and Kadla 2014).

Today's active packaging of food items has very broad range of antimicrobial activity. However, many of the microorganisms are non-pathogenic and beneficial to consumer. Nonetheless, these microorganisms are necessity of dairy industry for production and flavouring. So, the need of the hour is to develop a selective and specific target-oriented packaging material that could fulfil the requirement of being antimicrobial as well as selective to pathogens only. In this regard bacteriophages are propitious. The stability of phages is a crucial aspect of their application under different conditions. The packaging materials used in food packaging should be compatible to the survival of phages and uses thereof. In addition to survivability of

Table 7.3 Common techniques used in food industries for food preservation and their limitations

Techniques	Limitations	Year	References
Heat pasteurization	Fresh food	2018	Moye et al. (2018)
High pressure processing	Fresh food	2012	Bajovic et al. (2012)
Irradiation	Organoleptic quality	2014	Suklim et al. (2014)
Chemical sterilization	Corrosive	2016	Sohaib et al. (2016)

phages, their absorption and release rate need to be taken into account for better results.

7.3.6.2 Bacteriophage in Food Preservation

Food items, be it a fresh produce or frozen meat, need to be preserved until their consumption. During this preservation, these items tend to get spoilt. *Listeria monocytogenes* one of the pathogenic bacteria could stay alive at refrigerating temperature especially in ready to eat food. A phage (Listex™ p100) preparation specific to *L. monocytogenes* was found more effective while treating the sliced ham (Figueiredo and Almeida 2017) and deli meat (Chibeu et al. 2013) in comparison to Nisin (bacteriocin) at 4–8 °C. One species of the bacteria can be targeted by many bacteriophages. The mixture of the different phages is called phage cocktail. The use of Phage cocktails is more effective than single phage in terms of wide range within a species and to thwart resistance development by bacteria. Phage cocktails have also been used along with other antimicrobial agents such as sodium diacetate and potassium lactate which demonstrated better outcomes (Kim et al. 2019). Similarly, ListShield™ a phage cocktail targeting *L. monocytogenes* is an another example of commercially available bio-control agent (Moye et al. 2018).

7.3.7 *Control and Prevention of Biofilm in Food Industry Using Bacteriophage*

Food contamination happens gradually and intensifies while passing through several hands, equipment, surfaces and units from field to plate. *Staphylococcus* and *Streptococcus* are often found on food contact surfaces and coliform bacteria in water. Eradication of these contaminating bacteria becomes more challenging in presence of biofilms. Biofilms provide a good support and protective environment to bacteria by their tough surface properties. Biofilms as biological advantage provide a niche for multiple species to thrive which could not be possible in free-floating culture (Donlan 2002). These films are composed of extracellular matrix (Huang et al. 2019) consisting a mixture of different biomolecules such as proteins, lipids, carbohydrates and nucleic acids. These biofilms act as channels to keep the microbes close to each other and facilitate the exchange of nutrients and gases. Along with these advantages it provides protection from environmental damage, antimicrobial agents and host immune system (Yin et al. 2019).

Biofilm formation could be induced by the procedures used by food processing industries. In these industries process design revolves around a number of parameters such as temperature, oxygen availability pH, osmolarity, nutrient availability and surface properties. Higher salt concentration and lower pH have been reported as an enhancing factor for the biofilm formation for *L. monocytogenes* in cheese industries (Latorre et al. 2010). Similarly, the surface properties, hydrophobicity, roughness and charge, also govern the biofilm formation. Hydrophobic surface is more favourable to *L. monocytogenes* to make biofilm whereas; *S. aureus* could make biofilms irrespective of hydrophobicity.

Biofilms are a menace to food industries since they are capable of causing blocking of the tubing and filters and damage the equipment surface. They also hinder the heat transfer during the process. Cleaning protocols followed by industries such as dairy, poultry, meet and sea food, are not often foolproof. *Vibreo spp, L. monocytogene, Salmonella* and *Aeromonas hydrophilla* are the most common pathogens that form biofilms. *Salmonella* spp. isolated from animal feed and fish meal factories have demonstrated high biofilm forming ability thereof and could persist in the industry premises for years (Vestby et al. 2009). There are many tactics to get rid of biofilms and problems associated with it, a few of them have been categorized in the following flow chart in Fig. 7.5 (Gutiérrez et al. 2016).

Bacteriophage can be used as a promising antibacterial agent to counter biofilms formation. Bacteriophage PVP-SE2 was used against *Salmonella enteritidis* biofilm formed on different surfaces, which come in contact with food. This phage demonstrated its potential to remove the 48 h old biofilm from stainless steel and

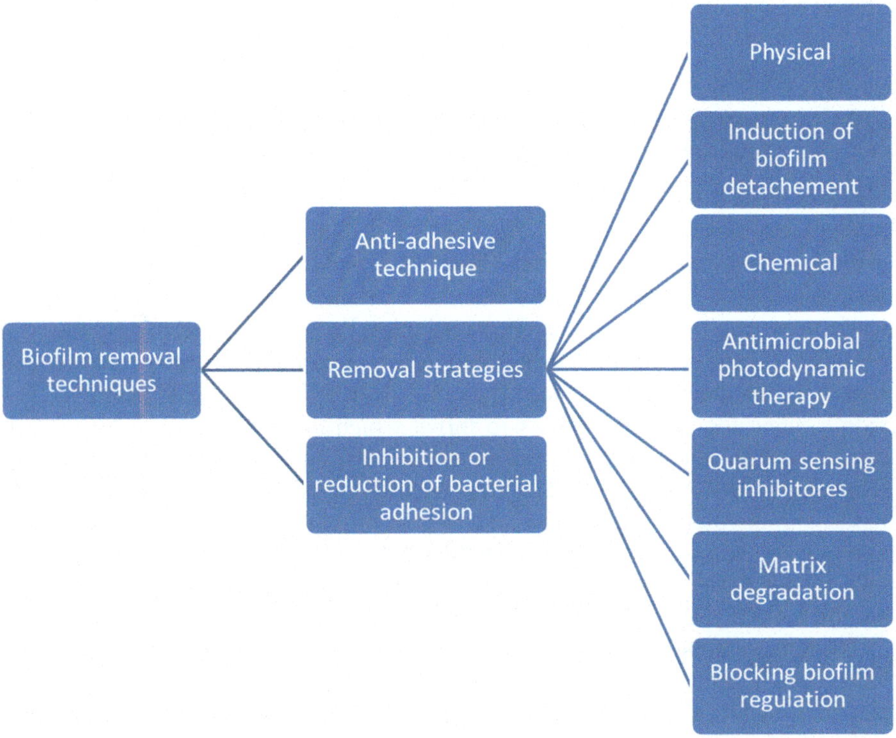

Fig. 7.5 Representation of different approaches in a flow chart to counter the biofilm associated problems

polystyrene surface successfully. This phage was also found to be amply potent to reduce the salmonella load on poultry skin in room temperature and frozen condition (Milho et al. 2018). Similarly, three different phages LiMN4L, LiMN4p and LiMN17 were assayed against biofilm produced by *L. monocytogenes* on food contact stainless steel surface. The study was carried out on 7 day old biofilm using individual phage as well as cocktail of phage. The phage cocktail was found to be more effective against biofilm as it was capable of reducing the biofilm up to undetectable levels compared to that of the individual phage (Ganegama Arachchi et al. 2013). Two newly isolated bacteriophages, vB_EfaS zip a shiphophage and vB_EfaP-max a podophage against enterococci were able to reduce the biofilm in cocktail mixture up to 2.5log cfu/mL within 3 h of treatment (Melo et al. 2019). In an another study bacteriophage cocktail Listex p100 regarded as GRAS demonstrated the removal of biofilm on the machinery surface along with the elimination of bacteria population in broths and dried cured hem against 5 different strain of listeria (Iacumin et al. 2016).

7.3.8 Bacteriophage Encoded Lytic Enzymes as Disinfectant

Bacteriophages are parasites that need to infect a host bacterial cell to propagate and thrive. In order to do that, phage has to inject the genetic material into the cell at first and needs to break the host cell wall to escape, later. Therefore, bacteriophage genetic material encodes some lytic enzymes which help them break the cell wall (Fernandes and São-José 2018). Bacterial cells consisting cytoplasmic membrane and cell wall fall under monodermic category whereas, the didermic bacteria possess extra layer of lipids. Both the type of bacteria have the ability to secret polysaccharides capsule which makes the phage entry challenging. Thus, besides the use of the phage as such, an alternative way to counter the pathogens by using phage derived lytic enzymes as bactericidal agents exists. Bacteriophage encoded lytic enzymes are capable of degrading the cell wall and cell membrane by breaking the bonds between monomers of peptidoglycans (murein) (Fernandes and São-José 2018). Bacteriophages lyse the bacterial cell using endolysins or called lysins; (i) endolysins, (ii) holins and (iii) spanins. Endolysins act on peptidoglycan whereas holins create pores/ holes in plasma membrane by depolarization of lipid bilayer. These holes facilities the diffusion of endolysin and pave accessibility to peptidoglycan layer (Matamp and Bhat 2019; Young 2013). There is a special class of holins reported as pinholins. They do not create large pores like holins but make heptameric channels and in a cascade of reaction, activation and refolding of accessory enzymes to degrade peptidoglycans. Spanins have been reported in case of gram negative bacteria to disrupt the outer membrane (Berry et al. 2012). The action of spanins can be classified into three mechanisms, (i) inner and outer membrane fusion (Berry et al. 2010), (ii) pore formation and (iii) enzymatic action which depend on the components, o-spanin and i-spanin (Berry et al. 2010). A few of the

Table 7.4 A list of endolysins and respective phage along with experimental effects

Phage	Enzyme	Bacteria	Effect	References
Vibrio phage qdvp001	Lysqdvp001	*Vibrio alginolyticus* and *V. parahaemolyticus*	Sea food contamination prevention	Matamp and Bhat (2019)
Escherichia coli prophage	PlyE146	*E. coli K12*	Reduce load by 2 $\log_{10}$ CFU/mL in 2 hours	Larpin et al. (2018)
vB_SepiS-phiIPLA7	EPS depolymerase (Dpo7)	*Staphylococcus aureus*	24 h-biofilm biomass reduced to 53–85% on polystyrene surface	Gutiérrez et al. (2015)
Salmonella phage phi68	Endolysin (Lys68)	*Salmonella typhimurium*	Reduce 3–5 log cfu in 2 hr	Oliveira et al. (2014)
phi-SauS-IPLA88	Endolysin LysH5	*Staphylococcus aureus*	Reduce 1–3 log units	Gutiérrez et al. (2014)

bacteriophage encoding endolysins, their source, host and reported effects have been summarised in Table 7.4.

7.4 Formulation and Encapsulation of Bacteriophage

Bacteriophage application in the arena of food preservation and packaging industry and technology in the form of spray, absorbent pads, applied on the packaging material and mixed with preservative agents are a few of the common ways. Bacteriophages are entities made-up of biomolecules such as proteins and nucleic acid which makes them vulnerable to various physiochemical environments such as low or high pH, temperature, UV radiation and various salts. These harsh conditions may result in inactivation of phage particles and lead to inefficiency in clearing the pathogens (González-Menéndez et al. 2018). Phages are more stable in buffer at refrigerator temperature rather than at room temperature. This causes a problem in storage as well as in transportation of the phages.

Encapsulation of phage particles could improve the sturdiness and viability for longer time. Encapsulation can overcome the limitations put by the environment on the use of phages (Anal and Singh 2007). Along with stability, sturdiness and survivability, encapsulation also controls the release of encapsulated phage particles, which is an important parameter to be considered. Table 7.5 lists various encapsulation methods applied to entrap bacteriophages.

Properties of encapsulated phase formulation should not,

(i) Cause aggregation of the phage particles
(ii) Damage the morphology of phage
(iii) Hamper the activity of the phage
(iv) The titre of phage particles should not decrease drastically

Table 7.5 Encapsulation methods applied on various bacteriophages

Phage	Encapsulation	Application	significance	References
ZCEC5	Chitosan–alginate bead with a honey and gelatin matrix	Against zoonotic pathogen, *E. coli*	Stable in water and complete release of phage in 4–5 h	Abdelsattar et al. (2019)
(UAB_Phi20, UAB_Phi78, and UAB_Phi87	Alginate/$CaCO_3$	Against *Salmonella* I poultry	Rescue commercial broilers from Salmonella	Colom et al. (2017)
ΦKAZ14	Chitosan nanoparticles	Against avian pathogenic *Escherichia coli*	Decreased mortality to 16%	Kaikabo et al. (2017)
phiIPLA-RODI	Liposome Nanovesicles (like phospholipids and surfactants)	food biopreservatives and food processing industry	Infectivity was maintained for 6 months at 4 °C	González-Menéndez et al. (2018)
K phages and T3 phages	Microfluidics loposome	Against *S. aureus* and *E. coli*	Non tail phage survived more than tail phage	Cinquerrui et al. (2018)
(MRSA) phage cocktail	Transfersomes	Restrict *S. aureus*	Showed more stability than free phage	Chhibber et al. (2017)
PEV2 – Podovirus and PEV40 – Myovirus	Microfluidic liposome	*P. aeruginosa*	59% and 50% efficiency of encapsulation	Leung et al. (2018)
Listeria phage A511	Sodium alginate, gum and gelatin	*L. monosytogene*	Maximize the stability and viability in thermal processing	Ahmadi et al. (2018)

(v) The binding of formulation material to phage particle should be tight enough to hold but loose enough to release slowly
(vi) Last but not the least, the material used to encapsulate phage should not be toxic or hazardous

Bacteriophage ZCEC5 against *E. coli* was encapsulated using chitosan – alginate and evaluated for the stability and viability. Over the period of 8 weeks, encapsulated phage was assessed for the leakage in distilled water and no leakage was found. These phage containing beads showed the slow release of phage particle over the period of 5 h with a rate 5.3 log PFU/mL per h at low pH. The viability of the encapsulated versus free phage was tested at pH 2. The free phage count dropped below the detection level within 10 min of incubation, whereas encapsulated phage showed a reduction in phage titer to 1 log PFU unit only in 1 h at 37 °C (Abdelsattar et al. 2019).

Some of the techniques used in formulation and encapsulation listed below.

(i) Freeze drying of bacteriophage for storage and encapsulation
(ii) Freeze drying of encapsulated phage

(iii) Spray freeze drying of phage
(iv) Spray drying of bacteriophage for storage and encapsulation
(v) Drying bacteriophage on filter paper
(vi) Liposome formation

Phage formulation and encapsulation can be taken up a notch in terms of stability, survivability and uniformity by incorporating new methods and techniques. There is more scope in this field to improve and implement the techniques such as stimuli (temperature, radiation, light, enzymes and pH) based polymerization, membrane based emulsification, nanoparticles and microfluidic emulsification (Malik et al. 2017). The new materials and techniques can also improve the controlled release of phage in different environmental conditions.

7.5 Bacteriophage Market and Approval

Antibiotics are the most prescribed among all kind of medicines world-wide. Thus, the market of the antibiotics is huge and has been thriving since decades. Globally, antibiotics market has raised 39 billion in 2015, 40 billion in 2017 and 42.6 billion in 2018 and expected to cross 56 billion by 2025 with the CAGR (compound annual growth rate) of 4.1%. With the patents having expired globally for most of the antibiotics, almost 80% of them have become generic (https://www.mordorintelligence.com/industry-reports/antibiotics-market; https://www.alliedmarketresearch.com/antibiotics-market). These generic drugs are now available to all the pharma companies for production, which facilitates the cheap and ample availability of antibiotics in the market. This incriminates use of antibiotics gave birth to a problem- resistance development in pathogenic bacteria.

The Staphage lysate is a product re-launched into the market for the use of veterinarians on dogs to control *Staphylococcus* infection. Though this product was licensed for human use initially, now is being used for the treatment of a medical condition among canines called Pyoderma. Similarly, there are a number of products in market and many more to come in the near future. The implementation of phage and phage-based products gaining popularity around the globe is self-explanatory for its commercial potential and some of the commercially available phase-based products are listed out in Table 7.6. Many of the phage products are approved and certified as generally recognized as safe (GRAS) by authorised agencies like Ministry of health Canada and Israel, USA, Food and drug administration (FDA), USA department of agriculture (USDA), Goods receipt number (GRN), FASIS (Food Safety and Inspection Service), European food safety authority (EFSA), Food standard Australia New Zealand (FSANZ), Swiss Bundesamt für Gesundheit) BAG, US, environmental protection agency (EPA) and Code of Federal Regulations (FCR).

Table 7.6 The list of companies and institutes in the field of bacteriophage-based products

Company	Location	Stabilised in (year)	Product	Status	Information available on
Delmont laboratories	Pennsylvania, US	1952	Staphage lysate (1954)	In market	https://delmontlabs.com/
Omnilytics	Sandy, Utah, US	1954	AgriPhage AgriPhage- CMM AgriPhage- Fire Blight AgriPhage- citrus canker	In market	https://www.omnilytics.com/about-us/
AmpliPhi Biosciences	Virginia, US	1989	–	–	ampliphibio.com
Eliava institute	Tibilisi, Republic of Georgia	1916	Elimers Elipyoge Phage CF Elicoli Bugltser Elicosali	–	https://web.archive.org/web/20160302070442/http://www.eliavaphageny.com/about.html
Armata Pharmaceuticals	California, US	1989	AP-PA02	In Pipe line	https://www.armatapharma.com/
Phage tech	California, US	1997	Phage based diagnostics	–	https://www.phagetech.com/
Intralytics	Columbia, US	1998	ListShield EcoShild SalmoFresh Shigashield Salmolyse ListPhage	In market	http://www.intralytix.com/
iNtRON Bio	Korea	1999	N-Rephasin® SAL200	In pipe line	http://intodeworld.com/
Gangagen	Banglore, India	2000	P128	–	http://www.gangagen.com/

(continued)

Table 7.6 (continued)

Company	Location	Stabilised in (year)	Product	Status	Information available on
Phage Biotech	Israel	2000	–	–	www.phage-biotech.com
Clan cells	Bouffere, France	2000	Phagoburn	In pipe line	www.clean-cells.com
Novolytics	Lancashire, UK	2002	–	–	www.novolytics.co.uk/
Technophage	Lisbon, Portugal	2005	Chronic ulcers (TP-102) Respiratory (TP-122) Urinary tract infection (TP-164)	In Pipe line	http://www.technophage.pt/
Micreos EBI	Netherlands	2005	Listex Salmonelex Staphefekt	–	https://www.micreos.com/
Innophage Ltd	Portugal	–	–	–	http://www.innophage.com/
Jafral	Slovinia	2011			www.jafral.com
phageLux	Shanghai, China	2013	Lexia Agariphage		http://www.phagelux.com
Adaptive phage therapeutics	Maryland, US	2016	–		http://www.aphage.com/
PhagePro	Boston, US	2016	ProphaLytic-VC		https://www.phageproinc.com/
Phagomed	Vienna	2017	–		https://www.phagomed.com/

7.6 Conclusions

The lytic property and selective nature of the bacteriophages have demonstrated extraordinary outcomes against the pathogenic food spoiler bacteria. These selective bacteriophages have been successfully incorporated as antibacterial agents into the pre harvest such as poultry, aquaculture, fruits and vegetables as well as post harvested including meat, eggs, milk and milk products. Bacteriophages could be considered for their use in food process industries during food packaging, food preservation and sanitization; however, more detailed research needs to be done for better application. Interdisciplinary research including the experts in phage biology, polymer science, biotechnology, material science and food technology is the dire need to improve the phage utility and efficacy by inventing novel methods and compatible materials of encapsulation. Bacteriophage use in the dairy industry has more beneficial effect due to its specificity for the host which can be innocuous to the desired bacteria, which cannot be achieved by the use of antibiotics or other non-specific antimicrobials. Biofilm removal and restricting the formation has been efficiently achieved by bacteriophage application. The use of bacteriophage and lytic enzymes could also curb the problem raised by antibiotic resistant bacteria. Bacteriophage and its products provide the researchers with a promising future to come up with more alternative tools to combat resistant pathogenic bacteria and problems associated with them.

Acknowledgments The first author likes to extend his warm gratitude towards Indian Council for Medical Research (ICMR), Government of India for providing the Senior Research Fellowship stipend. The authors also thank the Department of Science and Technology, Government of India, and VIT, Vellore for providing the facilities. Authors would like to express special thanks to Ms. Divya G, Senior Scientist (Biocon Research limited) for manuscript editing and formatting.

References

Abdelsattar AS, Abdelrahman F, Dawoud A, Connerton IF, El-Shibiny A (2019) Encapsulation of E. coli phage ZCEC5 in chitosan–alginate beads as a delivery system in phage therapy. AMB Express 9: 87. https://doi.org/10.1186/s13568-019-0810-9

Abuladze T, Li M, Menetrez MY, Dean T, Senecal A, Sulakvelidze A (2008) Bacteriophages reduce experimental contamination of hard surfaces, tomato, spinach, broccoli, and ground beef by *Escherichia coli* O157:H7. Appl Environ Microbiol 74:6230–6238. https://doi.org/10.1128/AEM.01465-08

Ackermann H (2011) Bacteriophage taxonomy. Microbiol Aust 32:90–94. https://health.uni-hohenheim.de/fileadmin/einrichtungen/gesundheitswissenschaften/Downloads/Bacteriophages_Taxonomy_2011-Ackermann.pdf

Ahmadi H, Wang Q, Lim LT, Balamurugan S (2018) Encapsulation of Listeria phage A511 by alginate to improve its thermal stability. Methods Mol Biol 1681:89–95. https://doi.org/10.1007/978-1-4939-7343-9_7

Alcaine SD, Pacitto D, Sela DA, Nugen SR (2015) Phage & phosphatase: a novel phage-based probe for rapid, multi-platform detection of bacteria. Analyst 140:7629–7636. https://doi.org/10.1039/c5an01181g

Amit SK, Uddin MM, Rahman R, Islam SMR, Khan MS (2017) A review on mechanisms and commercial aspects of food preservation and processing. Agric Food Secur 6:51. https://doi.org/10.1186/s40066-017-0130-8

Anal AK, Singh H (2007) Recent advances in microencapsulation of probiotics for industrial applications and targeted delivery. Trends Food Sci Technol 18:240–251. https://doi.org/10.1016/j.tifs.2007.01.004

Atterbury RJ, Connerton PL, Dodd CER, Rees CED, Connerton IF (2003) Application of host-specific bacteriophages to the surface of chicken skin leads to a reduction in recovery of *Campylobacter jejuni*. Appl Environ Microbiol 69:6302–6306. https://doi.org/10.1128/AEM.69.10.6302-6306.2003

Bajovic B, Bolumar T, Heinz V (2012) Quality considerations with high pressure processing of fresh and value added meat products. Meat Sci 92:280–289. https://doi.org/10.1016/j.meatsci.2012.04.024

Baños A, García-López JD, Núñez C, Martínez-Bueno M, Maqueda M, Valdivia E (2016) Biocontrol of *Listeria monocytogenes* in fish by enterocin AS-48 and *Listeria* lytic bacteriophage P100. LWT Food Sci Technol 66:672–677. https://doi.org/10.1016/j.lwt.2015.11.025

Berry J, Savva C, Holzenburg A, Young R (2010) The lambda spanin components Rz and Rz1 undergo tertiary and quaternary rearrangements upon complex formation. Protein Sci 19:1967–1977. https://doi.org/10.1002/pro.485

Berry J, Rajaure M, Pang T, Young R (2012) The spanin complex is essential for lambda lysis. J Bacteriol 194:5667–5674. https://doi.org/10.1128/JB.01245-12

Bigot B, Lee WJ, McIntyre L, Wilson T, Hudson JA, Billington C, Heinemann JA (2011) Control of *Listeria monocytogenes* growth in a ready-to-eat poultry product using a bacteriophage. Food Microbiol 28:1448–1452. https://doi.org/10.1016/j.fm.2011.07.001

Bigwood T, Hudson JA, Billington C, Carey-Smith GV, Heinemann JA (2008) Phage inactivation of foodborne pathogens on cooked and raw meat. Food Microbiol 25:400–406. https://doi.org/10.1016/j.fm.2007.11.003

Borie C, Albala I, Sànchez P, Sánchez ML, Ramírez S, Navarro C, Morales MA, Retamales J, Robeson J (2008) Bacteriophage treatment reduces *Salmonella* colonization of infected chickens. Avian Dis 52:64–67. https://doi.org/10.1637/8091-082007-reg

Boyacioglu O, Sulakvelidze A, Sharma M, Goktepe I (2016) Effect of a bacteriophage cocktail in combination with modified atmosphere packaging in controlling *Listeria monocytogenes* on fresh-cut spinach. Irish J Agric Food Res 55:74. https://doi.org/10.1515/ijafr-2016-0007

Bren L (2007) Bacteria-eating virus approved as food additive. FDA Consum 41:20–22. https://pubmed.ncbi.nlm.nih.gov/17342833/

Burnham S, Hu J, Anany H, Brovko L, Deiss F, Derda R, Griffiths MW (2014) Towards rapid on-site phage-mediated detection of generic Escherichia coli in water using luminescent and visual readout. Anal Bioanal Chem 406:5685–5693. https://doi.org/10.1007/s00216-014-7985-3

Carlton RM, Noordman WH, Biswas B, De Meester ED, Loessner MJ (2005) Bacteriophage P100 for control of *Listeria monocytogenes* in foods: genome sequence, bioinformatic analyses, oral toxicity study, and application. Regul Toxicol Pharmacol 43:301–312. https://doi.org/10.1016/j.yrtph.2005.08.005

Chen J, Griffiths MW (1996) *Salmonella* detection in eggs using lux+ bacteriophages. J Food Prot 59:908–914. https://doi.org/10.4315/0362-028X-59.9.908

Chhibber S, Shukla A, Kaur S (2017) Transfersomal phage cocktail is an effective treatment against methicillin-resistant *Staphylococcus aureus*-mediated skin and soft tissue infections. Antimicrob Agents Chemother 61:e02146–e02116. https://doi.org/10.1128/AAC.02146-16

Chibani CM, Farr A, Klama S, Dietrich S, Liesegang H (2019) Classifying the unclassified: a phage classification method. Viruses 11:195. https://doi.org/10.3390/v11020195

Chibeu A, Agius L, Gao A, Sabour PM, Kropinski AM, Balamurugan S (2013) Efficacy of bacteriophage LISTEX™P100 combined with chemical antimicrobials in reducing *Listeria monocytogenes* in cooked Turkey and roast beef. Int J Food Microbiol 167:208–214. https://doi.org/10.1016/j.ijfoodmicro.2013.08.018

Chin BA, Suh S-J, Chen I-H, Xi J, Liu Y, Du S, Horikawa S, Huang T-S (2018) Isolation of highly selective phage-displayed oligopeptide probes for detection of *Listeria monocytogenes* in ready-to-eat food. In Proceedings of the SPIE 10665, sensing for agriculture and food quality and safety X, 106650N (15 May 2018). https://doi.org/10.1117/12.2305132

Cinquerrui S, Mancuso F, Vladisavljevic GT, Bakker SE, Malik DJ (2018) Nanoencapsulation of bacteriophages in liposomes prepared using microfluidic hydrodynamic flow focusing. Front Microbiol 9:2172. https://doi.org/10.3389/fmicb.2018.02172

Colom J, Cano-Sarabia M, Otero J, Aríñez-Soriano J, Cortés P, Maspoch D, Llagostera M (2017) Microencapsulation with alginate/$CaCO_3$: a strategy for improved phage therapy. Sci Rep 7:41441. https://doi.org/10.1038/srep41441

Donlan RM (2002) Biofilms: microbial life on surfaces. Emerg Infect Dis 8:881–890. https://doi.org/10.3201/eid0809.020063

Ferguson S, Roberts C, Handy E, Sharma M (2013) Lytic bacteriophages reduce *Escherichia coli* O157: H7 on fresh cut lettuce introduced through cross-contamination. Bacteriophage 3:e24323. https://doi.org/10.4161/bact.24323

Fernandes S, São-José C (2018) Enzymes and mechanisms employed by tailed bacteriophages to breach the bacterial cell barriers. Viruses 10:396. https://doi.org/10.3390/v10080396

Fernández L, Escobedo S, Gutiérrez D, Portilla S, Martínez B, García P, Rodríguez A (2017) Bacteriophages in the dairy environment: from enemies to allies. Antibiotics 6:27. https://doi.org/10.3390/antibiotics6040027

Figueiredo ACL, Almeida RCC (2017) Antibacterial efficacy of nisin, bacteriophage P100 and sodium lactate against *Listeria monocytogenes* in ready-to-eat sliced pork ham. Brazilian J Microbiol 48:724–729. https://doi.org/10.1016/j.bjm.2017.02.010

Fiorentin L, Vieira ND, Barioni W (2005) Oral treatment with bacteriophages reduces the concentration of *Salmonella Enteritidis* PT4 in caecal contents of broilers. Avian Pathol 34:258–263. https://doi.org/10.1080/01445340500112157

Fortier LC, Sekulovic O (2013) Importance of prophages to evolution and virulence of bacterial pathogens. Virulence 4:354–365. https://doi.org/10.4161/viru.24498

Franche N, Vinay M, Ansaldi M (2017) Substrate-independent luminescent phage-based biosensor to specifically detect enteric bacteria such as *E. coli*. Environ Sci Pollut Res 24:42–51. https://doi.org/10.1007/s11356-016-6288-y

Franks I (2011) Probiotics: probiotics and diarrhea in children. Nat Rev Gastroenterol Hepatol 8:602. https://doi.org/10.1038/nrgastro.2011.177

Ganegama Arachchi GJ, Cridge AG, Dias-Wanigasekera BM, Cruz CD, McIntyre L, Liu R, Flint SH, Mutukumira AN (2013) Effectiveness of phages in the decontamination of *Listeria monocytogenes* adhered to clean stainless steel, stainless steel coated with fish protein, and as a biofilm. J Ind Microbiol Biotechnol 40:1105–1116. https://doi.org/10.1007/s10295-013-1313-3

García P, Madera C, Martínez B, Rodríguez A (2007) Biocontrol of *Staphylococcus aureus* in curd manufacturing processes using bacteriophages. Int Dairy J 17:1232–1239. https://doi.org/10.1016/j.idairyj.2007.03.014

Gigante A, Atterbury RJ (2019) Veterinary use of bacteriophage therapy in intensively-reared livestock. Virol J 16:155. https://doi.org/10.1186/s12985-019-1260-3

Gill JJ, Sabour PM, Leslie KE, Griffiths MW (2006) Bovine whey proteins inhibit the interaction of *Staphylococcus aureus* and bacteriophage K. J Appl Microbiol 101:377–386. https://doi.org/10.1111/j.1365-2672.2006.02918.x

Giraffa G, Zago M, Carminati D (2017) Lactic acid bacteria bacteriophages in dairy products: problems and solutions. In: Microbiological Opportunities and Challenges in the Dairy Industry, pp 233–250. https://doi.org/10.1002/9781119115007.ch13

González-Menéndez E, Fernández L, Gutiérrez D, Pando D, Martínez B, Rodríguez A, García P (2018) Strategies to encapsulate the *Staphylococcus aureus* bacteriophage phiIPLA-RODI. Viruses 10:495. https://doi.org/10.3390/v10090495

Goode D, Allen VM, Barrow PA (2003) Reduction of experimental *Salmonella* and *Campylobacter* contamination of chicken skin by application of lytic bacteriophages. Appl Environ Microbiol 69:5032–5036. https://doi.org/10.1128/AEM.69.8.5032-5036.2003

Gouvêa DM, Mendonça RCS, Lopez MES, Batalha LS (2016) Absorbent food pads containing bacteriophages for potential antimicrobial use in refrigerated food products. LWT Food Sci Technol 67:159–166. https://doi.org/10.1016/j.lwt.2015.11.043

Greer GG, Dilts BD (2002) Control of Brochothrix thermosphacta spoilage of pork adipose tissue using bacteriophages. J Food Prot 65:861–863. https://doi.org/10.4315/0362-028X-65.5.861

Guenther S, Huwyler D, Richard S, Loessner MJ (2009) Virulent bacteriophage for efficient biocontrol of *Listeria monocytogenes* in ready-to-eat foods. Appl Environ Microbiol 75:93–100. https://doi.org/10.1128/AEM.01711-08

Guenther S, Herzig O, Fieseler L, Klumpp J, Loessner MJ (2012) Biocontrol of *Salmonella typhimurium* in RTE foods with the virulent bacteriophage FO1-E2. Int J Food Microbiol 154:66–72. https://doi.org/10.1016/j.ijfoodmicro.2011.12.023

Gutiérrez D, Ruas-Madiedo P, Martínez B, Rodríguez A, García P (2014) Effective removal of *Staphylococcal* biofilms by the endolysin LysH5. PLoS One 9:e107307. https://doi.org/10.1371/journal.pone.0107307

Gutiérrez D, Briers Y, Rodríguez-Rubio L, Martínez B, Rodríguez A, Lavigne R, García P (2015) Role of the pre-neck appendage protein (Dpo7) from phage vB_SepiS-phiIPLA7 as an anti-biofilm agent in *Staphylococcal* species. Front Microbiol 6:1315. https://doi.org/10.3389/fmicb.2015.01315

Gutiérrez D, Rodríguez-Rubio L, Martínez B, Rodríguez A, García P (2016) Bacteriophages as weapons against bacterial biofilms in the food industry. Front Microbiol 7:825. https://doi.org/10.3389/fmicb.2016.00825

Gutiérrez D, Fernández L, Rodríguez A, García P (2019) Role of bacteriophages in the implementation of a sustainable dairy chain. Front Microbiol 10:12. https://doi.org/10.3389/fmicb.2019.00012

Hall GM (2010) Preservation by curing (drying, salting and smoking). In: Fish processing: sustainability and new opportunities. Wiley, pp 51–76. https://doi.org/10.1002/9781444328585.ch3

Harada LK, Silva EC, Campos WF, Del Fiol FS, Vila M, Dąbrowska K, Krylov VN, Balcão VM (2018) Biotechnological applications of bacteriophages: state of the art. Microbiol Res 212–213:38–58. https://doi.org/10.1016/j.micres.2018.04.007

Hooton SPT, Atterbury RJ, Connerton IF (2011) Application of a bacteriophage cocktail to reduce *Salmonella Typhimurium* U288 contamination on pig skin. Int J Food Microbiol 151:157–163. https://doi.org/10.1016/j.ijfoodmicro.2011.08.015

Huang H, Peng C, Peng P, Lin Y, Zhang X, Ren H (2019) Towards the biofilm characterization and regulation in biological wastewater treatment. Appl Microbiol Biotechnol 103:1115–1129. https://doi.org/10.1007/s00253-018-9511-6

Huff WE, Huff GR, Rath NC, Balog JM, Xie H, Moore PA, Donoghue AM (2002) Prevention of *Escherichia coli* respiratory infection in broiler chickens with bacteriophage (SPR02). Poult Sci 81:437–441. https://doi.org/10.1093/ps/81.4.437

Iacumin L, Manzano M, Comi G (2016) Phage inactivation of *Listeria monocytogenes* on san Daniele dry-cured ham and elimination of biofilms from equipment and working environments. Microorganisms 4:4. https://doi.org/10.3390/microorganisms4010004

Jamet A, Touchon M, Ribeiro-Gonçalves B, Carriço JA, Charbit A, Nassif X, Ramirez M, Rocha EPC (2017) A widespread family of polymorphic toxins encoded by temperate phages. BMC Biol 15:75. https://doi.org/10.1186/s12915-017-0415-1

Kaikabo AA, Abdulkarim SM, Abas F (2017) Evaluation of the efficacy of chitosan nanoparticles loaded 4ΦKAZ14 bacteriophage in the biological control of colibacillosis in chickens. Poult Sci 96:295–302. https://doi.org/10.3382/ps/pew255

Kim S, Kim M, Ryu S (2014) Development of an engineered bioluminescent reporter phage for the sensitive detection of viable *Salmonella typhimurium*. Anal Chem 86:5858–5864. https://doi.org/10.1021/ac500645c

Kim J, Kim M, Kim S, Ryu S (2017) Sensitive detection of viable *Escherichia coli* O157:H7 from foods using a luciferase-reporter phage phiV10lux. Int J Food Microbiol 254:11–17. https://doi.org/10.1016/j.ijfoodmicro.2017.05.002

Kim YH, Lim JY, Yoon KS (2019) Effect of water activity, Yuza (Citrus junos Sieb. ex Tanaka) powder and the mixture of sodium lactate and sodium acetate on quality and safety in beef Jerky. Food Nutr Sci 10:588–605. https://doi.org/10.4236/fns.2019.106043

Kocharunchitt C, Ross T, McNeil DL (2009) Use of bacteriophages as biocontrol agents to control *Salmonella* associated with seed sprouts. Int J Food Microbiol 128:453–459. https://doi.org/10.1016/j.ijfoodmicro.2008.10.014

Korehei R, Kadla JF (2014) Encapsulation of T4 bacteriophage in electrospun poly(ethylene oxide)/cellulose diacetate fibers. Carbohydr Polym 100:150–157. https://doi.org/10.1016/j.carbpol.2013.03.079

Kumar Y, Tiwari S, Belorkar SA (2015) Drying: an excellent method for food preservation. Int J Eng Stud Tech Approach 1:1–17. https://www.semanticscholar.org/paper/Drying%3A-An-Excellent-Method-for-Food-Preservation-Kumar-Tiwari/d36651c13f4844523d9d0d2b935dabde23b8776e#citing-papers

Lakshmanan RS, Guntupalli R, Hu J, Petrenko VA, Barbaree JM, Chin BA (2007) Detection of *Salmonella typhimurium* in fat free milk using a phage immobilized magnetoelastic sensor. Sens Actuat B Chem 126:544–550. https://doi.org/10.1016/j.snb.2007.04.003

Larpin Y, Oechslin F, Moreillon P, Resch G, Entenza JM, Mancini S (2018) In vitro characterization of PlyE146, a novel phage lysin that targets gram-negative bacteria. PLoS One 13:e0192507. https://doi.org/10.1371/journal.pone.0192507

Latorre AA, Van Kessel JS, Karns JS, Zurakowski MJ, Pradhan AK, Boor KJ, Jayarao BM, Houser BA, Daugherty CS, Schukken YH (2010) Biofilm in milking equipment on a dairy farm as a potential source of bulk tank milk contamination with *Listeria monocytogenes*. J Dairy Sci 93:2792–2802. https://doi.org/10.3168/jds.2009-2717

Leung SSY, Morales S, Britton W, Kutter E, Chan HK (2018) Microfluidic-assisted bacteriophage encapsulation into liposomes. Int J Pharm 545:176–182. https://doi.org/10.1016/j.ijpharm.2018.04.063

Leverentz B, Conway WS, Alavidze Z, Janisiewicz WJ, Fuchs Y, Camp MJ, Chighladze E, Sulakvelidze A (2001) Examination of bacteriophage as a biocontrol method for Salmonella on fresh-cut fruit: a model study. J Food Prot 64:1116–1121. https://doi.org/10.4315/0362-028X-64.8.1116

Leverentz B, Conway WS, Camp MJ, Janisiewicz WJ, Abuladze T, Yang M, Saftner R, Sulakvelidze A (2003) Biocontrol of *Listeria monocytogenes* on fresh-cut produce by treatment with lytic bacteriophages and a bacteriocin. Appl Environ Microbiol 69:4519–4526. https://doi.org/10.1128/AEM.69.8.4519-4526.2003

Li M, Lin H, Khan MN, Wang J, Kong L (2014) Effects of bacteriophage on the quality and shelf life of *Paralichthys olivaceus* during chilled storage. J Sci Food Agric 94:1657–1662. https://doi.org/10.1002/jsfa.6475

Lone A, Anany H, Hakeem M, Aguis L, Avdjian AC, Bouget M, Atashi A, Brovko L, Rochefort D, Griffiths MW (2016) Development of prototypes of bioactive packaging materials based on immobilized bacteriophages for control of growth of bacterial pathogens in foods. Int J Food Microbiol 217:49–58. https://doi.org/10.1016/j.ijfoodmicro.2015.10.011

Madera C, Monjardín C, Suárez JE (2004) Milk contamination and resistance to processing conditions determine the fate of *Lactococcus lactis* bacteriophages in dairies. Appl Environ Microbiol 70:7365–7371. https://doi.org/10.1128/AEM.70.12.7365-7371.2004

Malik DJ, Sokolov IJ, Vinner GK, Mancuso F, Cinquerrui S, Vladisavljevic GT, Clokie MRJ, Garton NJ, Stapley AGF, Kirpichnikova A (2017) Formulation, stabilisation and encapsulation of bacteriophage for phage therapy. Adv Colloid Interf Sci 249:100–133. https://doi.org/10.1016/j.cis.2017.05.014

Matamp N, Bhat S (2019) Phage Endolysins as potential antimicrobials against multidrug resistant *Vibrio alginolyticus* and *Vibrio parahaemolyticus*: current status of research and challenges ahead. Microorganisms 7:84. https://doi.org/10.3390/microorganisms7030084

Mc Grath S, Fitzgerald GF, van Sinderen D (2007) Bacteriophages in dairy products: pros and cons. Biotechnol J 2:450–455. https://doi.org/10.1002/biot.200600227

McKenna F, El-Tarabily KA, Hardy GESTJ, Dell B (2001) Novel in vivo use of a polyvalent *Streptomyces* phage to disinfest Streptomyces scabies-infected seed potatoes. Plant Pathol 50:666–675. https://doi.org/10.1046/j.1365-3059.2001.00648.x

Melo LDR, Ferreira R, Costa AR, Oliveira H, Azeredo J (2019) Efficacy and safety assessment of two E*nterococci* phages in an in vitro biofilm wound model. Sci Rep 9:6643. https://doi.org/10.1038/s41598-019-43115-8

Milho C, Silva MD, Melo L, Santos S, Azeredo J, Sillankorva S (2018) Control of *Salmonella enteritidis* on food contact surfaces with bacteriophage PVP-SE2. Biofouling 34:753–768. https://doi.org/10.1080/08927014.2018.1501475

Miller RW, Skinner J, Sulakvelidze A, Mathis GF, Hofacre CL (2010) Bacteriophage therapy for control of necrotic enteritis of broiler chickens experimentally infected with *Clostridium perfringens*. Avian Dis Dig 54:33–40. https://doi.org/10.1637/9256.1

Modi R, Hirvi Y, Hill A, Griffiths MW (2001) Effect of phage on survival of *Salmonella Enteritidis* during manufacture and storage of Cheddar cheese made from raw and pasteurized milk. J Food Prot 64:927–933. https://doi.org/10.4315/0362-028X-64.7.927

Montaño A, Sánchez AH, Beato VM, López-López A, de Castro A (2015) Pickling. Encyclopedia of Food and Health, In, pp 369–374. https://doi.org/10.1016/B978-0-12-384947-2.00545-6

Morozova VV, Vlassov VV, Tikunova NV (2018) Applications of bacteriophages in the treatment of localized infections in humans. Front Microbiol 9:1696. https://doi.org/10.3389/fmicb.2018.01696

Moye ZD, Woolston J, Sulakvelidze A (2018) Bacteriophage applications for food production and processing. Viruses 10:205. https://doi.org/10.3390/v10040205

O'Flaherty S, Coffey A, Meaney W, Fitzgerald GF, Ross RP (2005) The recombinant phage lysin LysK has a broad spectrum of lytic activity against clinically relevant staphylococci, including methicillin-resistant *Staphylococcus aureus*. J Bacteriol 187:7161–7164. https://doi.org/10.1128/JB.187.20.7161-7164.2005

O'Flynn G, Ross RP, Fitzgerald GF, Coffey A (2004) Evaluation of a cocktail of three bacteriophages for biocontrol of *Escherichia coli* O157:H7. Appl Environ Microbiol. https://doi.org/10.1128/AEM.70.6.3417-3424.2004

O'Sullivan D, Paul Ross R, Fitzgerald GF, Coffey A (2000) Investigation of the relationship between lysogeny and lysis of *Lactococcus lactis* in cheese using prophage-targeted PCR. Appl Environ Microbiol 66:2192–2198. https://doi.org/10.1128/AEM.66.5.2192-2198.2000

Obeso JM, García P, Martínez B, Noé Arroyo-López F, Garrido-Fernández A, Rodriguez A (2010) Use of logistic regression for prediction of the fate of *Staphylococcus aureus* in pasteurized milk in the presence of two lytic phages. Appl Environ Microbiol 76:6038–6046. https://doi.org/10.1128/AEM.00613-10

Obradovic A, Jones JB, Momol MT, Balogh B, Olson SM (2004) Management of tomato bacterial spot in the field by foliar applications of bacteriophages and SAR inducers. Plant Dis 88:736–740. https://doi.org/10.1094/PDIS.2004.88.7.736

Oliveira H, Thiagarajan V, Walmagh M, Sillankorva S, Lavigne R, Neves-Petersen MT, Kluskens LD, Azeredo J (2014) A thermostable salmonella phage endolysin, Lys68, with broad bactericidal properties against gram-negative pathogens in presence of weak acids. PLoS One 9:e108376. https://doi.org/10.1371/journal.pone.0108376

Pao S, Rolph SP, Westbrook EW, Shen H (2006) Use of bacteriophages to control *Salmonella* in experimentally contaminated sprout seeds. J Food Sci 69:M127–M130. https://doi.org/10.1111/j.1365-2621.2004.tb10720.x

Park MK, Li S, Chin BA (2013) Detection of Salmonella typhimurium grown directly on tomato surface using phage-based Magnetoelastic biosensors. Food Bioprocess Technol 6:682–689. https://doi.org/10.1007/s11947-011-0708-2

Pilet MF, Leroi F (2010) Applications of protective cultures, bacteriocins and bacteriophages in fresh seafood and seafood products. In: Protective cultures, antimicrobial metabolites and bacteriophages for food and beverage biopreservation. pp 324–347. https://doi.org/10.1533/9780857090522.3.324

Pires DP, Cleto S, Sillankorva S, Azeredo J, Lu TK (2016) Genetically engineered phages: a review of advances over the last decade. Microbiol Mol Biol Rev 80:523–543. https://doi.org/10.1128/mmbr.00069-15

Pouillot F, Chomton M, Blois H, Courroux C, Noelig J, Bidet P, Bingen E, Bonacorsi S (2012) Efficacy of bacteriophage therapy in experimental sepsis and meningitis caused by a clone O25b: H4-ST131 Escherichia coli strain producing CTX-M-15. Antimicrob Agents Chemother 56:3568–3575. https://doi.org/10.1128/AAC.06330-11

Ravi Y, Pooja MK, Krushna Yadav DK (2017) Review- bacteriophages in food preservation. Int J Pure Appl Biosci 5:197–205. https://doi.org/10.18782/2320-7051.2873

Rawat S (2015) Food spoilage: microorganisms and their prevention. Pelagia Res Libr Asian J Plant Sci Res 5:47–56. https://www.imedpub.com/articles/food-spoilage-microorganisms-and-their-prevention.pdf

Sain A, Jayaprakash NS (2020) Draft genome sequence data of a T7like phage 3A_8767 isolated from wastewater of a butcher house near Palar River. Data Br 30:105446. https://doi.org/10.1016/j.dib.2020.105446

Sain A, Dubey V, Ghosh AR (2018) *Enterococcus Faecium* strain AVG44 - a potential probiotic isolated from human Faecal sample. Int J Pharma Bio Sci 9:85–93. https://doi.org/10.22376/ijpbs.2018.9.2.p85-93

Sharma M (2013) Lytic bacteriophages: potential interventions against enteric bacterial pathogens on produce. Bacteriophage 3:e25518. https://doi.org/10.4161/bact.25518

Sharma M, Patel JR, Conway WS, Ferguson S, Sulakvelidze A (2009) Effectiveness of bacteriophages in reducing *Escherichia coli* O157:H7 on fresh-cut cantaloupes and lettuce. J Food Prot 72:1481–1485. https://doi.org/10.4315/0362-028X-72.7.1481

Sharp NJ, Vandamm JP, Molineux IJ, Schofield DA (2015) Rapid detection of *Bacillus anthracis* in complex food matrices using phage-mediated bioluminescence. J Food Prot 78:963–968. https://doi.org/10.4315/0362-028X.JFP-14-534

Sklar IB, Joerger RD (2001) Attempts to utilize bacteriophage to combat *Salmonella enterica* serovar *enteritidis* infection in chickens. J Food Saf 21:15–29. https://doi.org/10.1111/j.1745-4565.2001.tb00305.x

Smartt AE, Xu T, Jegier P, Carswell JJ, Blount SA, Sayler GS, Ripp S (2012) Pathogen detection using engineered bacteriophages. Anal Bioanal Chem 402:3127–3146. https://doi.org/10.1007/s00216-011-5555-5

Sohaib M, Anjum FM, Arshad MS, Rahman UU (2016) Postharvest intervention technologies for safety enhancement of meat and meat based products; a critical review. J Food Sci Technol 53:19–30. https://doi.org/10.1007/s13197-015-1985-y

Soni KA, Nannapaneni R, Hagens S (2010) Reduction of *Listeria monocytogenes* on the surface of fresh channel catfish fillets by bacteriophage listex p100. Foodborne Pathog Dis 7:427–434. https://doi.org/10.1089/fpd.2009.0432

Suklim K, Flick GJ, Vichitphan K (2014) Effects of gamma irradiation on the physical and sensory quality and inactivation of *Listeria monocytogenes* in blue swimming crab meat (Portunas pelagicus). Radiat Phys Chem 103:22–26. https://doi.org/10.1016/j.radphyschem.2014.05.009

Tagliaferri TL, Jansen M, Horz HP (2019) Fighting pathogenic Bacteria on two fronts: phages and antibiotics as combined strategy. Front Cell Infect Microbiol 9:22. https://doi.org/10.3389/fcimb.2019.00022

Tanaka C, Yamada K, Takeuchi H, Inokuchi Y, Kashiwagi A, Toba T (2018) A lytic bacteriophage for controlling *Pseudomonas lactis* in raw cow's milk. Appl Environ Microbiol 84:e00111–e00118. https://doi.org/10.1128/AEM.00111-18

Thouand G, Vachon P, Liu S, Dayre M, Griffiths MW (2008) Optimization and validation of a simple method using P22::luxAB bacteriophage for rapid detection of *Salmonella enterica* serotypes A, B, and D in poultry samples. J Food Prot 71:380–385. https://doi.org/10.4315/0362-028X-71.2.380

Tomat D, Mercanti D, Balagué C, Quiberoni A (2013) Phage biocontrol of enteropathogenic and Shiga toxin-producing *Escherichia coli* during milk fermentation. Lett Appl Microbiol 57:3–10. https://doi.org/10.1111/lam.12074

Toro H, Price SB, McKee S, Hoerr FJ, Krehling J, Perdue M, Bauermeister L (2005) Use of bacteriophages in combination with competitive exclusion to reduce *Salmonella* from infected chickens. Avian Dis 49:118–124. https://doi.org/10.1637/7286-100404r

Ul Haq I, Chaudhry WN, Akhtar MN, Andleeb S, Qadri I (2012) Bacteriophages and their implications on future biotechnology: a review. Virol J 9:9. https://doi.org/10.1186/1743-422X-9-9

Varzakas T, Tzia C (2015) Handbook of food processing: food preservation. CRC Press. https://doi.org/10.1201/b19397

Vestby LK, Møretrø T, Langsrud S, Heir E, Nesse LL (2009) Biofilm forming abilities of *Salmonella* are correlated with persistence in fish meal- and feed factories. BMC Vet Res 5:20. https://doi.org/10.1186/1746-6148-5-20

Vinay M, Franche N, Grégori G, Fantino JR, Pouillot F, Ansaldi M (2015) Phage-based fluorescent biosensor prototypes to specifically detect enteric bacteria such as *E. coli* and *Salmonella enterica typhimurium*. PLoS One 10:e0131466. https://doi.org/10.1371/journal.pone.0131466

Wang F, Horikawa S, Hu J, Wikle HC, Chen IH, Du S, Liu Y, Chin BA (2017) Detection of *Salmonella typhimurium* on spinach using phage-based magnetoelastic biosensors. Sensors (Switzerland) 17:386. https://doi.org/10.3390/s17020386

Wei S, Chelliah R, Rubab M, Oh DH, Uddin MJ, Ahn J (2019) Bacteriophages as potential tools for detection and control of salmonella spp. in food systems. Microorganisms 7: 570. https://doi.org/10.3390/microorganisms7110570

Wernicki A, Nowaczek A, Urban-Chmiel R (2017) Bacteriophage therapy to combat bacterial infections in poultry. Virol J 14:179. https://doi.org/10.1186/s12985-017-0849-7

Wisuthiphaet N, Yang X, Young GM, Nitin N (2019) Rapid detection of Escherichia coli in beverages using genetically engineered bacteriophage T7. AMB Express 9:55. https://doi.org/10.1186/s13568-019-0776-7

Yin W, Wang Y, Liu L, He J (2019) Biofilms: the microbial "protective clothing" in extreme environments. Int J Mol Sci 20:3423. https://doi.org/10.3390/ijms20143423

Young R (2013) Phage lysis: do we have the hole story yet? Curr Opin Microbiol 16:790–797. https://doi.org/10.1016/j.mib.2013.08.008

Chapter 8
Food Applications of Cyclodextrins

Yogesh Kumar and Somya Singhal

Abstract Environmental conditions of food may degrade the biological activity of the principal compounds such as antioxidants, antimicrobial agents, vitamins, colorants, and flavors present in the food. However, these compounds are beneficial to human health in many ways such as reducing blood sugar level, weight loss, reduction in cholesterol level, and coronary heart disease. Therefore, to preserve the bioactive compounds, they need to be protected by a formulation that can deliver them to target sites without losing any bioactivity. Cyclodextrins are cyclic oligosaccharides produced from the degradation of starch with a hydrophobic interior and a hydrophilic exterior, capable of formation of inclusion with the guest molecule. Due to the inclusion complex property of cyclodextrin act as a delivery system and can improve the physical, chemical, and biological properties of the bioactive compounds in food. Therefore, this chapter is a narrative review on the cyclodextrin with emphasis given physico-chemical properties and ability to form inclusion complex. Also, the current state-of-the-art on their utilization in the food industry as an encapsulating material for bioactive compounds is reviewed.

Keywords Cyclodextrin · Encapsulation · Inclusion complex · Micro-/nanoencapsulation · Health · Vitamins

Abbreviations

CGTase	Glucosyltransferase/glucanotranferase
HI	Hydrogen iodide
H_3PO_4	Phosphoric acid
TCE	Trichloroethene
CD-NS	Cyclodextrin based nanosponges

Y. Kumar (✉)
Department of Food Science and Technology, National Institute of Food Technology Entrepreneurship and Management, Sonipat, Haryana, India

S. Singhal
Department of Food Engineering and Technology, Tezpur University, Tezpur, Assam, India

V. K. Maurya et al. (eds.), *Sustainable Agriculture Reviews 55*, Sustainable Agriculture Reviews 55, https://doi.org/10.1007/978-3-030-76813-3_8

BSA	Bovine serum albumin
PAA-NS	Poly (amidoamine) nanosponges
MCF-7 cells	Michigan cancer foundation-7
RH	Relative humidity
PAA	Polyacrylic acid
AITC	Allyl isothiocyanate complex
HTST	Hight temperature short time

8.1 Introduction

In starch, enzymatic degradation usually results in a production of several products such as glucose, maltotriose, and maltose that forms a long series of linear or branched chain malto-oligomers, known as dextrins. Starch degradation takes place by the action of glucosyltransferase enzyme (CGTase) resulting in the splitting of the chain. The primary cyclic structure called cyclodextrin containing α 1,4-linkage obtained from the intermolecular reaction in the absence of H_2O in the resulting chain. Commercially, the commonly used cyclodextrins are the α-cyclodextrin (6 glucose units), β-cyclodextrin (7 glucose units) and γ-cyclodextrin consisting of 8 glucose units. The primary property of cyclodextrin is to form inclusion complexes along with multiple compounds (Crini et al. 2018). Cyclodextrin containing torus- / ring-shaped structures bearing a hydrophobic cavity and hydrophilic exterior surface. This hydrophobicity in cyclodextrin interacts with the non-polar organic compounds or some part of organic compounds resulting in the formation of inclusion complexes.

In 1891, cyclodextrins were first discovered by Villier in the name of "cellulosine" during investigating the digestion of potato starch by *Bacillus amylobacter* (Szejtli 2013a). After 12 years, Schardinger (1902), encountered two crystalline polysaccharides like "cellulosine" during his study on the synthesis or degradation of starch using a different microorganism, that he termed as "dextrin α" and "dextrin β." He specified the isolated microorganism as *Bacillus macerans*. Moreover, he suggested that 25–30% starch was sufficient to prepared crystalline and amorphous dextrins (Szejtli 2013a, b). During the 1930s, Freudenberg along with his colleagues discovered that the crystalline Schardinger dextrins contain only maltose units and α-1, 4-glycosidic linkages. In 1936, they asserted the cyclic structure of the crystalline dextrins (Szejtli 2013a, b; Ueda 2002). During early 1942, the structures of both α- and β-cyclodextrin were confirmed with the help of X-ray crystallography. In 1948, the structure of γ-cyclodextrin got defined. In 1953, Freudenberg along with Camer and Plieinger received a patent based on the application of cyclodextrins complexation in drug formulations for protection from oxidation, stabilizing volatile substance, enhancing solubility, and many more (Szejtli 2013a, b).

The use of semi-systematic names for cyclodextrins was suggested by the "Joint Commission on Biochemical Nomenclature" in 1996 "by citing the prefix cyclo, followed by terms indicating the type of inter-saccharidic linkages, the number of units and the termination '-ose' (like "malto" for α-1,4 linked glucose units; "hexa" for six)". The semi-systematic names, such as cyclomaltohexaose for the cyclodextrin consisting of six α-1,4-linked glycosyl units, have been nearly consistently used as descriptors for the small cyclodextrins in addition to the Greek letter prefix version. It should be observed that the ending "-ose" signifies a free anomeric center, which is absent in cyclodextrins. Proposal of a systematic nomenclature was done where cyclic oligosaccharides composed of a single type of residue could be named "by giving the systematic name of the glycosyl residue, preceded by the linkage type in parentheses, preceded in turn by 'cyclo-' with a multiplicative suffix" such as cyclohexakis-(1,4)-α-D-glycosyl for α-cyclodextrin (Larsen 2002). The schematic representation in the development of cyclodextrin showed in Table 8.1.

8.1.1 Structure of Cyclodextrin

The three cyclodextrins (α-, β- and γ-cyclodextrins) are crystalline, non-hygroscopic substances and homogeneous in nature and have torus-like macro-rings composed of 6, 7 and 8 glucopyranose units, respectively (Fig. 8.1a, b and c). The ring that combines the cyclodextrins is a conical cylinder, which resembles a wreath-shaped truncated cone or doughnut (Szejtli 2013a, b; Saito et al. 2004). The cavity in the ring is lined by the hydrogen atoms and the glycosidic oxygen bridges. The non-bonding electron pairs of the glycosidic oxygen bridges are focused on the interior of the cavity resulting in a high electron density and depicting some Lewis base characteristics (Saito et al. 2004). In cyclodextrins, each glucopyranose unit has three free hydroxyls (OH) groups. Among these three free OH groups, one is primary (C-6) and two are secondary (C-2 and C-3). Each of these free OH groups can be altered by substituting the hydrogen atom or the OH group by multiple substituents such as hydroxyalkyl-, amino-, carboxyalkyl and several more to increase the solubility of the cyclodextrin derivatives obtained, to affix the certain catalytic group to the binding site in case of enzymatic modelling, to develop insoluble and immobilized structure like for chromatography or to improve the cyclodextrin and host interaction (Szejtli 2004).

In X-ray structures of cyclodextrin, it is observed that the 2° -OH groups (C-2 and C-3) are present on the broad edge of the ring and the 1° -OH groups (C-6) on the other edge. Cyclodextrin cavity contains apolar C-3 and C-5 hydrogens and ether-like oxygens. The structure of cyclodextrin consists of a hydrophilic region outside, which attracts water and hydrophobic region inside consisting of a polar cavity described as a "micro heterogeneous environment." The C–2–OH group of one glucopyranose unit can form a hydrogen bond with the C–3–OH group of the adjacent glucopyranose unit (Saito et al. 2004).

In the cyclodextrin structure, the entire secondary band is synthesized by H-bonds which form a rigid structure of β-cyclodextrin. This might be the reason that the β-cyclodextrin has the lowest water solubility among all cyclodextrins. In the

Table 8.1 Schematic representation in the development of cyclodextrins

Advancement	References
In 1891, Viller discovered cyclodextrins and named "cellulosine"	Szejtli (1988), Szejtli (2004), Ueda (2002)
In 1903, Schardinger found the crystalline dextrin and named dextrin A and B	
In the 1930s, Freudenberg and co-workers postulated the cyclic structure	
In 1942, the structure of α- and β-cyclodextrin were determined by X-ray crystallography	
In 1948, it was recognized that cyclodextrins can form inclusion complexes	
1996 semi-systematic names of cyclodextrins were recommended by the Joint Commission on Biochemical Nomenclature	Larsen (2002)
Use of cyclodextrin for encapsulation of food products	Hedges et al. (1995)
Cyclodextrin used as encapsulating material for the development of antimicrobial packaging material	Appendini and Hotchkiss (2002)
Cyclodextrin complexes in food: flavors and vitamins; physical property modifiers; taste modifiers; selective complexation and sequestration	Szejtli (2004)
The molecular encapsulation of lipophilic food ingredients with cyclodextrin improves the stability of flavors, vitamins, colorants, and unsaturated fats both in a physical and chemical sense leading to extended product shelf-life	Szente and Szejtli (2004)
Food applications include encapsulation of flavors using cyclodextrin; protection from oxidative degradation; elimination of odd taste from food; cholesterol sequestrant and food preservation	Astray et al. (2009)
Inclusion of polyphenols in cyclodextrins improves the water solubility of less water-soluble phytochemicals	Fang and Bhandari (2010)
Cyclodextrin in conjunction with nanoparticles used for oral delivery of proteins	Kanwar et al. (2011)
Depicted cyclodextrin as a secondary antioxidant due to which reduces browning of food	Lopez-Nicolas et al. (2014)
Multi applications of cyclodextrin in different streams of science (food, textile, cosmetic, pharmaceuticals, drug delivery, chemical)	Sharma and Baldi (2016)
Cyclodextrin as an encapsulation material for flavor and aroma	Kfoury et al. (2014a)
Nanoencapsulation of flavors and aromas by cyclodextrins in food processing and packaging	Fenyvesi and Szente (2016)
Encapsulations of selected antioxidants by cyclodextrins	Zarzycki and Głód (2016)
Cyclodextrin based nanosponges used in the purification of water	Sherje et al. (2017)
Hydroxypropyl-β-cyclodextrin used for encapsulating guava leaf oil which enhances its antioxidant and antimicrobial activity	Rakmai et al. (2018)
Cyclodextrin used as pre-encapsulating material along with the incorporation of the drug in a liposomal core which improves the loading efficiency of drug	Bhatt et al. (2018)
Cyclodextrin based polyrotaxanes used for the development of macroscopic functional materials such as slide ring gel, macroscopic assemblies, self-healing materials	Hashidzume et al. (2019)
β-cyclodextrin used as a solvent in ultrasound-assisted extraction in green pepper extracts which improves its antioxidant activity	Favre et al. (2020)

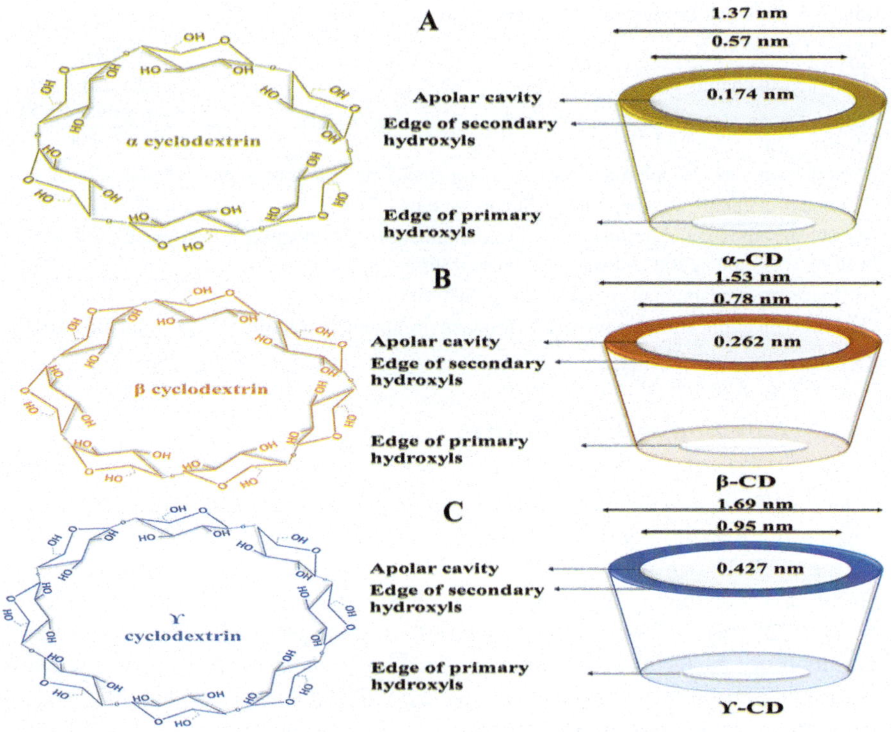

Fig. 8.1 Structure of cyclodextrins **(a)** α-cyclodextrin containing 6-glucopyaronse units, **(b)** β-cyclodextrin containing 7-glucopyaronse units and **(c)** γ-cyclodextrin containing 8-glucopyaronse units

α-cyclodextrin structure, there is one glucopyranose unit in a contorted position resulting in the incomplete H-bond belt. Therefore, only four are stable rather than the six possible H-bonds. The γ-cyclodextrin is a non-coplanar and a more flexible structure. Therefore, it is the most soluble among the three cyclodextrins. The diameter of the cavity is more on the side having 2° -OH groups than compared to the side with 1° -OH, as a free rotation of the latter reduces the diameter of the cavity (Saito et al. 2004). Besides, the solid-state structures of cyclodextrin 9, cyclodextrin 10, cyclodextrin 14, and cyclodextrin 26 have also been reported. The structure of cyclodextrin 9 illustrated a contorted elliptical boat-like shape, however, it retains a somewhat similar structure to regular cyclodextrins. In cyclodextrin 10 and cyclodextrin 14, they show a more elliptical macrocyclic kind of ring folded in a saddle-like shape. While the structure of cyclodextrin 26 is very different from the regular cyclodextrins as it possesses channel-like cavities containing two short V-amylose helices arranged in an anti-parallel direction (Larsen 2002; Ueda 2002). Selected books listed in Table 8.2 contain information on other cyclodextrins.

Table 8.2 Selected key books on cyclodextrins

Title	References
Cyclodextrin chemistry	Bender and Komiyama (1978)
Cyclodextrin technology	Szejtli (1988)
Cyclodextrin materials photochemistry, photophysics, and photobiology	Douhal (2006)
Cyclodextrin chemistry: preparation and application	Jin (2013)
Novel macromolecular architectures via a combination of cyclodextrin host/guest complexation and RAFT polymerization	Schmidt (2014)
Cyclodextrin fundamentals, reactivity, and analysis	Crini (2018)
Cyclodextrin applications in medicine, food, environment, and liquid crystals	Fourmentin (2018)

8.1.2 Isolation of Cyclodextrin

Viller was the first to discover cyclodextrin glucanotranferase (CGTase) from potato starch using *Bacillus amylobacter* for the production of cyclodextrin (Larsen 2002). During cyclodextrin production at the industrial level, a large number of bacteria can be used for the synthesis of CGTase such as *Bacillus circulars and Bacillus megaterium* (aerobic mesophilic bacteria), *Bacillus stearothermophilus* (aerobic thermophilic bacteria), *Thermoanaerobacterium thermosulfurigenes* (anaerobic thermophilic bacteria), *Bacillus circulars, Bacillus fat* (aerobic alkaliphilic bacteria) and *Halophilic bacilli* (aerobic halophilic bacteria). The main products of CGTase enzyme are different: α-cyclodextrin, β-cyclodextrin, and γ-cyclodextrin.

According to a study conducted by Yampayont et al. (2006), soil samples were procured from areas nearby to starch factories and were screened for cyclodextrin producing bacteria. Primarily, amylolytic activity on medium I agar plate containing soluble starch stained with iodine solution was tested. As a result, positive clones as a clear yellowish zone were visible against the deep blue background. Colonies having the ratio of a clear zone to colony size exceeding three were further tested for CGTase activity (Fig. 8.2a). Moreover, these colonies were inoculated on Horikoshi medium plate having phenolphthalein for cyclodextrin production. Isolated clones delivering CGTase can modify the starch present in the medium to cyclodextrin. Therefore, β-cyclodextrin can encapsulate phenolphthalein and produce a yellow zone contrary to a red background (Fig. 8.2b). Among the clones producing yellow zones, three were selected and confirmed for cyclodextrin formation through cyclodextrin-TCE assay.

At 45 °C, isolate producing cyclodextrin was identified and named as *BT01*. *Paenibacillus sp. BT01* was confirmed as rod-shaped gram-positive *Bacillus*. For producing maximal cyclodextrin forming activity, 40 °C for 72 h, at pH 10.0 in Horikoshi broth containing 0.5% soluble starch was found to be optimum culturing conditions. With the help of starch absorption, CGTase was partially purified, resulting in 64% recovery with a purification fold of 27. The enzyme showed optimum

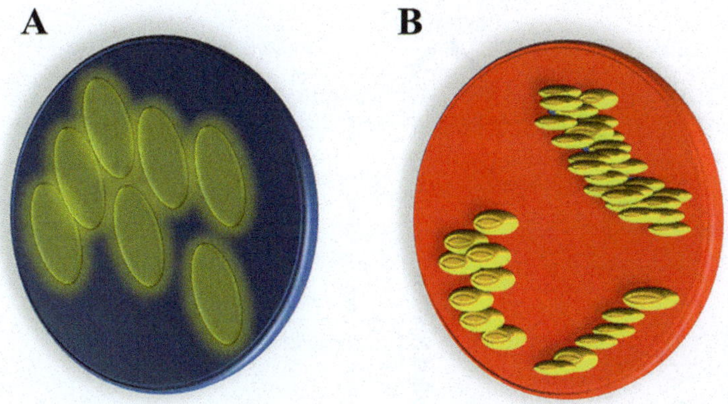

Fig. 8.2 Screening of cyclodextrins producing bacteria. (**a**) Dextrinizing activity on solid medium I stained with iodine solution where light shade = yellowish color of iodine solution. Dark shade = dark brown color of starch-iodine complex. (**b**) Cyclodextrins-forming activity on solid Horikoshi medium with phenolphthalein where light shade = colorless cyclodextrins-phenolphthalein complex on methyl orange background. Dark shade = methyl orange+phenolphthalein background (Yampayont et al. 2006)

temperature for dextrinizing were ought to be 70 °C and pH 6.0; and 50–55 °C and pH 7.0 for cyclodextrin forming activity, respectively.

8.1.3 Preparation of Cyclodextrins

The preparation of different cyclodextrins could be done using two methods: control and non-control system. The only difference between these processes is that in a non-control system, organic solvents can be added to prepare the different cyclodextrin while in the control system, no solvent is required. The purity of α-, β- and γ- cyclodextrins with the purity of >99% can be obtained using procedure showed in Figs. 8.3a, b, and c respectively (Szejtli 2013a, b).

8.1.4 Analysis of Cyclodextrins

8.1.4.1 UV Spectrophotometry

Colored reagents such as phenolphthalein, methyl orange, and bromocresol green were added to cyclodextrins resulting in an increase or decrease in the maximum absorbance thus, depicting a linear relation between cyclodextrin concentration and absorbance in a certain range. The concentration of α-, β- and γ-cyclodextrins are

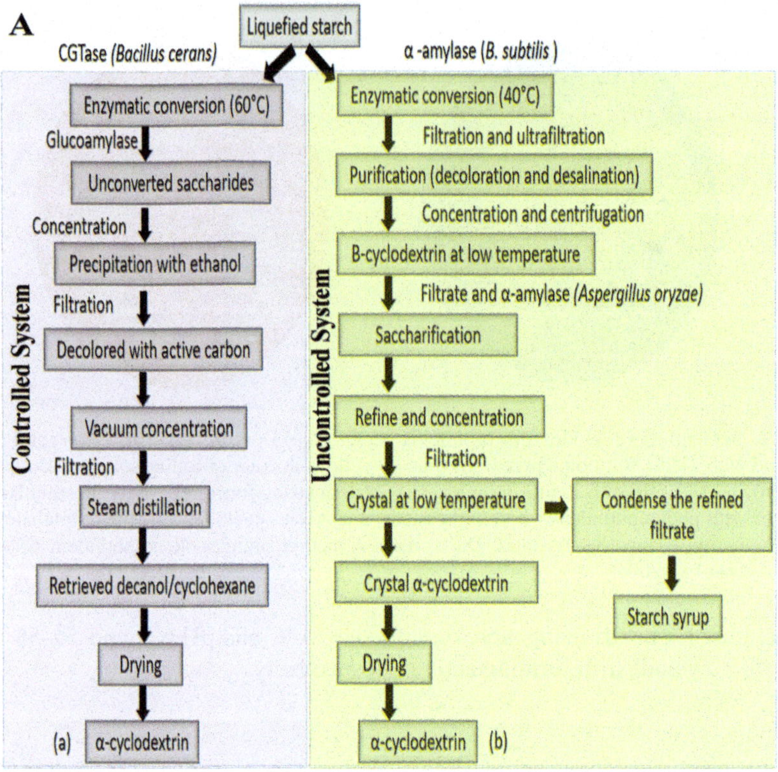

Fig. 8.3 (**a**) Preparation for α-cyclodextrin under controlled and uncontrolled systems. (**b**) Preparation for β-cyclodextrin under controlled and uncontrolled systems. (**c**) Preparation for γ-cyclodextrin under controlled and uncontrolled systems

quantified by UV spectrophotometry using colored reagents. The detection conditions are described in Table 8.3 (Szejtli 2013a, b).

8.1.4.2 High-Performance Liquid Chromatography

According to Yampayont et al. (2006), 0.5 ml of enzyme sample was mixed with 2.5 ml of the starch substrate (0.2% soluble potato starch in 0.2 M phosphate buffer maintained at pH 6.0) and left for incubation for 24 h at 40 °C. After incubation, the mixture was boiled in water for 5 min and then cooled. Further, the mixture was reacted with 20 units of β-amylase at 25 °C for 1 h and then again heated in boiling water to stop the reaction. Before injection, the mixture was filtered using a 0.45μm membrane filter. The mixture was injected and eluted using acetonitrile-water (70:30 v/v) at 1 ml/min flow rate. The cyclodextrin peaks were quantified by comparing the sample peaks with the retention time of standard cyclodextrins

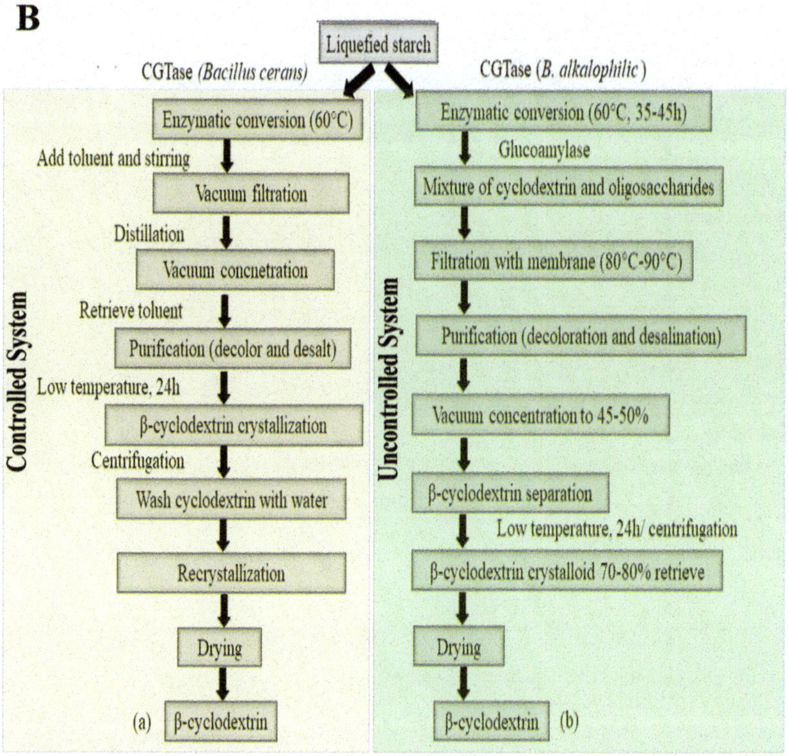

Fig. 8.3 (continued)

8.1.4.3 Thin-Layer Chromatography

The solution (5–10μL) composed of 30–70μg of cyclodextrin is applied on a silica gel plate (Macherey-Nagel Polygram Syl G'''). The chromatogram is developed for 3.5–4 h using n-butanol-ethanol-water (4,3,3) mixture to a height of 15–18 cm. After drying, the plate is exposed to iodine vapor for 1–2 min. The observations are shown in Table 8.4 (Szejtli 2013a, b).

8.1.4.4 Gas Chromatography

α, β, and γ-cyclodextrin and their mixtures can be investigated using gas chromatography. The samples are primarily prepared by disintegrating the cyclodextrin-solvent complexes and transforming them into volatile dimethyl silyl ethers. The initial column oven temperature of 325–405 °C was constantly maintained until γ-cyclodextrin was eluted. Moreover, the temperature of the injector and detector was set at 370 °C in addition to the 45–50 ml/min flow rate of carrier gas (helium) (Beadle 1969).

C

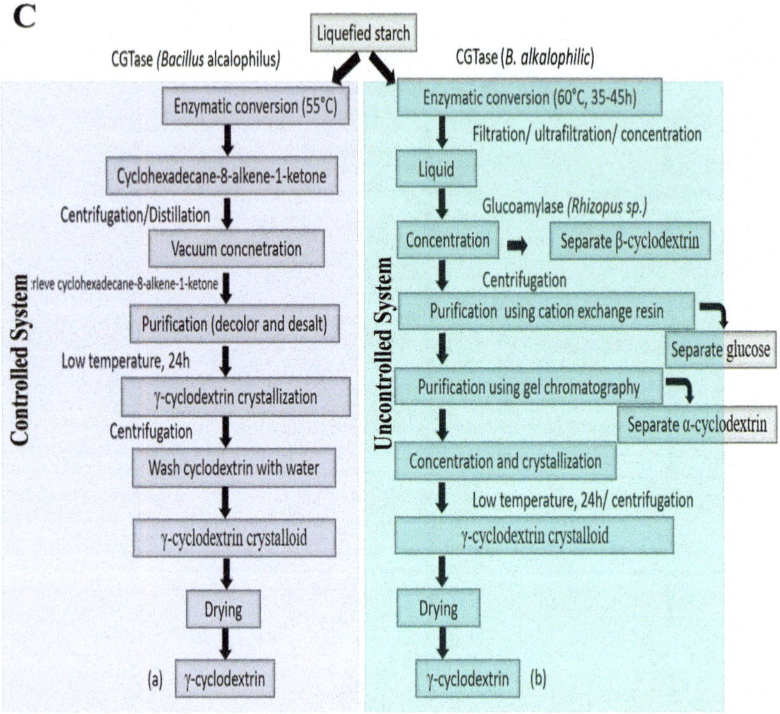

Fig. 8.3 (continued)

Table 8.3 Analysis of various cyclodextrin using UV Spectrophotometry

Component	Wavelength (nm)	Solution for detection
α-cyclodextrin	503	Methyl orange and α-cyclodextrins
β-cyclodextrin	553	Phenolphthalein and β-cyclodextrins
γ -cyclodextrin	630	Bromocresol and γ -cyclodextrins

Szejtli (2013a, b)

Table 8.4 Analysis of various cyclodextrin using thin layer chromatography

Component	R_f	Color reaction
Amylose	0.0	Blue-Violet
Dextrin	0.0–0.3	Brownish-Violet
α cyclodextrin	0.35	Yellow-Orange
β cyclodextrin	0.39	Lemon-Yellow
γ cyclodextrin	0.5–0.7	Brown

R_f: Retention time
Szejtli (2013a, b)

8.2 Physico-Chemical Properties of Cyclodextrins

8.2.1 Chemical Reactivity

There are no reducing end-groups in cyclodextrin, modification reactions take place at the hydroxyl (-OH) groups. One glucose unit of cyclodextrin contains three hydroxyl groups, the hydroxyl groups at carbon 2, 3 are 2° hydroxyl groups and at carbon 6 is 1° hydroxyl group. The 1° hydroxyl group at position 6 is the least acidic and most accessible, 2° hydroxyl groups at position 2 are most acidic and at position 3 are least accessible. Cyclodextrin-base reaction deprotonated all the hydroxyl groups, the hydroxyl group at position 6 selectively reacted with electrophilic reagents due to its easy accessibility. Some reactive agents also react with hydroxyl groups present at positions 2 and 3. An example of this type of reaction is the synthesis of 6-*O*-tosyl-cyclodextrin. Strong base-cyclodextrin reactions lead to the substitution of the hydroxyl group at position 2 due to its most acidic nature. But at position 3 substitution of the hydroxyl group is most difficult but β-cyclodextrin and cinnamyl bromide reaction allow the substitution at position 3 of the hydroxyl group. Therefore, with hydroxyl groups substitution at positions 2, 3, and 6 of cyclodextrin produced various multi-substituted by-products (Rezanka 2018).

8.2.2 Radiolysis

Cyclodextrins form supramolecular assemblies due to aggregations of cyclodextrin, aggregations of cyclodextrin inclusion complexes, cyclodextrin rotaxanes, and poly-rotaxanes, cyclodextrin nanotubes and their secondary assembly which may be responsible for the synthesis of nanoparticles by ionizing radiation. When an aqueous solution containing cyclodextrins is irradiated by ionizing radiation, OH° radicals formed due to ionization which interacts with hydrogen atoms of the hydroxyl group on carbon 1 and 5 position of cyclodextrin. Due to this interaction, the reaction between aqueous electrons and cyclodextrin remains weak which causes less formation of nanoparticles. Therefore, a higher dose of β-cyclodextrin (8.0×10^{-3} mol/L) could prevent this interaction, and the reduction product of Cu $(NO_3)_2$ available in aqueous solution could be converted to Cu_2O to Cu-nanoparticles. This was the first report depicting the formation of metal nanoparticles such as Cu-nanoparticles with the assistance of β-cyclodextrin. Further reported that Cu nanoparticles should be stabilized in a hydrophobic condition and in the presence of oxygen it was converted to CuO-nanoparticles. Therefore, the radiolytic synthesis of nanoparticles in assistance with cyclodextrins can be an efficient method in the formation of nanoparticles for functional food and nutraceuticals (Chen et al. 2010).

8.2.3 Acid Hydrolysis

It is observed that the acid hydrolysis of one glycosidic bond of β-cyclodextrin is slower than the linear oligosaccharides. It is due to the formation of inclusion complexes which can slow down the rate of acid hydrolysis. Therefore, it is noticed that the rate of the reactions depends only on the concentration of the catalyst H^+ ion and length of the alkyl chain of guest molecules. However, the presence of guest molecules still not confirmed for the interruption of acid hydrolysis. But, reaction of hydrolysis of α-cyclodextrin with 0.1 mol/L hydrochloric acid at 90 °C in the presence of guest molecules such as 1-butanol and 2-propanol, decelerates the acid hydrolysis reaction in both cases. However,1-butanol decelerates the acid hydrolysis more as compared to 2-propanol because of the formation of inclusion complex with guest and non-availability of oxygen of glycosidic bond in the cyclodextrin cavity and having long alkyl chain. Therefore, the concentration of the catalyst H^+ ion may have difficulties to attach oxygen in the presence of inclusion complex with guest molecules. With this property, cyclodextrin can be complexed with long chain oligosaccharides and may develop higher oligosaccharides from cyclodextrin (Vaitkus et al. 2011).

8.2.4 Crystal Structure

In the crystal lattice, molecules of cyclodextrin are packed in either of the modes *viz.* cage or channel structure. In a cage-type structure, the cavity of one cyclodextrin is blocked by the adjacent cyclodextrins from both sides resulting in isolated cavities. Thus, the molecules of cyclodextrins can be either packed in a brick-wall trend or herringbone trend (usually seen in α-, β- and γ-cyclodextrins). While for the crystal structures belonging to the channel-type, molecules of cyclodextrins are arranged like coins in a roll or stacked on top of each other. The guest molecules are enclosed in "limitless" channels, developed by the linearly aligned cavities (Alston et al. 1985). This arrangement can be either "head-to-head" type or "head-to-tail" type as shown in Fig. 8.4. Cyclodextrin crystallized from water does not contain an empty cavity, rather it is filled with water molecules, and rest formed an integral part of the crystal structure. During inclusion complex formation the guest molecule is substituted with the included water. Cyclodextrins exists in different crystal form which depends on the conditions.

α-cyclodextrin exists in three different crystal forms with herringbone structure; α-cyclodextrin.6H_2O (from I), α-cyclodextrin.6H_2O (form II) and α-cyclodextrin.7.5H_2O (form III). β-cyclodextrin exists in β-cyclodextrin.12H_2O and β-cyclodextrin.11H_2O whereas γ-cyclodextrin has γ-cyclodextrin.13.3H_2O crystal form with herringbone structure. In crystal form of α-cyclodextrin.6H_2O, a total of six water molecules are present; two inside the cavity and four are outside. In the β-cyclodextrin.11H_2O, the 11 water molecules are distributed at 16 position;

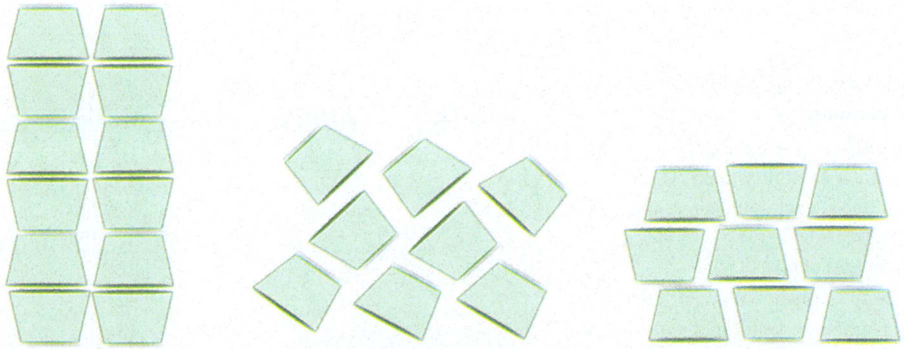

Fig. 8.4 Alignment of cyclodextrin rings in their complex crystal structures
Channel (**a**), herringbone (**b**) and brick (**c**) type

eight in the cavity (6.12 water molecules) and eight in the interstices (4.88 water molecules) whereas β-cyclodextrin.12H_2O have 6.5 water molecules in the cavity and 5.5 water molecules are in the interstices. The water molecules present in the cavity are associated with guest molecules during the inclusion complex whereas others interact with cyclodextrin crystal form. The other characteristics of cyclodextrin are present in Table 8.5.

Cyclodextrins do not have a defined melting point however, its thermo-analytical properties depend on the water content, heating rate, atmospheric condition, and crystal structure. The cyclodextrins show broad endothermic peaks due to the loss of water molecules. The hydrated α-cyclodextrin show endothermic peak at 80 °C, 106 °C and 129 °C while β- and γ-cyclodextrin giving peaks at 30 °C and 50 °C respectively which reflecting absorbed and bound water molecules. For anhydrous α- and β-cyclodextrins, small endothermic peaks are observed at 230 °C, 225 °C respectively and for γ-cyclodextrin at 167 °C and 152 °C (Szejtli 2013a, b).

8.2.5 Solubility

The water solubility of various cyclodextrins differ from each other and the values of cyclodextrins shown in Table 8.5. Cyclodextrins has low solubility as compared to linear saccharides due to the presence of inimical enthalpies of a solution and highly favorable entropies of solution. As compared to α- and γ-cyclodextrins, β-cyclodextrin is nine times less soluble. The α- and γ-cyclodextrins have similar thermodynamic properties. A decrease in solubility of β-cyclodextrin in water is due to the marked structure of water originating from the water–β-cyclodextrin interactions, resulting in compensation of the less favorable enthalpy by the less favorable entropy of solution (Saito et al. 2004). The thermodynamic characteristics for α-, β- and γ-cyclodextrins respectively; enthalpy as 7.67, 8.31, 7.73 kcal/mol, entropy as 13.8, 11.7,

Table 8.5 The main characteristics of three cyclodextrins

Cyclodextrin	α	β	γ
Glucopyranose units	6	7	8
Formulae	$C_{36}H_{60}O_{30}$	$C_{42}H_{70}O_{35}$	$C_{48}H_{80}O_{40}$
Molecular weight (g/mol)	972.9	1135.0	1297.1
Water solubility at 25 °C (g/L)	145	18.5	232
Central cavity diameter: external/internal (Å)	5.3/4.7	6.5/6.0	8.3/7.5
Height of torus (Å)	7.9	7.9	7.9
Approximate volume of cavity (Å)	174	262	427
Number of water molecules within the cavity	6–8	11–12	13–17
pKa	12.3	12.2	12.1
Crystal form (from water)	Hexagonal plates	Monoclinic parallelograms	Quadratic prisms
Crystal water weight (%)	10.2	13.2–14.5	8.13–17.7
Hydrolysis by *Aspergillus oryzae*, α-amylase	none	Slow	Fast

Szejtli (2013a, b)

14.7 J/K. Moreover, temperature also plays an important factor in the solubility of cyclodextrins. With the increase in temperature, the aqueous solubility of the cyclodextrins increases (Astray et al. 2009). Cyclodextrins solubility also decreases in the presence of organic molecules due to the formation of the inclusion complex.

8.3 Inclusion Complexes of Cyclodextrins as Encapsulation

8.3.1 Formation of Inclusion Complex

"Complexation is a simple structural phenomenon in which one host molecule of cyclodextrin accommodates another guest molecule to associate and form a complex" (Rajewski and Stella 1996). Cyclodextrins' lipophilic cavity at the interior side and hydrophilic part at the exterior surface help it in binding the guest molecules. During inclusion formation, the less polar guest molecules easily interact with the lipophilic cavity where the guest molecules replace the bound water molecules of the cavity. The process is firmly favored by the guest molecule-host (solvated hydrophobic/lipophilic cavity) interactions (Fig. 8.5a). During this process, change in entropy and enthalpy play a key role in inclusion formation (Saito et al. 2004). Inclusion of the guest in host molecules generally depends on their sizes, one guest molecules can interact with one or more cyclodextrins (host: guest complexes 1:1 and 2:1) and the two or more guest molecules can interact with one or more cyclodextrins (host: guest

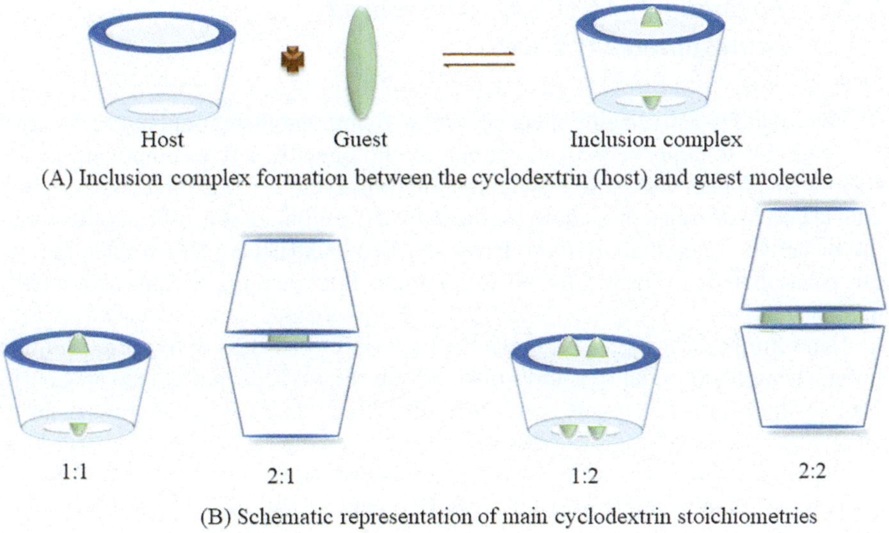

Fig. 8.5 Schematic representation of inclusion complex formation between cyclodextrin and guest molecules

complexes 1:2 and 2:2) as shown in Fig. 8.5b. Interactions between host and guest molecules take place through various possible reasons such as:

(a) Substitution of the strongly unfavored polar–apolar interactions (simultaneously between the included water and the cyclodextrin cavity, and between the water and the guest) by the more favored polar–polar interaction (between bulk water and the released cavity-water molecules) and apolar–apolar interaction (between the guest and the cavity).
(b) Release of cyclodextrin-ring strain on complexation.
(c) Van der Waals and hydrogen bonds between guest and host.

The guest and the host form a non-covalent bond in the inclusion complex. Several non-covalent interactions like dipole–dipole interaction, hydrophobic interactions, hydrogen bonding, van der Waal forces, London dispersion forces, and many others, subject to the formation of a stable inclusion complex. The beneficial effects of the guest-cyclodextrin complex include the increased guest solubility; prevent volatilization by stabilization of the guest molecule, prevention from degradation and oxidation due to exposure of heat and light; elimination or reduction of undesired odors or taste; prevention of harmful chemical reaction; directed chemical synthesis, separation and isolation of numerous chemicals (Saito et al. 2004).

8.3.2 *Formation of Cyclodextrins Based Nanosponges (CD-NS)*

The biologically active compounds present in functional food could not be functionally available to target sites. To functionalize biologically active compounds to their specific sites, the nanoparticles with amphiphilic cyclodextrins molecules could be considered to design a procedure for the delivery, solubilization, and stabilization of the bioactive compounds in food. However, cyclodextrins are less soluble in aqueous solution and inorganic solvents which limits their uses in the formulation (Crini et al. 2018).

Nanosponges is the part of nanotechnology which is a class of hyper cross-linked polymer-based colloidal structures made of sub-microscopic particles with cavities. Nanosponges can incorporate large molecules within their cavity. Therefore, several cross-linking agents bind cyclodextrin to form a polymer of the cyclodextrin-based nanosponges. The inner central cavity can incorporate substances in it. The term cyclodextrin-nanosponges was given by De Quan Li and Min Ma in 1998 but the use of nanosponges reported a long time ago. The polymerized cyclodextrin is less soluble and more stable, the less soluble cyclodextrin polymers are synthesized as a chain by cross-linking other molecules such as epichlorohydrin, epoxides, dialdehydes, diacyl chlorides to parent cyclodextrins. The cross-linkers are very reactive agents with two electrophilic sites capable to interact with the nucleophilic hydroxyl group on cyclodextrins. Thus, cross-linkers help to generate the cyclodextrin-nanosponges in which the lipophilic cavities and hydrophilic part able to incorporate the large molecules through inclusion and non-inclusion complexes. The structure of cyclodextrin nanosponges is shown in Fig. 8.6.

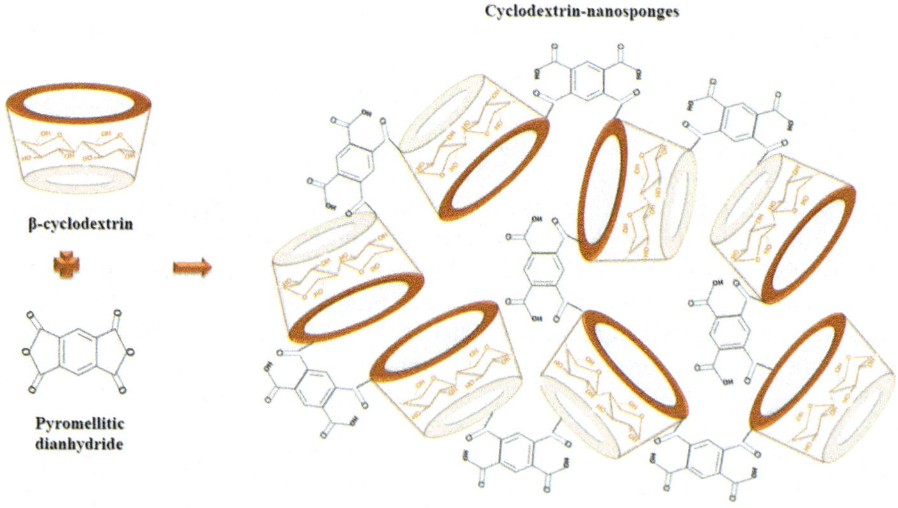

Fig. 8.6 Cross-linker reacted to cyclodextrin polymers to form cyclodextrin nanosponges

Table 8.6 Different cross-linkers used in the formation of cyclodextrin nanosponges

Class	Examples
Dicarboxylic acid chlorides	Glutaryl chloride, adipoyl chloride, sebacoyl, terephthaloyl chloride
Chlorhydrins	Epichlorohydrin
Acid anhydrides	Glutaric anhydride, maleic anhydride, phthalic anhydride, pyromellitic anhydride
Alkyl dihalides	Dichlorodimethyl siloxane, dichloromethane
Diisocyanates	Hexamethylene diisocyanate, isophorone diisocyanate, polydiisocyanate
Dicarboxylic acids	Succinic acid, 2,3-napthalene dicarboxylic acid, 2,2-bis(acryamido) acetic acid

Sherje et al. (2017)

The cross-linkers have their properties which shows the effect on the solubility of cyclodextrin polymer. Water-soluble or insoluble cyclodextrin polymers can be produced by controlling the reaction conditions of the cross-linkers. The cross-linkers play a major role in the synthesis of cyclodextrin polymers, various cross-linkers with polymers given in Table 8.6. The cyclodextrins-nanosponges are used in a variety of applications such as prevention of degradation of drugs, drug delivery, volatile oils, and water purification (Sherje et al. 2017).

8.4 Applications of Cyclodextrins in Food and Pharmacology

8.4.1 As Cyclodextrin Based Nanosponges

Cyclodextrin based nanosponges (CD-NS) have major applications in the field of drug delivery by preventing the degradation of drugs (Ansari et al. 2011), controlled-release (Deshmukh et al. 2016) and volatile oils (Montazer and Mehr 2010). Various researchers are also studying the action of CD-NS on cancer and tumor (Daga et al. 2016; Minelli et al. 2012; Swaminathan et al. 2010). Also, it can be used as a diagnostic tool (Chen et al. 2012), purification of water (Euvrard et al. 2016), agrochemistry (Seglie et al. 2012), and flame retardant (Alongi et al. 2010).

8.4.1.1 Solubility Enhancement

For any drug to be effective, it has to be in the form of a solution to get absorbed by the gastrointestinal tract for systemic circulation. Hence, to increase the water solubility and bioavailability of lipophilic drugs, the inclusion complexation of drugs with cyclodextrin can be a beneficial course of action. Chemical interaction of CD-NS and drug leads to a reduction in drug crystallinity resulting in enhancement of solubility or dissolution rate. This also helps in forming hydrophilic complex by rendering hydrophilic compounds on the outer side while masking the hydrophobic compounds in the inner side of the complex. However, this technique is comparatively less suitable for hydrophilic drugs with moderately polar nature (Alongi et al. 2011). Methylated cyclodextrins exhibit low molar substitution and are potential solubilizers among available cyclodextrin derivatives. It also increases the efficiency of drug release (Vyas et al. 2008; Shende et al. 2015; Sherje et al. 2017).

8.4.2 Modulating Drug Release

Modified drug release dosage draws more benefits over conventional dosage as it aids in preventing frequent dosing. The dosage forms are modified by optimizing the drug regimen resulting in drug release at a slow and steady rate for the entire dosing interval. This approach also helps in decreasing the side effects of the drug on the host. CD-NS enhances the absorption of drugs through biological hurdles by acting as a drug carrier in immediate release dosage forms. While CD-NS having hydrophobic nature can be used in formulating the sustainable release dosage form of water-soluble drugs in addition to peptides and proteins (Trotta et al. 2012).

For instance, *in vitro* release of drug flurbiprofen exhibited a gradual release of approximately less than 10% after 1 h 10 min from β-CD-NS. Another study has been seen on *in vitro* release of calcium. The study showed a prolonged release of calcium from CD-NS (Shende et al. 2013). Thus, CD-NS can be added to secure the drug from the gastric environment and efficiently releasing the drug into the intestinal tract of the host (Sherje et al. 2017).

8.4.3 Drug Delivery

There are various limitations such as low permeability, poor solubility, low stability, short half-life, and increased molecular weight in recent drugs resulting in challenges in formulations. Poor dissolution leads to poor solubility which hampers the absorption from the gastrointestinal tract resulting in limited bioavailability of the drug. Thus, to overcome such challenge, cyclodextrin based nanosponges can be used as it can lead to the formation of both inclusion and non-inclusion complex by interacting with both organic and inorganic molecules resulting in the efficient drug delivery of low water-soluble dosage form. CD-NS structure exhibits multiple interaction sites for incorporating drugs within. Moreover, it also exhibits cyclodextrin cavities, hydrophobic in nature enveloped by hydrophilic nanochannels which allow significant interaction of molecules with diverse lipophilic intensities and structure (Trotta et al. 2012; Sherje et al. 2017).

8.4.4 Protein Delivery

The proteins are quite difficult to administer as it has the property of aggregation, denaturation, short half-life, large molecular mass, rapid enzymatic degradation, and poor bioavailability. However, when proteins were encapsulated with CD-NS, they resulted to exhibit enhanced stability and improved pharmacological properties. For delivery of Bovine serum albumin (BSA) as a model protein, swellable cyclodextrin- based poly (amidoamine) nanosponges (PAA-NS) by cross-linking β-cyclodextrin with either 2,2-bis-acrylamidoacetic acid or with poly(amidoamine) chain were synthesized (Swaminathan et al. 2010). The nanosponges exhibited prolonged release of BSA for more than 24 h with excellent swelling capacity and 250–300 °C stability (Sherje et al. 2017).

8.4.5 Gas Delivery

Various gases can be stored easily in nanosponges. In a study, it is seen that β-cyclodextrin nanosponges can act as storage for a huge quantity of gases including oxygen, 1-methyl cyclopropane, and carbon dioxide. Moreover, ultrasound can be used to increase *in vitro* release and oxygen permeation. Sustainable release of the gas was noted with the nanosponge/hydrogel system (Sherje et al. 2017).

8.4.6 Protection of Drug from Enzymes or Light

Nanosponges can also act as carriers to secure the drug from chemical, enzyme, and light-induced degradation. Trotta et al. (2012) studied the protective effect of nanosponges encapsulated with 5-fluorouracil against MCF-7 cells. Another study reported that camptothecin molecule when encapsulated with CD-NS, showed increased shelf life with sustained release of the drug (Swaminathan et al. 2010). Moreover, it has also been marked that combination of CD-NS and 2-hydroxy-4(octyloxy)-benzophenone (UV stabilizer) enhanced the time of oxidation induction in polypropylene up to three times (Alongi et al. 2011; Sherje et al. 2017).

8.4.7 Miscellaneous

CD-NS can be used as a potential solution in various fields other than drug or protein delivery such as diagnostic tools, prostheses, and implants, cosmetics, agriculture, fillers for natural rubber, flame retardants as well as purification of water. Such molecules can be engineered in such a way that it can help in prevention, diagnosis as well as treatment of human diseases (Wang et al. 2009). An element of curing human diseases such as diabetes, cancer, or cardiac diseases is a way through prostheses and implants. These can also be used in repairing ruptured ligament or bone and even in providing the vision to impaired bionic challenged person. CD-NS such as γ-oryzanol loaded NS can also be used in gel preparation or oil-water emulsion to protect skin against photodegradation. It is also used as a body odor preventing agents by trapping and sustain the release of essential oil such as linalool. CD-NS in the presence of acid results in dehydration leading to water vapor and char. This phenomenon helps in protecting the co-polymer from combustion (Alongi et al. 2010; Enescu et al. 2012). In agriculture, CD-NS can be complexed with methyl anthranilate to prevent hydrolysis and hence, preventing the formation of anthranilic acid resulting in the peculiar smell. This smell protects the crop from birds by acting as a bird-repelling agent (Lien and Telford 2009). In recent studies, it is seen that cyclodextrin can be used as an effective absorption of cationic dyes and metals (Zhao et al. 2015). Moreover, it can absorb both organic and inorganic substances from water (Sherje et al. 2017).

8.5 Cyclodextrins as Shelf Life Enhancer of Food Products

Cyclodextrins can also be employed in food packaging materials as it acts as two-fold packaging material. It helps in the reduction of residual organic volatile contaminants in packaging materials. Moreover, it strengthens the barrier properties such as transmission rate and diffusion rate of the packaging material resulting in improved sensory properties of end products. For instance, it is used as a carrier to deliver antimicrobial compounds in packaged fresh-cut fruits or vegetables during high relative humidity (RH) conditions (Ayala-Zavala et al. 2008a). Besides, due to its property of producing an antifungal volatile during storage, it has been used for the reduction of post-harvest berry diseases (Almenar et al. 2007). Moreover, it is also seen that during the antioxidative active packaging, it limits the release of α-tocopherol from the same (Siro et al. 2006; Astray et al. 2009).

The residuals of organic volatile contaminants present in the packaging materials can be reduced. The undesired flavors released from foods can be removed or eliminated during storage conditions. Moreover, releasing behaviors of the guests included in the packing materials can be controlled for retaining the high-quality and safety of food (Ayala-Zavala et al. 2008a).

8.5.1 *Complementary Effect of Cyclodextrins with Antimicrobial Compounds*

Antimicrobial compounds can be complexed with cyclodextrins which provides beneficial effects to prevent microbial growth and oxidation of food products. In fruits and vegetable packaging this inclusion complex slowly releases the antimicrobial and antioxidant compounds when the humidity in the headspace of packaging material increases. β-cyclodextrin used to formed complex with antimicrobial compounds which enhances the shelf life of food products. The important antimicrobial compounds such as cinnamaldehyde encapsulate using polyacrylic acid (PAA) onto cellulose fibers that produce a long shelf life antimicrobial film of bread. To reduce strong odor and enhance the antimicrobial time and effect the cyclodextrins-AITC (Allyl Isothyocynate Complex) inclusion complex is used in meat and baking products (Hill et al. 2013).

8.6 Inhibitory Effect of Cyclodextrins on the Retrogradation of Starch and Starchy Products

The inclusion complex of hydroxyl propyl (HP) β-cyclodextrin reduces the retrogradation of rice amylose. HP β- cyclodextrin restricts the formation from V- to B-type during the recrystallization of amylase molecules and it gives rise to an intermediate crystalline pattern (V+B). In the presence of β-cyclodextrins V pattern is formed, it reduces the bread staling, hardness rate, and improves the texture of bread during storage. For fresh crumbs of bread, an A-pattern is prominent but in the presence of β-cyclodextrins, it changes to B- pattern and formed V+B type crystalline. β-cyclodextrin also facilitates a V+A pattern crystallite and reduces the transformation from V to A patterns of the aging crust in bread (Tian et al. 2010).

8.7 Protection Against Heat-Induced Decomposition

Various components of flavor are sensitive against heat thus, to improve the chemical stability of encapsulated agents during the extreme conditions, empty capsules entrap the heat-sensitive flavor components either partially or completely. Cyclodextrin complexes of volatile flavor withstand at high temperature without any degradation of flavor compounds. Essential oils (garlic and lemon oil) adsorbed onto lactose and complexed with β-cyclodextrin upon heating with nitrogen atmosphere. High stability of volatile compounds such as cinnamaldehyde and benzaldehyde has been achieved by employing the cyclodextrin complexes (Szente and Szejtli 2004). Therefore, cyclodextrin complexes prevent volatile flavor compounds from heat.

8.8 Protection Against Light and Oxidative Induced Decomposition

Several flavors inducing components such as citral (responsible for fresh citrus odor) and cinnamaldehyde are sensitive against irradiation. Under UV irradiation, the citral component transforms into cyclized form such as 'photocitral A' and 'photocitral B' and monoterpenes like *p*-cymene that further causes taste alteration in citrus containing juices. Thus, β-cyclodextrin molecules entrap the citral component and prevent the formation of the any above cyclic products resulting in the retention of original flavor even after 6 h exposure to UV radiation (Szente and Szejtli 2004).

Cyclodextrins forms a complex with polyphenol oxidase which is responsible for browning of fruit and vegetables which prevents polyphenolic bioactives from oxidation. Cyclodextrins also prevent lipophilic food constituents from light and oxygen (Del Valle 2004). Oxygen sensitive flavors and food ingredients entrapped completely or partially by cyclodextrins can improved the stability of the complex and prevent from oxidative reactions. Cyclodextrins used as encapsulating material for carotenoid pigments to enhance its functioning against oxygen and light (Pfitzner et al. 2000).

8.9 Encapsulation of Flavors

Flavor plays a crucial role in increasing the consumption of food. However, processing of food and storage conditions affects aroma both ways, directly and indirectly, thus generation to the off-flavor components in food (Astray et al. 2009). Thus, to overcome this loss of aroma and flavor, volatile ingredients should be encapsulated before processing in foods and beverages. Several commercial techniques are already in use for encapsulation including co-crystallization, coacervation, extrusion, fluidized-bed coating, freeze-drying, spray-cooling/chilling, emulsification, solvent evaporation, high-pressure homogenization, micro fluidization, dehydration/rehydration, film hydration/sonication, thin-film hydration, film dispersion, hot homogenization, precipitation, stirring, molecular complexation, co-solvent desolation, air-bath oscillation, nanoprecipitation, electrospinning and spray drying (Maurya et al. 2020). However, such techniques involving the formation of flavor/cyclodextrin molecular-inclusion complexes result in better retention of volatile components responsible for flavor development from various rigorous processing methods like microwaving, freezing, and thawing (Jouquand et al. 2004). If pre-extrusion flavoring is desired, then it can prove to be a great potential during high-temperature short time (HTST) food extrusion process (Bhandari et al., 2001). Among the encapsulating techniques, the addition of β-cyclodextrin leads to the most effective in preventing the loss of flavors during heat and evaporation treatment (Astray et al. 2009).

Cyclodextrins act like 'empty capsules' for the compounds of particular molecular size and can entrap the flavor resulting in the formation of flavor/cyclodextrin molecular-inclusion complexes. During the formation of complex, the most hydrophobic guest molecule will be complexed first followed by a hydrophilic guest molecule (Astray et al. 2009). The merit of this technique over other encapsulating techniques is that it protects every flavor constituent effectively in a multicomponent food system. This encapsulation at the molecular level limits the interaction between co-encapsulated constituents differing nature such as essential oils, flavor concentrates, and oleoresins (Szente and Szejtli 2004). Cyclodextrins is also commonly used for protecting flavors against heat, oxygen, and evaporation (Astray et al. 2009).

The β-cyclodextrin based encapsulations prevent the interactions of essential oils, natural and synthetic flavors that protect all types of flavors without altering in the food composition and its organoleptic properties (Szente and Szejtli 2004).

8.10 Elimination of Undesired Taste and Odor of Food Using Cyclodextrins

Taste and odor play a huge role in food products that are to be commercialized. Bitterness is avoided in most of the food products especially in citrus juices except in some foods and beverages such as wine, coffee, and beer. For this bitterness, particularly two classes of chemical compounds *viz.* limonoids (mainly limonin) and flavonoids (mainly naringin) are responsible. Similarly, some foods exhibit undesirable smell which can be overcome by cyclodextrins complexes. These cyclodextrins form cyclodextrin inclusion complexes resulting in minimizing or eliminating the undesirable smell from the food products (Astray et al. 2009). Moreover, in an aqueous cyclodextrin solution, the ratio of free to complexed guest molecules depends on various factors such as association or stability constant of the complex, concentration, and temperature of both constituents. In diluted warm solutions, the equilibrium is shifted towards guest molecules whereas, in concentrated cold solutions, it is shifted towards complexation. Thus, when cyclodextrin-flavor complex encounters the taste buds as dilute warm solution, somewhat elimination of taste and odor takes place. Moreover, at a lower temperature, higher cyclodextrin concentration is effective against undesired tastes and odor (Szente and Szejtli 2004).

For instance, cyclodextrins have been added in the manufacture of soybean protein, soybean milk, and fish products to deodorize them. However, in seafood and meat products, instead of the pure form of cyclodextrins such as α-cyclodextrin, β-cyclodextrin, γ-cyclodextrin, a mixture of these cyclodextrins is added along with the linear dextrin. When the mixture is added to such products, gel formation takes place resulting in retaining textural properties and preventing the leakage of oil and fat from the products. Cyclodextrins are also added in other food products including milk casein hydrolysate, orange juice, grapefruit juice, raw rice, and cooked rice to eliminate bitterness and unwanted smell as well as to improve the quality of the product. Also, cyclodextrins have been used as sweeteners and with a sweetener such as aspartame to improve the stability and taste of the desired product (Singh et al. 2002; Astray et al. 2009). Moreover, it can also be added in rice crackers to improve crunchiness and retard staling of the same.

β-cyclodextrin is also used to prevent bitterness of beverages, 0.3% of β-cyclodextrin retards the bitterness of canned juices. β-cyclodextrin also retards the bitterness of grape and mandarin juices. 10% of β-cyclodextrin used to prevent bitterness of the milk protein casein hydrolysate which is easy to digest (Astray et al. 2009).

8.11 Cyclodextrins as Cholesterol Sequestrant

Cyclodextrins have been employed by several researchers to reduce cholesterol content (up to 90–99%) and improving the nutritional value of foods and beverages. Examples of such foods and beverages such as milk (Kwak et al. 2004), mayonnaise (Jung et al. 2008), butter (Jung et al. 2005); lard (Kim et al. 2007); cheese (Kwak et al. 2001, 2003; Kim et al. 2005; Han et al. 2008); egg yolks (Astray et al. 2009) and cream (Shim et al. 2003; Astray et al. 2009) are shown in Table 8.7. In the dairy industry, β-cyclodextrin is used to remove the cholesterol from the cream which reduces the whipping time of cream (Shim et al. 2003). Tables 8.7 and 8.8 represents the application of different cyclodextrin in different food and beverages.

8.12 Limitation and Future Prospects of Cyclodextrins

Despite several benefits cyclodextrins also carry some limitations. For instance, β-cyclodextrin is one of the most explored cyclodextrins for toxicity studies, metabolism, and resorption. The price of β-cyclodextrin is commercially high because of its wide range of applications. Not all the drugs are suitable for cyclodextrin complexation. Inorganic compounds generally are not suitable for cyclodextrin complexation except HCl, HBr, HI, H_3PO_4, halogens, and gases such as CO_2, Kr, Xe. The strong hydrophilic molecule (small or large) can't be complexed with cyclodextrins. Moreover, ionized species form weaker complex due to its hydrated and soluble property (Szejtli 2013a, b). Therefore, for any of the above-mentioned limitations, the strong hydrophilic molecule should be investigated for the formation of specific inclusion complex in cyclodextrins which can be utilized for the development of functional food and nutraceuticals, encapsulation.

Table 8.7 Application of cyclodextrin in different food and food products

Active moiety	Cyclodextrin	Applications	References
Allyl isothiocyanate	β-	Antibacterial, stability	Aytac et al. (2014)
Trans- anethole	α-, β-, HP- β	Stability, solubility	Kfoury et al. (2014a)
	α-, β-, HP- β	Antioxidant, solubility	Kfoury et al. (2014b)
Camphor	α-, β-, γ-	Solubility	Yu et al. (2003)
	β-	Stability, release	Ciobanu et al. (2012)
Carvacrol	α-, β-, HP- β	Antibacterial, antifungal, solubility	Liang et al. (2012)
	β-	Antibacterial, solubility	Santos et al. (2015)
	β-	Pain management	Guimaraes et al. (2015)
Carvone	β-	Stability	Partanen et al. (2002)
	β-	Stability, solubility	Ajisaka et al. (2000)
Catfish oil	β-	Making odor	Haiyee et al. (2016)
Caryophyllene	β-	Bioavailability, dissolution	Liu et al. (2013)
	β-	Bioavailability	Liu et al. (2013)
Cinnamaldehyde	β-	Antibacterial, solubility	Hill et al. (2013)
	α-, β-	Antibacterial	Chun et al. (2015)
Cinnamon leaf	β-	Bioavailability, stability, solubility	Ayala-Zavala et al. (2008b)
Citronellal	β-	Stability, solubility	Ajisaka et al. (2000)
	β-	Mosquito repellant	Songkro et al. (2012)
	β-	Anti-hyperalgesic	Santos et al. (2016)
Curcumin	β-	Solubility	Jahed et al. (2014)
	β-	Stability, solubility	Mangolim et al. (2014)
	HP- β, M- β	Antiangiogenic anti-inflammatory, solubility	Yadav et al. (2009)
Eugenol	β-	Stability	Seo et al. (2010)
	β-, HP- β-	Stability	Choi et al. (2009)
	HP- β-	Solubility	Garg et al. (2010)
	β-	Antibacterial, stability	Wang et al. (2011)
	α-, β-, HP- β	Antibacterial, antifungal, solubility	Liang et al. (2012)
	β-	Antibacterial, solubility	Hill et al. (2013)
	α-, β-, HP- β	Antibacterial, solubility	Kfoury et al. (2014b)
	HP- β	Solubility	Garg et al. (2010)
	β-	Release, storage temperature	Chun et al. (2012)
	β-	Release, storage temperature	Seo et al. (2010)
Estragole	α-, β-, γ-, HP- β	Antioxidant, stability	Kfoury et al. (2015)
	α-, β-, HP- β	Antioxidant, solubility	Kfoury et al. (2014b)
Ethyl benzoate	HP- β	Stability, solubility	Yuan et al. (2014)
Follium artemisia argyi	β-	Stability	Jiang et al. (2016)

(continued)

Table 8.7 (continued)

Active moiety	Cyclodextrin	Applications	References
Fish oil	β-	Masking	Choi et al. (2010)
Garlic oil	β-	Bioavailability, stability, solubility	Ayala-Zavala et al. (2008a)
Geraniol	β-	Stability, solubility	Mourtzinos et al. (2008)
	β-	Stability, solubility	Ajisaka et al. (2000)
	β-	Anticancer, antimicrobial, insect repellant	Menezes et al. (2012)
Isoeugenol	α-, β-, HP- β	Antioxidant, solubility	Kfoury et al. (2014b)
Lemon oil	β-	Extraction, flavor	Padukka et al. (2000)
D-limonene	β-	Stability, flavor	Yuliani et al. (2006)
Limonene	β-	Stability	do Carmo et al. (2017)
	β-	Stability	Partanen et al. (2002)
	β-	Stability, solubility	Ajisaka et al. (2000)
Linalool	β-, HP-β	Stability, solubility	Numanoglu et al. (2007)
	β-	Anti-inflammatory, analgesic	Quintans-Junior et al. (2013)
	α-, β-, HP- β	Antibacterial, antifungal, solubility	Liang et al. (2012)
	β-	Pain management	Nascimento et al. (2014)
	β-	Stability, release	Ciobanu et al. (2012)
	β-	Antinociceptive	Quintans-Junior et al. (2013)
	β-	Gastric lesion	da Silva et al. (2016)
	β-	Food additive, flavor	Menezes et al. (2014)
Lippia grata	β-	Pain management	Siqueira-Lima et al. (2014)
Litsea cubeba	β-	Stability	Wang et al. (2009)
Lycopene	β-	Supercritical precipitation	Nerome et al. (2013)
Menthe piperita	β-	Complexation	Ciobanu et al. (2013)
Menthol	β-	Stability, solubility	Ajisaka et al. (2000)
Menthone	β-	Stability, solubility	Ajisaka et al. (2000)
Myrcene	β-	Stability, solubility	Ajisaka et al. (2000)
Nerol	β-	Stability, solubility	Ajisaka et al. (2000)
Pulegone	β-, γ-	Stability	Moon et al. (2008)
Starch	β-	Stability, flavor	Yuliani et al. (2006)
Salvia sclarea	β-	Stability	Tian et al. (2008)
Satureja montana	β-	Antifungal, antioxidant	Haloci et al. (2014)
Sweet orange	β-	Flavor	Zhu et al. (2014)
Terpineol	β-, HP- β	Stability, solubility	dos Santos et al. (2012)

(continued)

Table 8.7 (continued)

Active moiety	Cyclodextrin	Applications	References
	β-	Stability, solubility	Mazzobre et al. (2011)
	β-	Antibacterial, stability	Ajisaka et al. (2000)
Thyme	β-	Antimicrobial, antifungal	Del Toro-Sanchez et al. (2010)
Thymol	β-	Antimicrobial	Tao et al. (2014)
Thymus catharinae Camarda	β-	Antimicrobial	Delogu et al. (2016)
Vanillin	α-, β-, γ-	Stability	Kayaci and Uyar (2011)
	β-	Stability	Hundre et al. (2015)
Xiang-Fu-Si-Wu oil	β-	Bioavailability	Xi et al. (2015)

8.13 Conclusion

Various kind of encapsulation are present which entraps a fine particle of an active core with coating material. At molecular level encapsulation can be occurred using a category of oligosaccharides called cyclodextrins. Encapsulates made with cyclodextrins may possibly hold the key for many future encapsulated formulation solutions.

In this chapter, we presented the overview of cyclodextrins keeping the focus on its ability to form an inclusion complex with a range of guest molecules. This unique property of cyclodextrin could be used as encapsulation material that can accommodate different guest molecules into its lipophilic cavity and provide stability to the guest molecule. This type of molecular encapsulation will affect physicochemical properties of the guest molecules. The ability of cyclodextrin to form complexes with a wide variety of light, heat and oxygen sensitive compounds helps to change the solubility of the molecules, to increase the stability of compound in the presence of light, heat and oxidizing conditions and to decrease volatility of compound. Further cyclodextrin based nanosponges have shown better encapsulation ability, solubilization capacity, and biocompatibility concerning other molecules like cyclodextrins are less soluble in aqueous and inorganic solvents. Cyclodextrins offer protective effect for sensitive compounds such as flavor and aroma, ensure controlled release, reduce loss and volatility and provide superior handling of volatile compounds. This leads to maintaining food organoleptic properties and extending shelf life. Moreover, it has also found a crucial role in smart food packaging by sustain releasing the antimicrobial agents which prevent from microbial spoilage. The wide applications of all three forms of cyclodextrin (α, β, and γ) indicate that there might be an increase in the utilization of cyclodextrin in the food industry due to its health beneficial properties. However, there is less consumption of the same due to high production cost, thus, biotechnological advancements may be improved in the efficient manufacture of cost effective and highly purified cyclodextrins and its derivatives. more work should be done on making the production cost-effective.

Table 8.8 Application of cyclodextrin in beverages

Substrate	Application	References
Apple juice	Browning reduction and natural antioxidant capacity	Lopez-Nicolas et al. (2007a)
Bitter gourd juice	Debittering juice	Deshaware et al. (2018)
Broccoli juice	Glucoraphanin preservation	Martinez-Hernandez et al. (2019)
Carrot-orange juice	Enhanced carotene concentration	Karangwa et al. (2012)
Cheese	Mask catechin bitterness	Ho et al. (2019)
Cream	Cholesterol reduction	Lee et al. (2012)
Coffee	Encapsulation of natural antioxidants	Aguiar et al. (2016)
	Encapsulation of caffeic, quinic and chlorogenic acids for enhancing antioxidant activity and masking bitterness	Aree (2019)
Coffee extracts	Improve chlorogenic acid and decrease caffeine concentration	Budryn et al. (2014)
	Reduction in protein nutritional quality status	Budryn et al. (2015)
Functional food and beverage	Microencapsulation of refined kenaf seed oil	Chew et al. (2018)
Grape juice	Anthocyanin degradation reduction	Shao et al. (2014)
Homogenized milk	Cholesterol removal	Han et al. (2005)
	Cholesterol reduction	Lee et al. (2012), Tahir et al. (2013), Tahir and Lee (2013)
	Cholesterol removal	Kim et al. (2004)
	Mask catechin bitterness	Ho et al. (2019)
	Oxyresveratrol fortification	Matencio et al. (2020)
Juice models	Oxyresveratrol fortification	Matencio et al. (2020)
Lingonberry juice	Bioactive compounds protection and modification	Kelanne et al. (2019)
Milk fat	Cholesterol reduction	Alonso et al. (2009)
Mulberry juice	Improved polyphenols retention in hot processed food	Cheng et al. (2019)
Non-alcoholic lemon juice model	Aroma and shelf life enhancement	Saldanha do Carmo et al. (2017)
Peach juice	Browning reduction	Lopez-Nicolas et al. (2007b)
Pear juice	Color enhancement	Lopez-Nicolas and Garcia-Carmona (2007)
	Browning reduction	Lopez-Nicolas et al. (2009)
Peach juice	Water holding capacity, pH and color preservation	Watson et al. (2017)
Pomegranate juice (clear)	Color and antioxidant activity stabilization	Kulcan et al. (2019)

(continued)

Table 8.8 (continued)

Substrate	Application	References
Soft drinks and fruit beverage	Prolonged shelf life	Saldanha do Carmo et al. (2017), Lobo et al. (2018)
Yogurt	Masks goaty flavor	Young et al. (2012)
	Mask catechin bitterness	Ho et al. (2019)

References

Aguiar J, Estevinho BN, Santos L (2016) Microencapsulation of natural antioxidants for food application–The specific case of coffee antioxidants–A review. Trends Food Sci Technol 58:21–39. https://doi.org/10.1016/j.tifs.2016.10.012

Ajisaka N, Hara K, Mikuni K, Hara K, Hashimoto H (2000) Effects of branched cyclodextrins on the solubility and stability of terpenes. Biosci Biotechnol Biochem 64(4):731–734. https://doi.org/10.1271/bbb.64.731

Almenar E, Auras R, Rubino M, Harte B (2007) A new technique to prevent the main post harvest diseases in berries during storage: inclusion complexes β-cyclodextrin-hexanal. Int J Food Microbiol 118(2):164–172. https://doi.org/10.1016/j.ijfoodmicro.2007.07.002

Alongi J, Poskovic M, Frache A, Trotta F (2010) Novel flame retardants containing cyclodextrin nanosponges and phosphorus compounds to enhance EVA combustion properties. Polym Degrad Stab 95(10):2093–2100. https://doi.org/10.1016/j.polymdegradstab.2010.06.030

Alongi J, Poskovic M, Frache A, Trotta F (2011) Role of β-cyclodextrin nanosponges in polypropylene photooxidation. Carbohydr Polym 86(1):127–135. https://doi.org/10.1016/j.carbpol.2011.04.022

Alonso L, Cuesta P, Fontecha J, Juarez M, Gilliland SE (2009) Use of β-cyclodextrin to decrease the level of cholesterol in milk fat. J Dairy Sci 92(3):863–869. https://doi.org/10.3168/jds.2008-1452

Alston DR, Lilley TH, Stoddart JF (1985) The binding of cyclobutane-1, 1-dicarboxylatodiamineplatinum (II) by α-cyclodextrin in aqueous solution. J Chem Soc Chem Commun 22:1600–1602. https://doi.org/10.1039/C39850001600

Ansari KA, Vavia PR, Trotta F, Cavalli R (2011) Cyclodextrin-based nanosponges for delivery of resveratrol: in vitro characterisation, stability, cytotoxicity and permeation study. AAPS Pharm Sci Tech 12(1):279–286. https://doi.org/10.1208/s12249-011-9584-3

Appendini P, Hotchkiss JH (2002) Review of antimicrobial food packaging. Innov Food Sci Emerg Technol 3(2):113–126. https://doi.org/10.1016/S1466-8564(02)00012-7

Aree T (2019) Understanding structures and thermodynamics of β-cyclodextrin encapsulation of chlorogenic, caffeic and quinic acids: implications for enriching antioxidant capacity and masking bitterness in coffee. Food Chem 293:550–560. https://doi.org/10.1016/j.foodchem.2019.04.084

Astray G, Gonzalez-Barreiro C, Mejuto JC, Rial-Otero R, Simal-Gándara J (2009) A review on the use of cyclodextrins in foods. Food Hydrocoll 23:1631–1640. https://doi.org/10.1016/j.foodhyd.2009.01.001

Ayala-Zavala JF, Del-Toro-Sanchez L, Alvarez-Parrilla E, González-Aguilar GA (2008a) High relative humidity in-package of fresh-cut fruits and vegetables: advantage or disadvantage considering microbiological problems and antimicrobial delivering systems. J Food Sci 73(4):R41–R47. https://doi.org/10.1111/j.1750-3841.2008.00705.x

Ayala-Zavala JF, Soto-Valdez H, Gonzalez-Leon A, Alvarez-Parrilla E, Martin-Belloso O, Gonzalez-Aguilar GA (2008b) Microencapsulation of cinnamon leaf (Cinnamomum zeylanicum) and garlic (Allium sativum) oils in β-cyclodextrin. J Incl Phenom Macrocycl Chem 60(3–4):359–368. https://doi.org/10.1007/s10847-007-9385-1

Aytac Z, Dogan SY, Tekinay T, Uyar T (2014) Release and antibacterial activity of allyl isothiocyanate/β-cyclodextrin complex encapsulated in electrospun nanofibers. Colloids Surf B: Biointerfaces 120:125–131. https://doi.org/10.1016/j.colsurfb.2014.04.006

Beadle JB (1969) Analysis of cyclodextrin mixtures by gas chromatography of their dimethylsilyl ethers. J Chromatogr A 42:201–206. https://doi.org/10.1016/s0021-9673(01)80616-6

Bender ML, Komiyama M (1978) Reactivity and structure concepts in organic chemistry. In: Cyclodextrin chemistry, vol 6. Springer-Verlag, New York, pp 50–60. https://doi.org/10.1007/978-3-642-66842-5_6

Bhandari B, D'Arcy B, Young G (2001) Flavour retention during high temperature short time extrusion cooking process: a review. Int J Food Sci Technol 36(5):453–461. https://doi.org/10.1046/j.1365-2621.2001.00495.x

Bhatt P, Lalani R, Vhora I, Patil S, Amrutiya J, Misra A, Mashru R (2018) Liposomes encapsulating native and cyclodextrin enclosed paclitaxel: enhanced loading efficiency and its pharmacokinetic evaluation. Int J Pharm 536(1):95–107. https://doi.org/10.1016/j.ijpharm.2017.11.048

Budryn G, Nebesny E, Pałecz B, Rachwał-Rosiak D, Hodurek P, Miskiewicz K, Oracz J, Zyzelewicz D (2014) Inclusion complexes of β-cyclodextrin with chlorogenic acids (CHAs) from crude and purified aqueous extracts of green Robusta coffee beans (Coffea canephora L.). Food Res Int 61:202–213. https://doi.org/10.1016/j.foodres.2013.10.013

Budryn G, Zaczynska D, Rachwał-Rosiak D, Oracz J (2015) Changes in properties of food proteins after interaction with free and β-cyclodextrin encapsulated hydroxycinnamic acids. Eur Food Res Technol 240(6):1157–1166. https://doi.org/10.1007/s00217-015-2419-9

Chen Q, Shen X, Gao H (2010) Radiolytic synthesis of nanoparticles in supramolecular assemblies. Adv Colloid Interf Sci 159(1):32–44. https://doi.org/10.1016/j.cis.2010.05.002

Chen KJ, Garcia MA, Wang H, Tseng HR (2012) Supramolecular nanoparticles for molecular diagnostics and therapeutics. Supramolecular chemistry: from molecules to nanomaterials. https://doi.org/10.1002/9780470661345.smc194

Cheng JR, Xiang R, Liu XM, Zhu MJ (2019) The effects of thermal processing and β-cyclodextrin on extractable polyphenols in mulberry juice-enriched dried minced pork slices. LWT Food Sci Technol 116:108503. https://doi.org/10.1016/j.lwt.2019.108503

Chew SC, Tan CP, Nyam KL (2018) Microencapsulation of refined kenaf (Hibiscus cannabinus L.) seed oil by spray drying using β-cyclodextrin/gum arabic/sodium caseinate. J Food Eng 237:78–85. https://doi.org/10.1016/j.jfoodeng.2018.05.016

Choi MJ, Soottitantawat A, Nuchuchua O, Min SG, Ruktanonchai U (2009) Physical and light oxidative properties of eugenol encapsulated by molecular inclusion and emulsion–diffusion method. Food Res Int 42(1):148–156. https://doi.org/10.1016/j.foodres.2008.09.011

Choi MJ, Ruktanonchai U, Min SG, Chun JY, Soottitantawat A (2010) Physical characteristics of fish oil encapsulated by β-cyclodextrin using an aggregation method or polycaprolactone using an emulsion–diffusion method. Food Chem 119(4):1694–1703. https://doi.org/10.1016/j.foodchem.2009.09.052

Chun JY, You SK, Lee MY, Choi MJ, Min SG (2012) Characterization of β-cyclodextrin self-aggregates for eugenol encapsulation. Int J Food Eng 8(2). https://doi.org/10.1515/1556-3758.2590

Chun JY, Jo YJ, Bjrapha P, Choi MJ, Min SG (2015) Antimicrobial effect of α-or β-cyclodextrin complexes with trans-cinnamaldehyde against Staphylococcus aureus and Escherichia coli. Dry Technol 33(3):377–383. https://doi.org/10.1080/07373937.2014.957388

Ciobanu A, Mallard I, Landy D, Brabie G, Nistor D, Fourmentin S (2012) Inclusion interactions of cyclodextrins and crosslinked cyclodextrin polymers with linalool and camphor in Lavandula angustifolia essential oil. Carbohydr Polym 87(3):1963–1970. https://doi.org/10.1016/j.carbpol.2011.10.005

Ciobanu A, Landy D, Fourmentin S (2013) Complexation efficiency of cyclodextrins for volatile flavor compounds. Food Res Int 53(1):110–114. https://doi.org/10.1016/j.foodres.2013.03.048

Crini G, Fourmentin S, Fenyvesi E, Torri G, Fourmentin M, Morin-Crini N (2018) Cyclodextrins, from molecules to applications. Environ Chem Lett 16(4):1361–1375. https://doi.org/10.1007/s10311-018-0763-2

da Silva FV, de Barros FH, Oliveira IS, Viana AFSC, da Costa DS, Lopes MTP, de Lira KL, Quintans-Junior LJ, de Sousa AA, Oliveira RDCM (2016) Beta-cyclodextrin enhanced gastroprotective effect of (−)-linalool, a monoterpene present in rosewood essential oil, in gastric lesion models. NS Arch Pharmacol 389(11):1245–1251. https://doi.org/10.1007/s00210-016-1298-3

Daga M, Ullio C, Argenziano M, Dianzani C, Cavalli R, Trotta F, Ferretti C, Zara GP, Gigliotti CL, Ciamporcero ES, Pettazzoni P (2016) GSH-targeted nanosponges increase doxorubicin-induced toxicity "in vitro" and "in vivo" in cancer cells with high antioxidant defenses. Free Radic Biol Med 97:24–37. https://doi.org/10.1016/j.freeradbiomed.2016.05.009

Del Toro-Sanchez CL, Ayala-Zavala JF, Machi L, Santacruz H, Villegas-Ochoa MA, Alvarez-Parrilla E, Gonzalez-Aguilar GA (2010) Controlled release of antifungal volatiles of thyme essential oil from β-cyclodextrin capsules. J Incl Phenom Macrocycl Chem 67:431–441. https://doi.org/10.1007/s10847-009-9726-3

Del Valle EM (2004) Cyclodextrins and their uses: a review. Process Biochem 39(9):1033–1046. https://doi.org/10.1016/S0032-9592(03)00258-9

Delogu G, Juliano CCA, Usai M (2016) Thymus catharinae Camarda essential oil: β-cyclodextrin inclusion complexes, evaluation of antimicrobial activity. Nat Prod Res 30(18):2049–2057. https://doi.org/10.1080/14786419.2015.1107558

Deshaware S, Gupta S, Singhal RS, Joshi M, Variyar PS (2018) Debittering of bitter gourd juice using β-cyclodextrin: mechanism and effect on antidiabetic potential. Food Chem 262:78–85. https://doi.org/10.1016/j.foodchem.2018.04.077

Deshmukh K, Tanwar YS, Sharma S, Shende P, Cavalli R (2016) Functionalized nanosponges for controlled antibacterial and antihypocalcemic actions. Biomed Pharmacother 84:485–494. https://doi.org/10.1016/j.biopha.2016.09.017

do Carmo CS, Pais R, Simplício AL, Mateus M, Duarte CM (2017) Improvement of aroma and shelf-life of non-alcoholic beverages through cyclodextrins-limonene inclusion complexes. Food Bioprocess Technol 10(7):1297–1309. https://doi.org/10.1007/s11947-017-1897-0

dos Santos C, Buera MP, Mazzobre MF (2012) Influence of ligand structure and water interactions on the physical properties of β-cyclodextrins complexes. Food Chem 132(4):2030–2036. https://doi.org/10.1016/j.foodchem.2011.12.044

Douhal A (ed) (2006) Cyclodextrin materials photochemistry, photophysics and photobiology. Elsevier, Burlington. https://doi.org/10.1016/B978-0-444-52780-6.X5000-1

Enescu D, Alongi J, Frache A (2012) Evaluation of nonconventional additives as fire retardants on polyamide 6, 6: phosphorous-based master batch, α-zirconium dihydrogen phosphate, and β-cyclodextrin based nanosponges. J Appl Polym Sci 123(6):3545–3555. https://doi.org/10.1002/app.34874

Euvrard E, Morin-Crini N, Druart C, Bugnet J, Martel B, Cosentino C, Moutarlier V, Crini G (2016) Cross-linked cyclodextrin-based material for treatment of metals and organic substances present in industrial discharge waters. Beilstein J Org Chem 12(1):1826–1838. https://doi.org/10.3762/2Fbjoc.12.172

Fang Z, Bhandari B (2010) Encapsulation of polyphenols–a review. Trends Food Sci Technol 21(10):510–523. https://doi.org/10.1016/j.tifs.2010.08.003

Favre LC, Rolandelli G, Mshicileli N, Vhangani LN, dos Santos FC, van Wyk J, del Pilar BM (2020) Antioxidant and anti-glycation potential of green pepper (Piper nigrum): optimization of β-cyclodextrin-based extraction by response surface methodology. Food Chem 316:126280. https://doi.org/10.1016/j.foodchem.2020.126280

Fenyvesi E, Szente L (2016) Nanoencapsulation of flavors and aromas by cyclodextrins. In: Encapsulations, pp 769–792. https://doi.org/10.1016/B978-0-12-804307-3.00018-1

Fourmentin S, Crini G, Lichtfouse E (eds) (2018) Cyclodextrin applications in medicine, food, environment and liquid crystals, vol 17. Springer, Cham. https://doi.org/10.1007/978-3-319-76162-6

Garg A, Gupta B, Prakash R, Singh S (2010) Preparation and characterization of hydroxypropyl-β-cyclodextrin inclusion complex of eugenol: differential pulse voltammetry and 1H-NMR. Chem Pharm Bull 58(10):1313–1319. https://doi.org/10.1248/cpb.58.1313

Guimaraes AG, Oliveira MA, dos Santos AR, dos Passos MP, Serafini MR, de Souza Araujo AA, Bezerra DP, Junior LJQ (2015) Encapsulation of carvacrol, a monoterpene present in the essential oil of oregano, with β-cyclodextrin, improves the pharmacological response on cancer pain experimental protocols. Chem Biol 227:69–76. https://doi.org/10.1016/j.cbi.2014.12.020

Haiyee ZA, Yahya NI, Rashid NA, Hashim DM (2016) Characterisation of catfish (Clarias batrachus) oil: β-cyclodextrin inclusion complex. MJAS 20(4):838–843. https://doi.org/10.17576/mjas-2016-2004-17

Haloci E, Toska V, Shkreli R, Goci E, Vertuani S, Manfredini S (2014) Encapsulation of Satureja montana essential oil in β-cyclodextrin. J Incl Phenom Macrocycl Chem 80:147–153. https://doi.org/10.1007/s10847-014-0437-z

Han EM, Kim SH, Ahn J, Kwak HS (2005) Cholesterol removal from homogenized milk with crosslinked β-cyclodextrin by adipic acid. Asian Australas J Anim Sci 18(12):1794–1799. https://doi.org/10.5713/ajas.2005.1794

Han EM, Kim SH, Ahn J, Kwak HS (2008) Comparison of cholesterol-reduced cream cheese manufactured using crosslinked-cyclodextrin to regular cream cheese. Asian Australas J Anim Sci 21(1):131–137. https://doi.org/10.5713/ajas.2008.70189

Hashidzume A, Yamaguchi H, Harada A (2019) Cyclodextrin-based rotaxanes: from rotaxanes to polyrotaxanes and further to functional materials. Eur J Org Chem 21:3344–3357. https://doi.org/10.1002/ejoc.201900090

Hedges AR, Shieh WJ, Sikorski CT (1995) Use of cyclodextrins for encapsulation in the use and treatment of food products. In: Risch SJ, Reineccius GA (eds) ACS symposium series on encapsulation and controlled release of food ingredients, vol 590. American Chemical Soc, Washington, DC, pp 60–71. https://doi.org/10.1021/bk-1995-0590.ch006

Hill LE, Gomes C, Taylor TM (2013) Characterization of beta-cyclodextrin inclusion complexes containing essential oils (trans-cinnamaldehyde, eugenol, cinnamon bark, and clove bud extracts) for antimicrobial delivery applications. LWT-Food Sci Technol 51(1):86–93. https://doi.org/10.1016/j.lwt.2012.11.011

Ho S, Thoo YY, Young DJ, Siow LF (2019) Stability and recovery of cyclodextrin encapsulated catechin in various food matrices. Food Chem 275:594–599. https://doi.org/10.1016/j.foodchem.2018.09.117

Hundre SY, Karthik P, Anandharamakrishnan C (2015) Effect of whey protein isolate and β-cyclodextrin wall systems on stability of microencapsulated vanillin by spray–freeze drying method. Food Chem 174:16–24. https://doi.org/10.1016/j.foodchem.2014.11.016

Jahed V, Zarrabi A, Bordbar AK, Hafezi MS (2014) NMR (1H, ROESY) spectroscopic and molecular modelling investigations of supramolecular complex of β-cyclodextrin and curcumin. Food Chem 165:241–246. https://doi.org/10.1016/j.foodchem.2014.05.094

Jiang ZT, Tan J, Tan J, Li R (2016) Chemical components and molecular microcapsules of Folium *Artemisia argyi* essential oil with β-cyclodextrin derivatives. J Essent Oil Bear Plants 19(5):1155–1169. https://doi.org/10.1080/0972060X.2016.1185973

Jin ZY (2013) Cyclodextrin chemistry: preparation and application. World Scientific, Singapore. https://doi.org/10.1142/8630

Jouquand C, Ducruet V, Giampaoli P (2004) Partition coefficients of aroma compounds in polysaccharide solutions by the phase ratio variation method. Food Chem 85(3):467–474. https://doi.org/10.1016/j.foodchem.2003.07.023

Jung TH, Kim JJ, Yu SH, Ahn J, Kwak HS (2005) Properties of cholesterol-reduced butter and effect of gamma linolenic acid added butter on blood cholesterol. Asian Australas J Anim Sci 18(11):1646–1654. https://doi.org/10.5713/ajas.2005.1646

Jung TH, Ha HJ, Ahn JJ, Kwak HS (2008) Development of cholesterol-reduced mayonnaise with crosslinked β-cyclodextrin and added phytosterol. Korean J Food Sci Anim Resour 28(2):211–217. https://doi.org/10.5851/kosfa.2008.28.2.211

Kanwar JR, Long BM, Kanwar RK (2011) The use of cyclodextrins nanoparticles for oral delivery. Curr Med Chem 18(14):2079–2085. https://doi.org/10.2174/092986711795656243

Karangwa E, Hayat K, Rao L, Nshimiyimana DS, Foh MB, Li L, Ntwali J, Raymond LV, Xia S, Zhang X (2012) Improving blended carrot-orange juice quality by the addition of cyclodextrins during enzymatic clarification. Food Bioprocess Technol 5(6):2612–2617. https://doi.org/10.1007/s11947-011-0557-z

Kayaci F, Uyar T (2011) Solid inclusion complexes of vanillin with cyclodextrins: their formation, characterization, and high-temperature stability. J Agric Food Chem 59(21):11772–11778. https://doi.org/10.1021/jf202915c

Kelanne N, Laaksonen O, Seppala T, Yang W, Tuukkanen K, Loponen J, Yang B (2019) Impact of cyclodextrin treatment on composition and sensory properties of lingonberry (Vaccinium vitis-idaea) juice. LWT-Food Sci Technol 113:108295. https://doi.org/10.1016/j.lwt.2019.108295

Kfoury M, Auezova L, Greige-Gerges H, Ruellan S, Fourmentin S (2014a) Cyclodextrin, an efficient tool for trans-anethole encapsulation: chromatographic, spectroscopic, thermal and structural studies. Food Chem 164:454–461. https://doi.org/10.1016/j.foodchem.2014.05.052

Kfoury M, Landy D, Auezova L, Greige-Gerges H, Fourmentin S (2014b) Effect of cyclodextrin complexation on phenylpropanoids' solubility and antioxidant activity. Beilstein J Org Chem 10(1):2322–2331. https://doi.org/10.3762/bjoc.10.241

Kfoury M, Auezova L, Ruellan S, Greige-Gerges H, Fourmentin S (2015) Complexation of estragole as pure compound and as main component of basil and tarragon essential oils with cyclodextrins. Carbohydr Polym 118:156–164. https://doi.org/10.1016/j.carbpol.2014.10.073

Kim SH, Ahn J, Kwak HS (2004) Crosslinking of β-cyclodextrin on cholesterol removal from milk. Arch Pharm Res 27(11):1183–1187. https://doi.org/10.1007/BF02975126

Kim SH, Han EM, Ahn J, Kwak HS (2005) Effect of crosslinked β-cyclodextrin on quality of cholesterol-reduced cream cheese. Asian Australas J Anim Sci 18(4):584–589. https://doi.org/10.5713/ajas.2005.584

Kim SH, Kim HY, Kwak HS (2007) Cholesterol removal from lard with crosslinked β-cyclodextrin. Asian Australas J Anim Sci 20(9):1468–1472. https://doi.org/10.5713/ajas.2007.1468

Kulcan AA, Oziyci HR, Karhan M (2019) Quality stability of clear pomegranate juice treated with cyclodextrin. J Food Sci Technol 56(9):4139–4146. https://doi.org/10.1007/s13197-019-03884-6

Kwak HS, Nam CG, Ahn J (2001) Low cholesterol Mozzarella cheese obtained from homogenized and β-cyclodextrin-treated milk. Asian Australas J Anim Sci 14(2):268–275. https://doi.org/10.5713/ajas.2001.268

Kwak HS, Jung CS, Seok JS, Ahn J (2003) Cholesterol removal and flavor development in Cheddar cheese. Asian Australas J Anim Sci 16(3):409–416. https://doi.org/10.5713/ajas.2003.409

Kwak HS, Kim SH, Kim JH, Choi HJ, Kang J (2004) Immobilized β-cyclodextrin as a simple and recyclable method for cholesterol removal in milk. Arch Pharm Res 27(8):873–877. https://doi.org/10.1007/BF02980182

Larsen KL (2002) Large cyclodextrins. J Incl Phenom Macrocycl Chem 43:1–13. https://doi.org/10.1023/A:1020494503684

Lee YK, Ganesan P, Kwak HS (2012) Optimisation of cross-linking β-cyclodextrin and its recycling efficiency for cholesterol removal in milk and cream. Int J Food Sci Technol 47(5):933–939. https://doi.org/10.1111/j.1365-2621.2011.02924.x

Liang H, Yuan Q, Vriesekoop F, Lv F (2012) Effects of cyclodextrins on the antimicrobial activity of plant-derived essential oil compounds. Food Chem 135(3):1020–1027. https://doi.org/10.1016/j.foodchem.2012.05.054

Lien NR, Telford JR (2009) An investigation of the inclusion complex of cyclomaltoheptaose (β-cyclodextrin) with N-methylanthranilic acid in the solid state. Carbohydr Res 344(18):2606–2608. https://doi.org/10.1016/j.carres.2009.09.018

Liu H, Yang G, Tang Y, Cao D, Qi T, Qi Y, Fan G (2013) Physicochemical characterization and pharmacokinetics evaluation of β-caryophyllene/β-cyclodextrin inclusion complex. Int J Pharm 450(1–2):304–310. https://doi.org/10.1016/j.ijpharm.2013.04.013

Lobo FAT, Silva V, Domingues J, Rodrigues S, Costa V, Falcao D, de Lima Araujo KG (2018) Inclusion complexes of yellow bell pepper pigments with β-cyclodextrin: preparation, characterisation and application as food natural colorant. J Sci Food Agric 98(7):2665–2671. https://doi.org/10.1002/jsfa.8760

Lopez-Nicolas JM, García-Carmona F (2007) Use of cyclodextrins as secondary antioxidants to improve the color of fresh pear juice. J Agric Food Chem 55(15):6330–6338. https://doi.org/10.1021/jf070819x

Lopez-Nicolas JM, Nunez-Delicado E, Sanchez-Ferrer A, García-Carmona F (2007a) Kinetic model of apple juice enzymatic browning in the presence of cyclodextrins: the use of maltosyl-β-cyclodextrin as secondary antioxidant. Food Chem 101(3):1164–1171. https://doi.org/10.1016/j.foodchem.2006.03.018

Lopez-Nicolas JM, Perez-Lopez AJ, Carbonell-Barrachina A, Garcia-Carmona F (2007b) Use of natural and modified cyclodextrins as inhibiting agents of peach juice enzymatic browning. J Agric Food Chem 55(13):5312–5319. https://doi.org/10.1021/jf070499h

Lopez-Nicolas JM, Andreu-Sevilla AJ, Carbonell-Barrachina AA, García-Carmona F (2009) Effects of addition of α-cyclodextrin on the sensory quality, volatile compounds, and color parameters of fresh pear juice. J Agric Food Chem 57(20):9668–9675. https://doi.org/10.1021/jf901919t

López-Nicolás JM, Rodríguez-Bonilla P, García-Carmona F (2014) Cyclodextrins and antioxidants. Crit Rev Food Sci Nutr 54(2):251–276. https://doi.org/10.1080/10408398.2011.582544

Mangolim CS, Moriwaki C, Nogueira AC, Sato F, Baesso ML, Neto AM, Matioli G (2014) Curcumin–β-cyclodextrin inclusion complex: stability, solubility, characterisation by FT-IR, FT-Raman, X-ray diffraction and photoacoustic spectroscopy, and food application. Food Chem 153:361–370. https://doi.org/10.1016/j.foodchem.2013.12.067

Martínez-Hernandez GB, Venzke-Klug T, Carrion-Monteagudo MDM, Artes Calero F, Lopez-Nicolas JM, Artes-Hernandez F (2019) Effects of α-, β-and maltosyl-β-cyclodextrins use on the glucoraphanin–sulforaphane system of broccoli juice. J Sci Food Agric 99(2):941–946. https://doi.org/10.1002/jsfa.9269

Matencio A, Navarro-Orcajada S, Conesa I, Munoz-Sanchez I, Laveda-Cano L, Cano-Yelo D, García-Carmona F, Lopez-Nicolas JM (2020) Evaluation of juice and milk "food models" fortified with oxyresveratrol and β-Cyclodextrin. Food Hydrocoll 98:105250. https://doi.org/10.1016/j.foodhyd.2019.105250

Maurya VK, Aggarwal M, Ranjan V, Gothandam KM (2020) Improving bioavailability of vitamin A in food by encapsulation: an update. In: Daima HPNN, Ranjan S, Dasgupta N, Lichtfouse E (eds) Nanoscience in medicine, Environmental chemistry for a sustainable world, Vol 39, vol 1. Springer, Cham, pp 117–145. https://doi.org/10.1007/978-3-030-29207-2_4

Mazzobre MF, Dos Santos CI, del Pilar BM (2011) Solubility and stability of β-cyclodextrin–terpineol inclusion complex as affected by water. Food Biophys 6(2):274–280. https://doi.org/10.1007/s11483-011-9208-1

Menezes PP, Serafini MR, Santana BV, Nunes RS, Quintans LJ Jr, Silva GF, Medeiros IA, Marchioro M, Fraga BP, Santos MR, Araujo AA (2012) Solid-state β-cyclodextrin complexes containing geraniol. Thermochim Acta 548:45–50. https://doi.org/10.1016/j.tca.2012.08.023

Menezes PP, Serafini MR, Quintans-Junior LJ, Silva GF, Oliveira JF, Carvalho FMS, Souza JCC, Matos JDR, Alves PB, Matos IL, Hadaruga DI (2014) Inclusion complex of (−)-linalool and β-cyclodextrin. J Therm Anal Calorim 115(3):2429–2437. https://doi.org/10.1007/s10973-013-3367-x

Minelli R, Cavalli R, Ellis L, Pettazzoni P, Trotta F, Ciamporcero E, Barrera G, Fantozzi R, Dianzani C, Pili R (2012) Nanosponge-encapsulated camptothecin exerts anti-tumor activity in human prostate cancer cells. Eur J Pharm Sci 47(4):686–694. https://doi.org/10.1016/j.ejps.2012.08.003

Montazer M, Mehr EB (2010) Na-diclofenac β-cyclodextrin inclusion complex on cotton wound dressing. J Text Inst 101(5):373–379. https://doi.org/10.1080/00405000802439969

Moon TW, Lee JW, Jhee KH, Khang KW, Jeong HS, Yang SA, Kim HJ (2008) Supramolecular encapsulation of pulegone from oriental herb, schizonepeta tenuifolia briquet by β-and γ-cyclodextrins. Bull Kor Chem Soc 29(8):1579–1582. https://doi.org/10.5012/bkcs.2008.29.8.1579

Mourtzinos I, Kalogeropoulos N, Papadakis SE, Konstantinou K, Karathanos VT (2008) Encapsulation of nutraceutical monoterpenes in β-cyclodextrin and modified starch. J Food Sci 73(1):S89–S94. https://doi.org/10.1111/j.1750-3841.2007.00609.x

Nascimento SS, Camargo EA, DeSantana JM, Araujo AA, Menezes PP, Lucca-Junior W, Albuquerque-Junior RL, Bonjardim LR, Quintans-Junior LJ (2014) Linalool and linalool complexed in β-cyclodextrin produce anti-hyperalgesic activity and increase Fos protein expression in animal model for fibromyalgia. NS Arch Pharmacol 387(10):935–942. https://doi.org/10.1007/s00210-014-1007-z

Nerome H, Machmudah S, Fukuzato R, Higashiura T, Youn YS, Lee YW, Goto M (2013) Nanoparticle formation of lycopene/β-cyclodextrin inclusion complex using supercritical antisolvent precipitation. J Supercrit Fluids 83:97–103. https://doi.org/10.1016/j.supflu.2013.08.014

Numanoglu U, Şen T, Tarimci N, Kartal M, Koo OM, Önyüksel H (2007) Use of cyclodextrins as a cosmetic delivery system for fragrance materials: linalool and benzyl acetate. AAPS PharmSciTech 8(4):34–42. https://doi.org/10.1208/pt0804085

Padukka I, Bhandari B, D'Arcy B (2000) Evaluation of various extraction methods of encapsulated oil from β-cyclodextrin-lemon oil complex powder. J Food Compos Anal 13(1):59–70. https://doi.org/10.1006/jfca.1999.0820

Partanen R, Ahro M, Hakala M, Kallio H, Forssell P (2002) Microencapsulation of caraway extract in β-cyclodextrin and modified starches. Eur Food Res Technol 214(3):242–247. https://doi.org/10.1007/s00217-001-0446-1

Pfitzner I, Francz PI, Biesalski HK (2000) Carotenoid: methyl-bcyclodextrin formulations: an improved method for supplementation of cultured cells. Biochim Biophys Acta-Gen Subj 1474:163–168. https://doi.org/10.1016/S0304-4165(00)00014-3

Quintans-Junior LJ, Barreto RS, Menezes PP, Almeida JR, Viana AFS, Oliveira RC, Oliveira AP, Gelain DP, de Lucca JW, Araujo AA (2013) β-Cyclodextrin-complexed (−)-linalool produces antinociceptive effect superior to that of (−)-linalool in experimental pain protocols. Basic Clin Pharmacol Toxicol 113(3):167–172. https://doi.org/10.1111/bcpt.12087

Rajewski RA, Stella VJ (1996) Pharmaceutical applications of cyclodextrins. 2. In vivo drug delivery. J Pharm Sci 85(11):1142–1169. https://doi.org/10.1021/js960075u

Rakmai J, Cheirsilp B, Mejuto JC, Simal-Gándara J, Torrado-Agrasar A (2018) Antioxidant and antimicrobial properties of encapsulated guava leaf oil in hydroxypropyl-beta-cyclodextrin. Ind Crop Prod 111:219–225. https://doi.org/10.1016/j.indcrop.2017.10.027

Rezanka M (2018) Fundamentals and applications of cyclodextrins. In: Fourmentin S, Crini G, Lichtfouse E (eds) Environmental chemistry for a sustainable world, vol 1. Springer, Berlin, pp 1–56. https://doi.org/10.1007/978-3-319-76159-6_1

Saito Y, Cserhati T, Forgacs E (2004) Cyclodextrins in chromatography. Anal Bioanal Chem 379:6–7. https://doi.org/10.1007/s00216-004-2541-1

Saldanha do Carmo C, Maia C, Poejo J, Lychko I, Gamito P, Nogueira I, Bronze MR, Serra AT, Duarte CM (2017) Microencapsulation of α-tocopherol with zein and β-cyclodextrin using spray drying for colour stability and shelf-life improvement of fruit beverages. RSC Adv 7(51):32065–32075. https://doi.org/10.1039/C6RA25946D

Santos EH, Kamimura JA, Hill LE, Gomes CL (2015) Characterization of carvacrol beta-cyclodextrin inclusion complexes as delivery systems for antibacterial and antioxidant applications. LWT-Food Sci Technol 60(1):583–592. https://doi.org/10.1016/j.lwt.2014.08.046

Santos PL, Brito RG, Oliveira MA, Quintans JS, Guimaraes AG, Santos MR, Menezes PP, Serafini MR, Menezes IR, Coutinho HD, Araujo AA (2016) Docking, characterization and investigation of β-cyclodextrin complexed with citronellal, a monoterpene present in the essential oil of Cymbopogon species, as an anti-hyperalgesic agent in chronic muscle pain model. Phytomedicine 23(9):948–957. https://doi.org/10.1016/j.phymed.2016.06.007

Schardinger F (1902) Über das Verhalten der Kuhmilch gegen Methylenblau und seine Verwendung zur Unterscheidung von ungekochter und gekochter Milch. Zeitschrift für Untersuchung der Nahrungs-und Genußmittel, sowie der Gebrauchsgegenstände 5(22):1113–1121. https://doi.org/10.1007/BF02506750

Schmidt BV (2014) Novel macromolecular architectures via a combination of cyclodextrin host/guest complexation and RAFT polymerization, vol 1. Springer Science & Business, Cham, pp 1–202. https://doi.org/10.1007/978-3-319-06077-4

Seglie L, Spadaro D, Trotta F, Devecchi M, Gullino ML, Scariot V (2012) Use of 1-methylcylopropene in cyclodextrin-based nanosponges to control grey mould caused by Botrytis cinerea on Dianthus caryophyllus cut flowers. Postharvest Biol Technol 64(1):55–57. https://doi.org/10.1016/j.postharvbio.2011.09.014

Seo EJ, Min SG, Choi MJ (2010) Release characteristics of freeze-dried eugenol encapsulated with β-cyclodextrin by molecular inclusion method. J Microencapsul 27(6):496–505. https://doi.org/10.3109/02652041003681398

Shao P, Zhang J, Fang Z, Sun P (2014) Complexing of chlorogenic acid with β-cyclodextrins: inclusion effects, antioxidative properties and potential application in grape juice. Food Hydrocoll 41:132–139. https://doi.org/10.1016/j.foodhyd.2014.04.003

Sharma N, Baldi A (2016) Exploring versatile applications of cyclodextrins: an overview. Drug Deliv 3(3):729–747. https://doi.org/10.3109/10717544.2014.938839

Shende P, Deshmukh K, Trotta F, Caldera F (2013) Novel cyclodextrin nanosponges for delivery of calcium in hyperphosphatemia. Int J Pharm 456(1):95–100. https://doi.org/10.1016/j.ijpharm.2013.08.012

Shende PK, Gaud RS, Bakal R, Patil D (2015) Effect of inclusion complexation of meloxicam with β-cyclodextrin-and β-cyclodextrin-based nanosponges on solubility, in vitro release and stability studies. Colloids Surf B: Biointerfaces 136:105–110. https://doi.org/10.1016/j.colsurfb.2015.09.002

Sherje AP, Dravyakar BR, Kadam D, Jadhav M (2017) Cyclodextrin-based nanosponges: a critical review. Carbohydr Polym 173:37–49. https://doi.org/10.1016/j.carbpol.2017.05.086

Shim SY, Ahn J, Kwak HS (2003) Functional properties of cholesterol removed whipping cream treated by β-cyclodextrin. J Dairy Sci 86:2767–2772. https://doi.org/10.3168/jds.S0022-0302(03)73873-9

Singh M, Sharma R, Banerjee UC (2002) Biotechnological applications of cyclodextrins. Biotechnol Adv 20(5–6):341–359. https://doi.org/10.1016/S0734-9750(02)00020-4

Siqueira-Lima PS, Araujo AA, Lucchese AM, Quintans JS, Menezes PP, Alves PB, de Lucca JW, Santos MR, Bonjardim LR, Quintans-Junior LJ (2014) β-cyclodextrin complex containing lippia grata leaf essential oil reduces orofacial nociception in mice–evidence of possible involvement of descending inhibitory pain modulation pathway. Basic Clin Pharmacol 114(2):188–196. https://doi.org/10.1111/bcpt.12145

Siro I, Fenyvesi E, Szente L, De Meulenaer B, Devlieghere F, Orgovanyi J, Senyi J, Barta J (2006) Release of alpha-tocopherol from antioxidative low-density polyethylene film into fatty food simulant: influence of complexation in beta-cyclodextrin. Food Addit Contam 23(8):845–853. https://doi.org/10.1080/02652030600699064

Songkro S, Hayook N, Jaisawang J, Maneenuan D, Chuchome T, Kaewnopparat N (2012) Investigation of inclusion complexes of citronella oil, citronellal and citronellol with β-cyclodextrin for mosquito repellent. J Incl Phenom Macrocycl Chem 72(3–4):339–355. https://doi.org/10.1007/s10847-011-9985-7

Swaminathan S, Pastero L, Serpe L, Trotta F, Vavia P, Aquilano D, Trotta M, Zara G, Cavalli R (2010) Cyclodextrin-based nanosponges encapsulating camptothecin: physicochemical characterization, stability and cytotoxicity. Eur J Pharm Biopharm 74(2):193–201. https://doi.org/10.1016/j.ejpb.2009.11.003

Szejtli J (1988) Cyclodextrin inclusion complexes. In: Cyclodextrin technology. Topic in inclusion science. Springer, Dordrecht, pp 79–185. https://doi.org/10.1007/978-94-015-7797-7_2
Szejtli J (2004) Past, present and future of cyclodextrin research. Pure Appl Chem 76(10):1825–1845. https://doi.org/10.1351/pac200476101825
Szejtli J (2013a) *Cyclodextrin technology*. In: Szejtli J (ed) Topics in inclusion science, vol 1. Springer Science & Business Media, Dordrecht, pp 79–185. https://doi.org/10.1007/978-94-015-7797-7
Szejtli J (2013b) *Cyclodextrin technology*. In: Szejtli J (ed) Topics in inclusion science, vol 1. Springer Science & Business Media, Dordrecht, pp 1–78. https://doi.org/10.1007/978-94-015-7797-7
Szente L, Szejtli J (2004) Cyclodextrins as food ingredients. Trends Food Sci Technol 15:137–142. https://doi.org/10.1016/j.tifs.2003.09.019
Tahir MN, Lee Y (2013) Immobilisation of β-cyclodextrin on glass: characterisation and application for cholesterol reduction from milk. Food Chem 139(1–4):475–481. https://doi.org/10.1016/j.foodchem.2013.01.080
Tahir MN, Kwon C, Jeong D, Cho E, Paik SR, Jung S (2013) Cholesterol reduction from milk using β-cyclodextrin immobilized on glass. J Dairy Sci 96(7):4191–4196. https://doi.org/10.3168/jds.2012-6355
Tao F, Hill LE, Peng Y, Gomes CL (2014) Synthesis and characterization of β-cyclodextrin inclusion complexes of thymol and thyme oil for antimicrobial delivery applications. LWT-Food Sci Technol 59(1):247–255. https://doi.org/10.1016/j.lwt.2014.05.037
Tian XN, Jiang ZT, Li R (2008) Inclusion interactions and molecular microcapsule of Salvia sclarea L. essential oil with β-cyclodextrin derivatives. Eur Food Res Technol 227(4):1001. https://doi.org/10.1007/s00217-007-0813-7
Tian YQ, Li Y, Jin ZY, Xu XM (2010) Comparison tests of hydroxylpropyl β-cyclodextrin (HPβ-CD) and β-cyclodextrin (β-CD) on retrogradation of rice amylose. LWT-Food Sci Technol 43:488–491. https://doi.org/10.1016/j.lwt.2009.09.016
Trotta F, Zanetti M, Cavalli R (2012) Cyclodextrin-based nanosponges as drug carriers. Beilstein J Org Chem 8(1):2091–2099. https://doi.org/10.3762/bjoc.8.235
Ueda H (2002) Physicochemical properties and complex formation abilities of large-ring cyclodextrins. J Incl Phenom Macrocycl Chem 44(1–4):53–56. https://doi.org/10.1023/A:1023055516398
Vaitkus R, Grinciene G, Norkus E (2011) Inhibition of cyclodextrin acid hydrolysis by some inclusion complexes. J Incl Phenom Macrocycl Chem 69(3–4):345–347. https://doi.org/10.1007/s10847-010-9746-z
Vyas A, Saraf S, Saraf S (2008) Cyclodextrin based novel drug delivery systems. J Incl Phenom Macrocycl Chem 62(1-2):23–42. https://doi.org/10.1007/s10847-008-9456-y
Wang H, Wang S, Su H, Chen KJ, Armijo AL, Lin WY, Wang Y, Sun J, Kamei KI, Czernin J, Radu CG (2009) A supramolecular approach for preparation of size-controlled nanoparticles. Angew Chem 8(24):4344–4348. https://doi.org/10.1002/anie.200900063
Wang T, Li B, Si H, Lin L, Chen L (2011) Release characteristics and antibacterial activity of solid state eugenol/β-cyclodextrin inclusion complex. J Incl Phenom Macrocycl Chem 71(1–2):207–213. https://doi.org/10.1007/s10847-011-9928-3
Watson MA, Lea JM, Bett-Garber KL (2017) Spray drying of pomegranate juice using maltodextrin/cyclodextrin blends as the wall material. Food Sci Nutr 5(3):820–826. https://doi.org/10.1002/fsn3.467
Xi J, Qian D, Duan J, Liu P, Zhu Z, Guo J, Zhang Y, Pan Y (2015) Preparation, characterization and pharmacokinetic study of Xiangfu Siwu decoction essential oil/β-cyclodextrin inclusion complex. Molecules 20(6):10705–10720. https://doi.org/10.3390/molecules200610705
Yadav VR, Suresh S, Devi K, Yadav S (2009) Effect of cyclodextrin complexation of curcumin on its solubility and antiangiogenic and anti-inflammatory activity in rat colitis model. AAPS PharmSciTech 10(3):752. https://doi.org/10.1208/s12249-009-9264-8
Yampayont P, Iizuka M, Ito K, Limpaseni T (2006) Isolation of cyclodextrin producing thermotolerant Paenibacillus sp. from waste of starch factory and some properties of the cyclo-

dextrin glycosyltransferase. J Incl Phenom Macrocycl Chem 56(1–2):203–207. https://doi.org/10.1007/s10847-006-9084-3

Young OA, Gupta RB, Sadooghy-Saraby S (2012) Effects of cyclodextrins on the flavor of goat milk and its yogurt. J Food Sci 77(2):S122–S127. https://doi.org/10.1111/j.1750-3841.2011.02557.x

Yu SC, Bochot A, Le Bas G, Cheron M, Mahuteau J, Grossiord JL, Seiller M, Duchene D (2003) Effect of camphor/cyclodextrin complexation on the stability of O/W/O multiple emulsions. Int J Pharm 261(1–2):1–8. https://doi.org/10.1016/S0378-5173(03)00261-8

Yuan C, Lu Z, Jin Z (2014) Characterization of an inclusion complex of ethyl benzoate with hydroxypropyl-β-cyclodextrin. Food Chem 152:140–145. https://doi.org/10.1016/j.foodchem.2013.11.139

Yuliani S, Torley PJ, D'Arcy B, Nicholson T, Bhandari B (2006) Extrusion of mixtures of starch and d-limonene encapsulated with β-cyclodextrin: Flavour retention and physical properties. Food Res Int 39(3):318–331. https://doi.org/10.1016/j.foodres.2005.08.005

Zarzycki PK, Głód BK (2016) Cyclodextrins-based nanocomplexes for encapsulation of bioactive compounds in food, cosmetics, and pharmaceutical products: principles of supramolecular complexes formation, their influence on the antioxidative properties of target chemicals, and recent advances in selected industrial applications. In: Encapsulations, pp 717–767. https://doi.org/10.1016/B978-0-12-804307-3.00017-X

Zhao F, Repo E, Yin D, Meng Y, Jafari S, Sillanpaa M (2015) EDTA-cross-linked β-cyclodextrin: an environmentally friendly bifunctional adsorbent for simultaneous adsorption of metals and cationic dyes. Environ Sci Technol 49(17):10570–10580. https://doi.org/10.1021/acs.est.5b02227

Zhu G, Xiao Z, Zhou R, Zhu Y (2014) Study of production and pyrolysis characteristics of sweet orange flavor-β-cyclodextrin inclusion complex. Carbohydr Polym 105:75–80. https://doi.org/10.1016/j.carbpol.2014.01.060

Chapter 9
Biosensors: Potential in Food Industry

Varee Tyagi and Bhaswati Bhattacharya

Abstract The technology of biosensors is an interdisciplinary field encompassing engineering, chemistry, and biology, growing rapidly and finding use in different fields such as agriculture, medicine, and environmental science. Currently, a wide variety of biosensors are being utilized for the determination of food safety, quality, and authenticity in terms of detection of foodborne microorganisms, toxins, nutrients, and other harmful extraneous matter such as pesticides, heavy metals, and drugs. These biosensors have also proven to be helpful in defining the product freshness, thereby making the food product safe for consumers. However, the use of biosensors in the food industry at the commercial level is still at a nascent stage. Certain parameters such as improvement of analytical performance based on sensitivity, detection levels, reproducibility of results, and specificity towards target analyte are the need of the hour to avoid false positive outcomes thereby enhancing commercial acceptance. Another focus of concern is the simultaneous detection of target analytes in a matrix as well as the sample preparation of complex matrixes such as food to avoid non-specific interactions. In particular, the use of bacteriophage in phage-based sensors also requires the identification of new bacteriophages to encompass more target analytes for detection to improve their commercial acceptance. Optimized procedures with real sample analysis would aid in streamlining the technique enabling wider applications across various fields. Incorporation of new technologies such as nanotechnology, genetic engineering would further enhance the existing biosensor techniques in terms of their analytical performance as well as widening application scope, though their compatibility with target analyte and cost-effectiveness have to be kept in mind. In this chapter, we have reviewed various modern biosensing techniques being used in the food and agriculture sector focusing on their benefits, areas for improvement with the incorporation of other latest technologies.

V. Tyagi (✉) · B. Bhattacharya (✉)
Department of Basic and Applied Sciences, National Institute of Food Technology Entrepreneurship and Management (NIFTEM), Sonipat, Haryana, India

V. K. Maurya et al. (eds.), *Sustainable Agriculture Reviews 55*, Sustainable Agriculture Reviews 55, https://doi.org/10.1007/978-3-030-76813-3_9

Keywords Electrochemical sensors · Aptasensors · Immunosensors · Optical sensors · Phage-sensors · Nanotechnology · Food safety · Contaminants · Pathogens · Toxins

9.1 Introduction

The concerns related to food safety have significantly increased worldwide due to the inferior quality of foods. Prompt and timely determination and sensitive analysis of probable toxins and contaminants are of paramount importance in the agriculture and food industries. These industries are driven by multiple factors such as expanding preferences of consumers for chemical free and unprocessed foods, the short shelf life of fresh food products, waste minimization, cost reduction in processing operations, and therefore require low detection limits and pathogen removal from the supply chain that could lead to grave health concerns to consumers.

In the current society, high level of consumer awareness and safety anticipations have made it mandatory for the food manufacturers to meet the prerequisites of the contemporary users to help them formulate informed choices while purchasing, also keeping in mind their preference for food products meanwhile maintaining high-grade standards and assurance of product safety. These concerns are aggravated by the innate restrictions of traditional food analysis methods that include cumbersome, costly instrumentation leading to the shift towards the development of biosensors for food analysis. These biosensors aid in addressing three main kinds of food analysis concerns namely, safety, quality, and authenticity (Mehrotra 2016). The motivation behind food safety screening is to detect undesirable contaminants in food like pathogenic microbes, allergens, biological toxins, and pesticide and antibiotic residues. The nutritional value of a food product is established, approved, and endorsed on the basis of a similar kind of analysis. Analysis of authenticity aims to verify the origin of the product or its production process as well as providing information about the adulteration or counterfeiting of food products (Murugaboopathi et al. 2013; Bunney et al. 2017). The focus on biosensor technology for food analysis has boomed in the past decade to improve accuracy in target pursuit, quality from stakeholders like traders, safety regulators, and consumers as well as reducing scrutiny duration significantly. A simple search with keywords biosensors and biosensors in food and agriculture in google scholar and Science Direct from 1960 to the present times is depicted in Fig. 9.1. A similar trend can be observed from both the graphs, although search results from ScienceDirect did not show any outcomes in the 1960–1970 decade. There is abundant growth in the research results in the broad field of biosensors, and when specified for their application in the food and agriculture industry, their emergence significantly starts from the 1980s and is gradually on the rise.

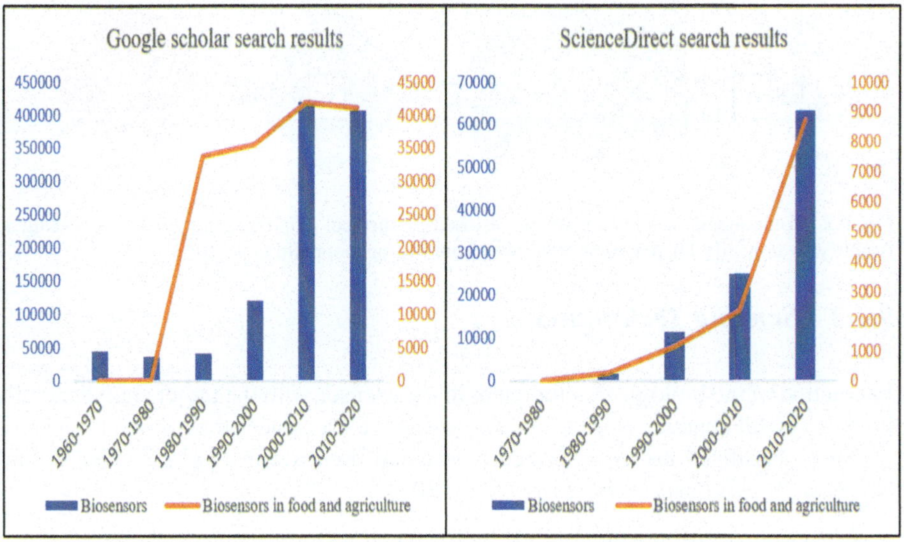

Fig. 9.1 Growth of biosensors and their application in food and agriculture since 1960–2020

9.1.1 *Fundamentals of Biosensors*

Biosensors, one of the various biotechnological tools to safeguard food in all aspects such as processing, storage, safety, and quality analysis, play a major role via its precise techniques, along with time and cost effectiveness. A biosensor is a diagnostic tool wherein a biological material explicitly interacts with a target analyte on specific recognition to produce a physical change that is detectable, quantified and transformed by a transducer into an electrical signal which is then, amplified, deduced and presented as target analyte concentration in the solution/matrix. The kind of interaction taking place between the biological material and the target analyte within a biosensor may be categorized into two: first being the conversion of the analyte into a different chemical molecule, and the second possibility of a simple binding between the analyte and the biological material (Bunney et al. 2017; Lozano et al. 2018; Malakar et al. 2020).

The process flow involved in the conversion of chemical information into electrical information in a biosensor comprises of few steps as below (Fig. 9.2) (Yunus 2019):

1. The target analyte interacts specifically on the biosensor surface.
2. Changes in the physico-chemical features of the transducer surface arise due to the occurrence of the interaction/reaction causing variations in the characteristics of the transducer.
3. These characteristic variations are quantified and transformed into electrical signals for further processing such as amplification and display.

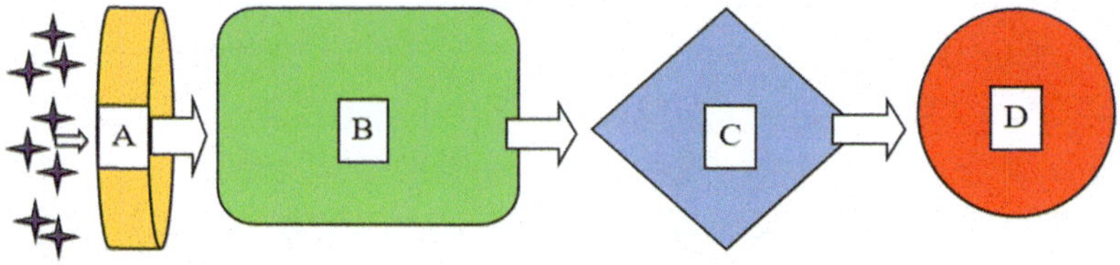

Fig. 9.2 Components of a biosensor- (**a**): Biosensor surface; (**b**): Transducer; (**c**): Processing & Amplifying unit; (**d**): Display unit (Redrawn from Murugaboopathi et al. 2013)

9.1.2 Sensing Techniques

Interaction of the biological component in a biosensor with the target analyte results in the physical changes close to the surface of the transducer that may fall into one of these classifications as described below and depicted in Fig. 9.2 (Thakur and Ragavan 2013; Lozano et al. 2018; Yunus 2019).

1. Absorption or dissipation of heat by the reaction- calorimetric biosensors.
2. Redox reaction causing electron movement & change in electron distribution resulting in electrical potential – basis for amperometric biosensors & potentiometric biosensors- electrochemical biosensors.
3. Absorption or production of light during the reaction -optical biosensors.
4. Change in the mass of the biological component as a result of the reaction – acoustic biosensors.

9.1.3 Properties

For the successful working of a biosensor, it should also possess the following fundamental characteristics (Bunney et al. 2017; Lozano et al. 2018; Yunus 2019):

1. High specificity for a target analyte.
2. Portable and biocompatible device.
3. Linear response over a useful range of target analyte concentration.
4. Cheap, small, and easy to use.
5. Durable and necessity of small volume of sample.
6. Quick, precise, and reproducible assay.
7. Robust, stable, and sterilizable device.

9.2 Classification of Biosensors

Biosensors can be classified on the basis of working principle and kind of application it is involved in. The biosensors described below are categorised on the basis of their biological recognition element which is an organic species that detects specific

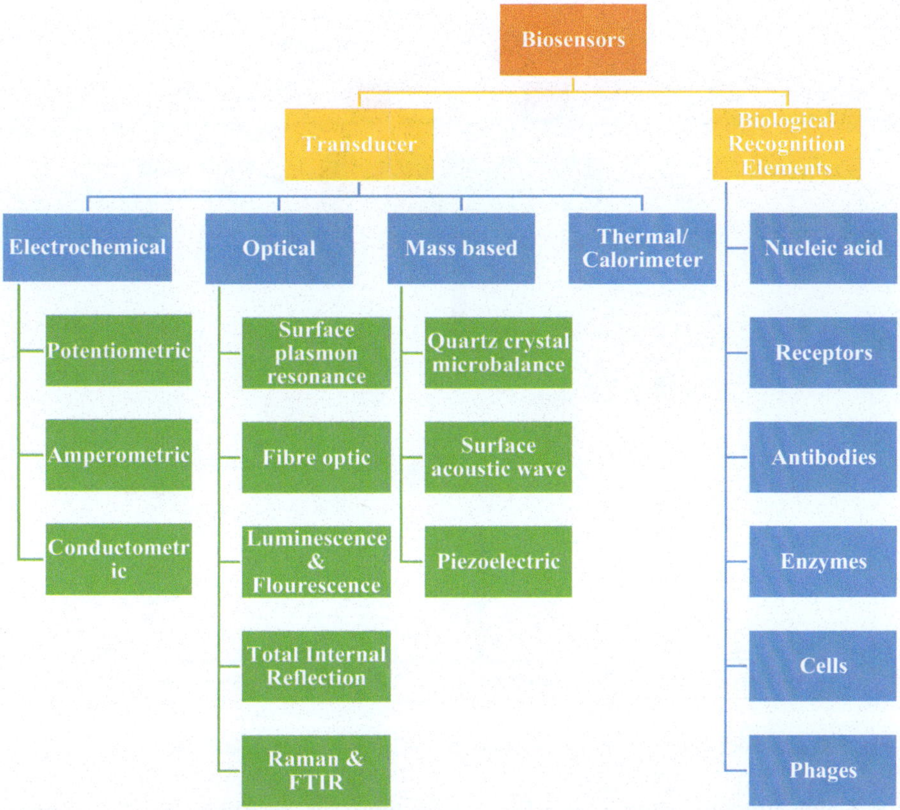

Fig. 9.3 Types of biosensors based on the physical change on interaction with the analyte and various types of biological recognition elements

target analyte from the sample, though at the same time is unresponsive to the presence of interfering species in the sample (Fig. 9.3). Since, the focus of this chapter is the application of various kinds of biosensors in food industry, some of the widely used and significant types of biosensors are discussed briefly.

9.2.1 Electrochemical Biosensors

Electrochemical transducers are utilized in case of these biosensors. During biochemical reactions, electrochemical signals are produced due to interaction between target molecule and receptor which are monitored via appropriate analysis systems (Fig. 9.4) (Bunney et al. 2017; Rubab et al. 2018; Rayappan et al. 2019; Campuzano et al. 2020).

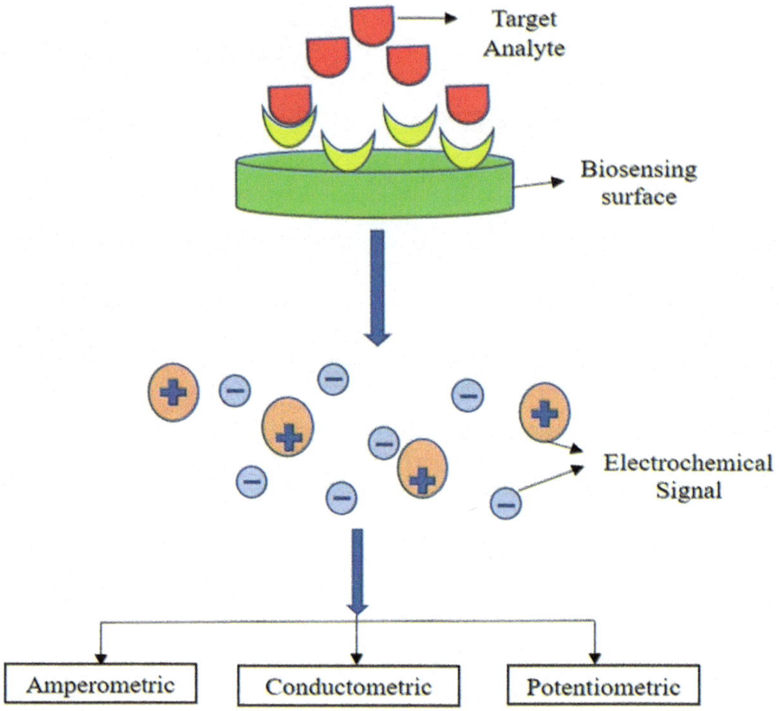

Fig. 9.4 Electrochemical biosensor (Redrawn from Campuzano et al. 2020)

1. Conductometric biosensor: The conductivity or resistivity of the solution changes as an electrochemical reaction produces ions or electrons. This change is measured by a conductiometric biosensor.
2. Amperometric biosensor: Electrochemical reduction/oxidation of an electroactive species produces current, which is monitored via an amperometric biosensor.
3. Potentiometric biosensor: Potential difference generated between the electrodes is measured by potentiometric biosensors when current flows due occurrence of electrochemical reactions as voltage is applied.

Further, classification of electrochemical biosensors includes enzymatic and non-enzymatic biosensors. Enzymatic biosensors are sensitive due to the involvement of immobilized enzyme via various methods such as covalent bonding, adsorption, entrapment and crosslinking. Therefore, these biosensors require appropriate operating conditions to maintain enzyme activity and stability, thereby restricting their use over a long period of time hampering response range as well as detection limits. Moreover, they are costly as well as complex in their construction. Due to these shortcomings of enzyme-based biosensors there has been a gradual shift towards non-enzymatic biosensors which are simple devices with high stability since they do not deal with enzymes requiring optimal conditions for their activity. These non-enzymatic biosensors usually, utilize nanomaterials to enhance their stability as well as sensitivity to the target (Revathi and Rajendra Kumar 2019). However, both enzymatic (Bollella and Gorton 2018; Gahlaut et al. 2019) and non-enzymatic (Luo et al. 2014; Ghanbari and Nejabati 2019; Gao et al. 2020) biosensors have been proven to contribute a great deal in food safety and quality assessment via the detection of various food contaminants- pathogens, adulterants and allergens (Baratella et al. 2018; Rubab et al. 2018; Rayappan et al. 2019; Vizzini et al. 2019; Campuzano et al. 2020; Riu and Giussani 2020).

With the inclusion of nanotechnology, analytical performance of electrochemical biosensors has been greatly improved in terms of detection levels, response range as well as better sensitivity and specificity, leading to wider applicability of this biosensor (Dervisevic et al. 2019; Gahlaut et al. 2019; Kuralay 2019; Muniandy et al. 2019; Pourakbari et al. 2019; Rayappan et al. 2019; Campuzano et al. 2020). Recent applications of electrochemical biosensors for the detection of various food contaminants are listed below (Table 9.1).

Over the years, electrochemical biosensors have been the most widely researched diagnostic tool in various fields, including food and agriculture. However, there needs to be some improvements in these biosensors for the better analysis of food and agricultural samples as the sample matrixes are usually complex in nature along with the development of multiple target analysis systems to save time, cost and sample requirement for analysis. Investigations on these aspects are underway and have been shown to have promising results (Vizzini et al. 2019), with the future

Table 9.1 Application of electrochemical biosensors for detection of various food contaminants

Target analyte	Sample	Biosensor type	References
Xanthine	Fish meat	Enzyme-based ultrasensitive electrochemical biosensor using poly(L-aspartic acid)/MWCNT bio-nanocomposite	Yazdanparast et al. (2019)
Xanthine	Fish meat	Nonenzymatic voltammetric xanthine biosensor with reduced graphene oxide/ polypyrrole/ CdO nanocomposite	Ghanbari and Nejabati (2019)
Xanthine, hypoxanthine	Fish meat	Triethylamine-controlled copper-BTC (benzenetricarboxylic acid) frameworks for electrochemical sensing	Li et al. (2019a)
Xanthine, hypoxanthine	Seafood (squid, large yellow croaker)	Xanthine oxidase immobilized electrochemical biosensor with copper-based metal–organic framework nanofiber film	Wang et al. (2019)
Penicillin, tetracyclin	Chicken and beef meat	Electrochemical biosensor based on hybrid nanowire/nanoparticle array	Li et al. (2019c)
Sulfadimethoxine	Fish, chicken, beef meat	Electrochemical sensor with reduced graphene oxide and gold nanoparticles	Mohammad-Razdari et al. (2019)
Antibiotic (Ceftiofur)	Turkey meat	Affinity-based electrochemical biosensor	Stevenson et al. (2019)
Salmonella enterica	Raw milk	Amperometric nanosensor	Saini et al. (2019)

focus on enhancing the space for testing various food and agriculture samples along with streamlining and improving optimizations, sensitivities, response ranges and reproduction of results.

9.2.2 Optical Biosensors

Optical biosensors are considered one of the most prevailing diagnostic devices amongst the biosensor technology till date. The underlying principle of these sensors is the measurement of signal (light) either by a luminescent process or via monitoring the variation in absorption of light within a reaction. Hence, the basis for optical biosensors are the optical properties such as absorption, fluorescence, bio- and chemi-luminescence, reflectance, refraction, dispersion, colorimetery and phosphorescence (Yunus 2019; Chen et al. 2019b; Chen and Wang 2020). Generally, within this biosensing system, the detection is broadly categorised into label- free and label- based. Label-free optical sensing aids in the detection of target molecule in its original form that is without altering the target analyte via any kind of interaction, unlike in label-based detection (Habimana et al. 2018).

Optical biosensors have been known to be better than their counterparts due to their low cost, higher sensitivity and specificity, along with the use of biodegradable electrodes. They also have reduced noise interference with the potential to be easily miniaturized such as a chip. Owing to better analytical performances (sensitivity), surface plasmon resonance (Fig. 9.5) and fluorescence based optical sensing systems are preferred, with fiberoptics, utilizing total internal reflection phenomenon, also gaining momentum in the food analysis arena (Gupta and Kant 2018; Habimana et al. 2018; Padilla and Thompson 2018; Yunus 2019; Chen et al. 2019b; Nabok et al. 2019; Pechprasarn et al. 2019; Zhou et al. 2019; Chen and Wang 2020; Younis et al. 2020).

Further improvements in optical biosensing systems have been made possible with the use of nanomaterials such as carbon nanostructures, magnetic nanoparticles and quantum dots (Dincer et al. 2019; Du et al. 2020; Younis et al. 2020). This has led to enhanced analytical performance of optical biosensors as well as

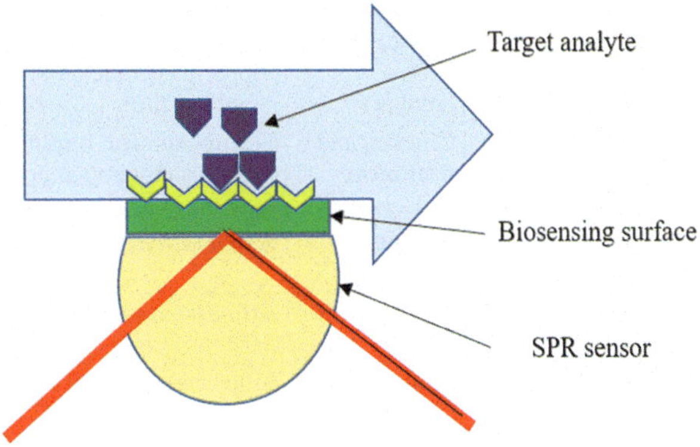

Fig. 9.5 Surface plasmon resonance (SPR) based-optical biosensor (Redrawn from Velasco-Garcia and Mottram 2003)

broadened and diversified the analyte list for detection encompassing various fields. In the food sector, optical biosensors have been used for detecting and analysing various toxins, pathogens, residual drugs and pesticides in various food matrixes (Sharma et al. 2018; Habimana et al. 2018; Padilla and Thompson 2018; Wang and Zhao 2018; Chen et al. 2019b; Nabok et al. 2019; Younis et al. 2020). Moreover, in the recent years this sensing technique has been in use for modelling hand-held/wearable devices also called point of care technology that substantially reduce analysis time, to almost seconds, along with the sample amount required without any additional pre-sample treatment (Habimana et al. 2018; Dincer et al. 2019). A few latest applications of optical biosensors in the field of food and agriculture industry are mentioned below (Table 9.2).

With the integration of technologies, optic biosensors have been upgraded to analyse multiple analytes with due precision and accuracy (Liao et al. 2018) and has been put to use for the detection of different milk and milk product contaminations (Pawar et al. 2020). This genre of biosensors is well scrutinised and are being probed further for optimization of systems and results to attain lower detection levels with better reproducibility and wider linearity. Extensive investigations are being carried to further improve the sensitivity and specificity towards various biological recognition elements as well as to reduce the cost of these biosensing systems for better commercial acceptance.

Table 9.2 Applications of optical biosensors for detection of various food contaminants

Target analyte	Sample	Biosensor type	References
Vitis vinifera varietal discrimination	*Vitis vinifera* leaf, must, wine	Label free DNA-based optical biosensor	Barrias et al. (2018)
Listeria monocytogenes	Lettuce	Optical biosensor with immunomagnetic separation, urease catalysis and pH indication	Chen et al. (2018)
Histophilus somni	Bovine and murine fluids	Nanomaterial optical fibre biosensor	Bandara et al. (2018)
Pesticide (parathion-methyl)	Tap water	Optical tyrosinase biosensor	Polatoglu and Ozkan (2019)
Insecticide (Pyrethroid)	Synthetic human fluids (plasma, urine)	Label- free optical whole-cell *E. coli* biosensor	Riangrungroj et al. (2019)
Salmonella spp.	Blueberries, chicken meat	Optical biosensor with oligonucleotide gold nanoparticles	Quintela et al. (2019)
Organophosphorous pesticides (chlorpyrifos-methyl, parathion, pirimiphos-methyl and diazinon)	Swine liver	Fiber optic biosensor based on covalent immobilization of acetylcholinesterase (AChE)	Yaneva et al. (2019)
Naphthalene	Water	Surface plasmon resonance (SPR)- plastic optical fiber (POF) biosensor	Cennamo et al. (2019)

9.2.3 Aptasensors (Aptamer Based)

Single-stranded oligonucleotide sequences with a wide recognition ability of numerous target molecules varying from large proteins to small ions with specificity and great affinity are aptamers. DNA, RNA or peptides are the building blocks of aptamers. In many diagnostic set-ups, these aptamers simulate antibody properties. After binding with their targets, aptamers go through structural changes. The in vitro process of selection of aptamers is called Systematic Evolution of Ligands by Exponential Enrichment (SELEX) (Duan et al. 2016; Li et al. 2019b; Wu et al. 2019b).

Aptamers provide chemical stability over a wide-ranging buffer conditions and withstand long term storages; they also resist the harsh treatments without diminishing its bioactivity. An interesting property of an aptamer is its reversible thermal denaturation, thereby making aptamers beneficial in the fabrication of biosensor devices. Aptamer enables the recognition of various molecular and therapeutic targets- metal ions, amino acids, drugs, any class of proteins (membrane proteins, immunoglobulins, growth factors and cytokines, enzymes, and viral proteins), whole cells and bio−/organic/inorganic small molecules. Aptamers are highly affinitive to targets with the dissociation constants (K_d) in the range of 10^{-6}–10^{-12} mol/L (Song et al. 2019). They are inexpensive, small sized and offer outstanding flexibility and ease in crafting their distinctive structure. Furthermore, combinatorial chemical synthesis delivers varied techniques for aptamer sequence alterations like the terminal tagging chemical groups. Various detailed reviews are available for aptasensor (Fig. 9.6) being used in food safety applications (Song et al. 2019) against targets such as food borne pathogens (Majdinasab et al. 2018; Kumar et al. 2019;

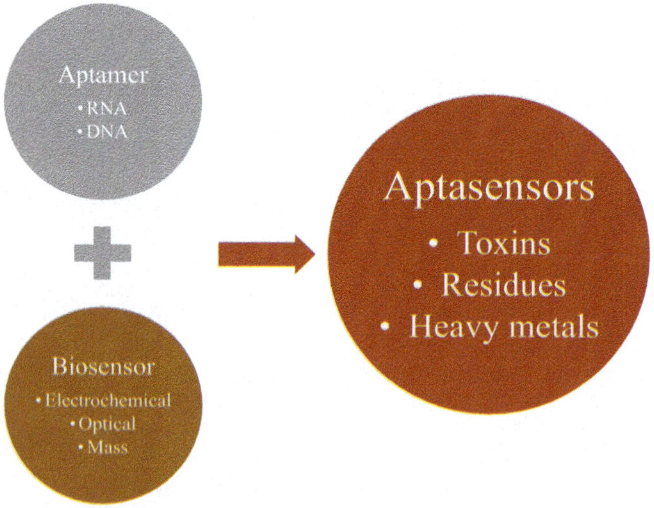

Fig. 9.6 Formation and applications of aptasensors in food analysis

Wu et al. 2019b), drug and pesticide residues (Liu et al. 2019; Gaudin 2020) and toxins (Evtugyn and Hianik 2019; Piecková et al. 2019; Ye et al. 2019).

Recently, microbes like *Listeria monocytogenes, S. typhimurium, Campylobacter jejuni* and toxins like ochratoxin A have been detected by quantitative polymerase chain reaction (qPCR) and iridium oxide nanoparticles in combination with aptamers (Sharma and Raghavarao 2018). This advantageous synergy of nanomaterials and aptasensors has been tapped into for the detection of numerous food contaminants (Duan et al. 2016; Sharma and Raghavarao 2018; Li et al. 2019b; Liu et al. 2019; Wu et al. 2019b). Some latest applications of aptasensors being used for the detection of various food contaminants are listed in Table 9.3.

Though, aptamers have high stability and are easily synthesized along with their wide applicability, their use for food analysis is restricted due to the complex food

Table 9.3 Application of aptasensors for detection of various food contaminants

Target analyte	Sample	Aptasensor type	Limit of detection	References
Salmonella typhimurium	Pork meat	Surface-enhanced Raman spectroscopy-based aptasensor with gold nanoparticles	4 cfu/mL	Ma et al. (2018b)
Egg white lysozyme; ß-conglutin lupine; Okadiac acid; Brevetoxin	Egg white; mussel tissue; sausages	Polydimethylsiloxane/paper microfluidic aptasensor functionalized by graphene oxide	–	Weng and Neethirajan (2018a)
Pseudomonas aeruginosa	Tap water; chicken meat	Bimodal aptasensor (surface-enhanced raman spectroscopy and colorimetric)	20–50 cfu/mL	Wu et al. (2018)
Malachite green	Fish meat	Colorimetric aptasensor with gold nanoparticles	15.95 nM	Jia et al. (2018)
Tobramycin	Milk; chicken eggs	Colorimetric aptasensor with gold nanoparticles	23.3 nM	Ma et al. (2018a)
Ochratoxin A	Red wine	RNase H-assisted fluorescence aptamer-based fluorescent biosensor	0.08 ng/mL	Wu et al. (2019a)
Histamine	Tuna meat	Aptasensor based on structure-switching mechanism	1μM	Dwidar and Yokobayashi (2019)
Kanamycin	Milk	Surface-enhanced Raman spectroscopy-based aptasensor	0.90 pg/mL	Jiang et al. (2019)
L. monocytogenes, *Salmonella* spp., and *E. coli*	Ham and chicken sausages	Colorimetric aptasensor with gold nanoparticles	10^5 cfu/mL	Ledlod et al. (2020)
Vanillin		Graphene oxide-based label-free capacitive aptasensor	9.91 pM	Mohan et al. (2020)

matrixes, false positive results due to non-specific binding with sample components, development and availability of aptamers specific to new contaminants, analysis of various contaminants simultaneously, and their vulnerability to surrounding conditions. Further research into these aspects of aptasensors are ongoing and need to be probed in the near future to have an all-in-one device for quick and real time monitoring of food samples.

9.2.4 Immunosensors

Immunosensors have not only emerged as an important diagnostic tool in the medical field but also proven to be effective in environmental and food safety applications. The basic working principle behind immunosensors is quite analogous with immunoassay technique that is the ability of an antibody to recognise specific antigens and form stable immune-complexes. The formation of these complexes causes change in either complex properties (density/mass changes) or signal responses (color/potential generation). The detection of these signals is possible with the use of specific transducers. Unlike the immunoassay technique, immunosensors facilitate quantification and label-free detection of the immuno- complexes. These sensors are, thereby, categorised on the basis of their detection principle such as electrochemical, microgravimetric and optical immunosensors (Asal et al. 2018; Azam et al. 2020).

In the recent times, immunosenors have been used for the detection of such various hazardous and undesirable compounds in environment (particularly water) and food samples. These sensors have gained attention as the means of rapid screening due to their high specificity, low cost, high throughput screening and sensitivity. The presence of drugs, toxins, pesticides (Capoferri et al. 2018; Reynoso et al. 2019) or pathogens in any matrix is considered unsafe, especially in case of food, which have been shown to be easily detected by various types of immunosensors with high sensitivity and low detection levels (Asal et al. 2018; Hosu et al. 2018; Daliri et al. 2019). Further advancement in the sensitivities and overall functioning of immunosensors has been possible with the use of nanomaterials such as metal nanoparticles, quantum dots, carbon nanotubes (Daliri et al. 2019; Azam et al. 2020). Latest applications utilizing immunosensors for the detection of different unwanted compounds are listed below (Table 9.4).

As can be seen, the amalgamation of various technologies with immunosenors has led to the detection of diverse components across several food and environmental samples. Moreover, detection of multiple compounds from a single matrix has also been shown to be successful leading to reductions in analysis cost and expenses. However, a few challenges remain to be addressed such as the sample preparation of complex samples (eg. food) and optimization to reduce non-target analyte intervention, robustness of immunosensors along with enhanced binding stability with target analyte to enhance detection efficiency, and lastly, compatibility of various

Table 9.4 Applications of immunosensors for detection of various food contaminants

Target analyte	Sample	Immunosensor type	References
Mycotoxins (aflatoxin B1, Ochratoxin A, Zearalenone)	Corn, rice, wheat	Surface enhanced raman scattering (SERS)- based immunosensor	Li et al. (2018)
Salmonella typhimurium	Chicken meat	Quartz-crystal microbalance (QCM)- based immunosensor	Fulgione et al. (2018)
Pesticides (Boscalid, Clothianidin, Nitenpyrem)	Vegetables (broccoli, cucumber, spinach, lettuce, welsh onion, tomato)	Surface plasmon resonance (SPR)- based simultaneous immunosensor	Hirakawa et al. (2018)
Avian coronavirus (infectious bronchitis virus)	Cotton thread, chicken whole blood	Molybdenum disulfide- based fluorescent immunosensor	Weng and Neethirajan (2018b)
Pesticides (Chlorfenapyr, Imazalil, Azoxystrobin, Isoxathion, Boscalid Nitenpyrem)	Tomato, eggplant, green pepper, lemon	Surface enhanced raman scattering (SERS)- based immunosensor	Miyake et al. (2020)
Pseudocercospora fijiensis	Banana leaf	Surface enhanced raman scattering (SERS)- based immunosensor	Luna-Moreno et al. (2019)
Botulinum	Milk, serum, phosphate buffered saline (PBS)	Nano-immunosensors	Cheng and Chuang (2019)
Antiviral drug (amantadine)	Chicken muscle, duck muscle, egg, pork	Label-free piezoelectric immunosensor	Yun et al. (2019)
Aflatoxin B1	Peanuts, rice, corn	Electrochemical immunosensor modified with ferrocene/ multi-walled carbon nanotube/ chitosan (Fc/ MWCNT/ CS)	Zhang et al. (2019)
Pesticides (carbaryl, dichlorodiphenyltri-choloroethane)	Honey	High Fundamental frequency quartz crystal microbalance (HFF-QCM)- based immunosenor	Cervera-Chiner et al. (2020)
Escherichia coli	Drinking water	Screen printed based impedimetric immunosensor	Cimafonte et al. (2020)
Estrogen (17β-estradiol)	Tap water	Localised surface plasmon resonance (LSPR)- based colorimetric immunosensor	Minopoli et al. (2020)
Melamine	Liquid milk, milk powder	Competitive electrochemical immunosensor based on branched polyethyleneimine functionalized reduced graphene oxide and gold nanoparticles modified electrode	Ren et al. (2020)
Cephalaxin	Milk, meat (beef, pawn, fish)	Electrochemical immunosensor based on carboxylated single-walled carbon nanotube-chitosan	Yu et al. (2020)

nanomaterials being used to improve immunosensor performance in terms of sensitivity, response range, detection levels thereby affecting reproducibility of results.

9.2.5 Sensors Using Bacteriophages

Phage- based sensors are the most recent addition to the biosensor technology. Bacteriophages are typically viruses that only infect bacteria, which makes them suitable for the detection of bacteria in various applications. This host specific nature as well as other beneficial properties such as tolerance towards environmental stress (temperature, pH etc.), easy bulk production and safe handling requirements along with the ability to discriminate between dead and live bacterial cells (since they infect only live bacterial cells) make them custom made for use in biosensors as biological recognition element (Singh 2018; Farooq et al. 2019).

These properties of bacteriophages have led to various new applications not only in the field of medicine but also food safety. In the food industry, phage therapy is used for ensuring growth of plant/animal during preharvest of production, whereas contamination by pathogens can be controlled during postharvest duration. Phages have not only been utilized to reduce and prevent formation of biofilms on equipments but also added to food products to extend shelf-life via controlling bacterial spoilage caused by *Pseudomonas, Salmonella, Streptococcus, Listeria* and many more (Richter et al. 2018; López-Cuevas et al. 2019; Połaska and Sokołowska 2019; Stone et al. 2019; Wei et al. 2019). Some recent advances pertaining to the use of bacteriophages in biosensors as biological recognition element (Fig. 9.7) are tabulated below (Table 9.5).

With the involvement of diverse technology prowess such as genetic engineering and nanotechnology, phage based-biosensors can further be utilized for a variety of new target analytes. This combination of technologies can also help in enhancing the sensitivity, specificity and robustness of the sensors. A major limitation that needs attention is the dearth of bacteriophage types that are in use as recognition elements for these sensors, restricting the scope of extensive applicability since phages are host specific.

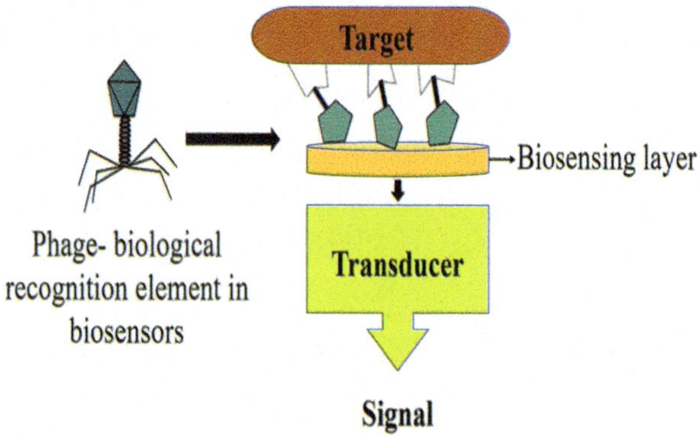

Fig. 9.7 Phage-based biosensor (Redrawn from Richter et al. 2018)

Table 9.5 Applications of phage-based biosensors in food safety

Target analyte	Sample	Phage-based biosensor type	References
Escherichia coli O157:H7, *E. coli* O45:H2, and *Salmonella*	Spinach, ground beef and chicken homogenates	Phage-based paper dipstick biosensor	Anany et al. (2018)
Bacillus cereus	–	Ferromagnetoelastic (FME) biosensor with *B. cereus* specific phage	Choi et al. (2018)
Pesticide (methyl viologen dichloride hydrate)	Apple peels	M13 bacteriophage/silver nanowire surface-enhanced raman scattering sensor	Koh et al. (2018)
Mycotoxin (Deoxynivalenol)	Wheat, corn	Phage displayed mimotope peptide-based immunosensor	Yan et al. (2019)
Escherichia coli O157:H7	Tomato	Millimeter- waves technology- based biosensor	Sultan et al. (2019)
Endocrine disrupting chemicals (bis-(2-ethylhexyl)-phthalate (BEHP), dibutyl phthalate (DBP), diethyl phthalate (DEP), and benzyl-butyl-phthalate (BBP))	–	Phage-based colorimetric sensor	Seol et al. (2019)
Escherichia coli	Simulated wash water	Nanophotonic device with T7 bacteriophage- based biosensor	Tilton et al. (2019)
Pesticide (Paraqaut)	–	Surface-enhanced raman scattering (SERS) sensors with M13 phage	Lee et al. (2019)
Salmonella	Tomato, spinach	Phage Magnetoelastic biosensor	Chen et al. (2019a)
Escherichia coli	Drinking water	Syringe-based biosensor with T7 bacteriophage	Hinkley et al. (2020)
Estrogen drugs (Mercilon, estradiol, estrone, gastodene) antibiotics (Duricef, citopcin, rifampin, amoxicillin)	–	Bacteriophage-based colorimetric sensor	Kim et al. (2020)

9.3 Nanotechnology in Biosensors

With current global situation, the need for safe and quality food is of utmost importance. Lifestyle changes have also led to enhanced consumer awareness about nutrition, safety and quality of food. Biosensors being diagnostic tools play a significant role in the food and agriculture sector by monitoring food and agri-produce safety and quality. Various biosensors have already been put to use for the same as discussed in previous sections, however, there is an urgent need for further improving the analytical performance of these biosensors along with their ability to detect multiple target analytes simultaneously within a food matrix. Rapid developments in the field of nanotechnology in the past two decades have unfolded various novel innovative solutions for many industrial and consumer sectors. Emergence of nanotechnology within food sector has led to numerous major impactful inventions linked to production, processing, storage, transportation, traceability, safety and security of food.

This overlap and merging of technologies into one another have not only helped the existing tools and processes to be upgraded to resolve problems but also facilitated the creation of new, state- of- the- art, compact techniques reducing usage of resources, time, and cost. Similar is the case with biosensing technology, where the introduction of nanotechnology in the form of various nanostructures such as nanoparticles, nanotubes, nanowires, carbon nanostructures, quantum dots, magnetic beads have brought about a revolution. These nanomaterials are quite different from the same material in bulk form in terms of their physicochemical properties, due to their dimensions being in nanoscale range. The incorporation of these into biosensors brings about all the difference in various aspects such as specific binding with the target, sensitivity mechanism, detection efficiency and response accuracy. Recent developments in the biosensing systems for the detection of food contaminants utilizing nanomaterials have been quoted in the different genre of biosensors in this chapter as well as in various other reports and reviews (Antonacci et al. 2017; Dede and Altay 2018; Lv et al. 2018; Di Pietrantonio et al. 2019; Dhole and Pitambara 2019; Jafarizadeh-Malmiri et al. 2019; Lu et al. 2019; Singh 2020; Du et al. 2020; Gouda et al. 2020; Lee and Moon 2020; Mohana et al. 2020). Further research on incorporating new target analytes such as illegal additives (sweeteners, preservatives), genetically modified foods, moisture are under way along with the existing ones, also exploring their form of commercialization (Denmark et al. 2019; Patel et al. 2020; Ramezani et al. 2020). Moreover, focus on utilizing variety of already existing and new nanomaterials along with their compatibility with target analyte and biosensors in entirety is also significantly increasing.

Use of nanotechnology in biosensing techniques has immensely aided in the all-round enhancement of biosensor performances. Various parameters such as response time, detection limits, sensitivity/resolution, selectivity and portability (point- of-care technology) of biosensors have greatly benefitted with the inclusion of nanomaterials. However, some features of this combination of technologies such as cost, specific sample preparation and protocol validation with real samples need to be worked around for their improved marketability and commercialization. Additionally, toxicity concerns related to use of nanomaterials have to be addressed in terms of their exposure to environment and humans along with risk assessment to determine permissible limits/concentrations. Finally, their interactions with biological target analytes have to be monitored and understood to prevent adverse/false positive results.

9.4 Conclusion and Future Scope

In the present scenario, food and agricultural industries are up against various difficulties, especially in terms of assuring safe and nutritious food to consumers. For ensuring the same, their primary obstacle is the lack of a rapid and cost-effective technique that is able to detect pathogens as well as allergenic constituents in food. For tackling this obstacle, biosensor technology is the best way forward. Biosensors enable rapid and precise detection of components within a matrix along with a pronounced level of sensitivity.

Usually, the chemical & microbiological analysis in the food and agriculture industries are carried out regularly by trained personnel which may turn out to be expensive, tedious, time consuming and may at times yield inaccurate results. The likely applications of this technology not only encompass the mentioned chemical and microbiological analysis of food products but also the detection of contaminants, product content verification, product freshness and monitoring of raw materials conversion.

Biosensors have the potential to bring about an analytical revolution by offering prompt, precise, non-destructive and inexpensive methods for quality control in the agriculture and food industries. This could be achieved by focusing on further integration and application of nanotechnology that has the capability of enhancing sensitivity, reproducibility and precision of biosensors. Also, the utilization of bacteriophages with proper care would be ornamental for devising accurate detection systems. Furthermore, this technique could serve a greater purpose by being a preventive detection measure by its incorporation into assembly lines right from determining the quality of raw materials to finished food product enabling the detection of risks/hazards at an early stage and thereby help in avoiding risks/damages to industries and consumers alike.

References

Anany H, Brovko L, El Dougdoug NK, Sohar J, Fenn H, Alasiri N, Jabrane T, Mangin P, Ali MM, Kannan B, Filipe CD (2018) Print to detect: a rapid and ultrasensitive phage-based dipstick assay for foodborne pathogens. Anal Bioanal Chem 410:1217–1230. https://doi.org/10.1007/s00216-017-0597-y

Antonacci A, Arduini F, Moscone D, Palleschi G, Scognamiglio V (2017) Nanostructured (bio) sensors for smart agriculture. TrAC – Trends Anal Chem 98:95–103. https://doi.org/10.1016/j.trac.2017.10.022

Asal M, Özen Ö, Şahinler M, Polatoğlu İ (2018) Recent developments in enzyme, DNA and immuno-based biosensors. Sensors (Switzerland) 18(6):1924. https://doi.org/10.3390/s18061924

Azam NFN, Lim SA, Ahmed MU (2020) Carbon nanomaterials for electrochemiluminescence-based immunosensors: recent advances and applications. In: Chandra P, Prakash R (eds) Nanobiomaterial engineering. Springer, Singapore, pp 71–90. https://doi.org/10.1007/978-981-32-9840-8_4

Bandara AB, Zuo Z, McCutcheon K, Ramachandran S, Heflin JR, Inzana TJ (2018) Identification of *Histophilus somni* by a nanomaterial optical fiber biosensor assay. J Vet Diagn Investig 30(6):821–829. https://doi.org/10.1177/1040638718803665

Baratella D, Bonaiuto E, Magro M, de Almeida RJ, Kanamori Y, Lima GPP, Agostinelli E, Vianello F (2018) Endogenous and food-derived polyamines: determination by electrochemical sensing. Amino Acids 50:1187–1203. https://doi.org/10.1007/s00726-018-2617-4

Barrias S, Fernandes JR, Eiras-dias JE, Brazão J (2018) University of Lisboa, Faculty of Sciences. BioISI – Biosyst Integrative Sci Food Chem. https://doi.org/10.1016/j.foodchem.2018.07.058

Bollella P, Gorton L (2018) Enzyme based amperometric biosensors. Curr Opin Electrochem 10:157–173. https://doi.org/10.1016/j.coelec.2018.06.003

Bunney J, Williamson S, Atkin D, Jeanneret M, Cozzolino D, Chapman J (2017) The use of electrochemical biosensors in food analysis. Curr Res Nutr Food Sci J 5:183–195. https://doi.org/10.12944/CRNFSJ.5.3.02

Campuzano S, Montiel VRV, Serafín V, Yáñez-Sedeño P, Pingarrón JM (2020) Cutting-edge advances in electrochemical affinity biosensing at different molecular level of emerging food allergens and adulterants. Biosensors 10(2):10. https://doi.org/10.3390/bios10020010

Capoferri D, Della Pelle F, Del Carlo M, Compagnone D (2018) Affinity sensing strategies for the detection of pesticides in food. Foods 7(9):148. https://doi.org/10.3390/foods7090148

Cennamo N, Zeni L, Ricca E, Isticato R, Marzullo VM, Capo A, Staiano M, D'Auria S, Varriale A (2019) Environmental monitoring exploiting optical fiber biosensors. The case of naphthalene detection in water. In: Di Francia G, Di Natale C, Alfano B et al (eds) Sensors and microsystems, proceeding. Springer, Cham, pp 65–70. https://doi.org/10.1007/978-3-030-37558-4_10

Cervera-Chiner L, March C, Arnau A, Jiménez Y, Montoya Á (2020) Detection of DDT and carbaryl pesticides in honey by means of immunosensors based on high fundamental frequency quartz crystal microbalance (HFF-QCM). J Sci Food Agric 100:2468. https://doi.org/10.1002/jsfa.10267

Chen C, Wang J (2020) Optical biosensors: an exhaustive and comprehensive review. Analyst 145(5):1605–1628. https://doi.org/10.1039/C9AN01998G

Chen Q, Huang F, Cai G, Wang M, Lin J (2018) Sensors and actuators B: chemical an optical biosensor using immunomagnetic separation, urease catalysis and pH indication for rapid and sensitive detection of listeria monocytogenes. Sensors Actuators B Chem 258:447–453. https://doi.org/10.1016/j.snb.2017.11.087

Chen I-H, Liu Y, Du S et al (2019a) Effects of different broth enrichment upon phage magnetoelastic biosensor for fast detecting low salmonella counts on problematic produce. Adv Microbiol 09:541–555. https://doi.org/10.4236/aim.2019.96033

Chen Y, Liu J, Yang Z, Wilkinson JS, Zhou X (2019b) Biosensors and bioelectronics optical biosensors based on refractometric sensing schemes: a review. Biosens Bioelectron 144:111693. https://doi.org/10.1016/j.bios.2019.111693

Cheng HP, Chuang HS (2019) Rapid and sensitive nano-immunosensors for botulinum. ACS Sens 4:1754–1760. https://doi.org/10.1021/acssensors.9b00644

Choi IY, Park JH, Gwak KM, Kim KP, Oh JH, Park MK (2018) Studies on lytic, tailed Bacillus cereus-specific phage for use in a ferromagnetoelastic biosensor as a novel recognition element. J Microbiol Biotechnol 28:87–94. https://doi.org/10.4014/jmb.1710.10033

Cimafonte M, Fulgione A, Gaglione R, Papaianni M, Capparelli R, Arciello A, Bolletti-Censi S, Borriello G, Velotta R, Della-Ventura B (2020) Screen printed based impedimetric immunosensor for rapid detection of Escherichia coli in drinking water. Sensors 20:1–17. https://doi.org/10.3390/s20010274

Daliri F, Aboagye AA, Kyei-Baffour V, Elahi F, Chelliah R, Daliri EBM (2019) Immunosensors for food safety: current trends and future perspectives. J Food Hyg Saf 34:509–518. https://doi.org/10.13103/jfhs.2019.34.6.509

Dede S, Altay F (2018) Biosensors from the first generation to nano-biosensors. Int Adv Res Eng J 02:200–207

Denmark DJ, Bustos-perez X, Swain A, Phan MH, Mohapatra S, Mohapatra SS (2019) Readiness of magnetic nanobiosensors for point-of-care commercialization. J Electron Mater 48:4749. https://doi.org/10.1007/s11664-019-07275-7

Dervisevic M, Dervisevic E, Şenel M (2019) Recent progress in nanomaterial-based electrochemical and optical sensors for hypoxanthine and xanthine. A review. Microchim Acta 186:1. https://doi.org/10.1007/s00604-019-3842-6

Dhole A, Pitambara M (2019) Nanobiosensors: a novel approach in precision agriculture. In: Panpatte DG, Jhala YK (eds) Nanotechnology for agriculture. Singapore Springer, pp. 241–262

Di Pietrantonio F, Cannatà D, Benetti M (2019) Biosensor technologies based on nanomaterials. In: Functional nanostructured interfaces for environmental and biomedical applications. Elsevier, Amsterdam, pp 181–242. https://doi.org/10.1016/b978-0-12-814401-5.00008-6

Dincer C, Bruch R, Costa-rama E, Fernández-Abedul MT, Merkoçi A, Manz A, Urban GA, Güder F (2019) Disposable sensors in diagnostics, food, and environmental monitoring. Adv Mater 31:1806739. https://doi.org/10.1002/adma.201806739

Du H, Li Z, Wang Y, Yang Q, Wu W (2020) Nanomaterial-based optical biosensors for the detection of foodborne bacteria. Food Rev Int:1–30. https://doi.org/10.1080/87559129.2020.1740733

Duan N, Wu S, Dai S, Gu H, Hao L, Ye H, Wang Z (2016) Advances in aptasensors for the detection of food contaminants. Analyst 141:3942–3961. https://doi.org/10.1039/c6an00952b

Dwidar M, Yokobayashi Y (2019) Development of a histamine aptasensor for food safety monitoring. Sci Rep 9:1–7. https://doi.org/10.1038/s41598-019-52876-1

Evtugyn G, Hianik T (2019) Aptamer-based biosensors for mycotoxin detection. In: Nanomycotoxicology, Academic press, London, pp 35–70. https://doi.org/10.1016/B978-0-12-817998-7.00003-3

Farooq U, Yang Q, Ullah MW, Wang S (2019) Principle and development of phage- based biosensors. In: Biosensors for environmental monitoring. IntechOpen, London, pp 1–19

Fulgione A, Cimafonte M, Della Ventura B, Iannaccone M, Ambrosino C, Capuano F, Proroga YT, Velotta R, Capparelli R (2018) QCM-based immunosensor for rapid detection of *Salmonella typhimurium* in food. Sci Rep 8:1–8. https://doi.org/10.1038/s41598-018-34285-y

Gahlaut A, Hooda V, Gothwal A, Hooda V (2019) Enzyme-based ultrasensitive electrochemical biosensors for rapid assessment of nitrite toxicity: recent advances and perspectives. Crit Rev Anal Chem 49:32–43. https://doi.org/10.1080/10408347.2018.1461551

Gao X, Du X, Liu D, Liu D, Gao H, Wang P, Yang J (2020) Core-shell gold-nickel nanostructures as highly selective and stable nonenzymatic glucose sensor for fermentation process. Sci Rep 10:1–10. https://doi.org/10.1038/s41598-020-58403-x

Gaudin V (2020) The growing interest in development of innovative optical aptasensors for the detection of antimicrobial residues in food products. Biosensors 10(3):21. https://doi.org/10.3390/bios10030021

Ghanbari K, Nejabati F (2019) Construction of novel nonenzymatic xanthine biosensor based on reduced graphene oxide/polypyrrole/CdO nanocomposite for fish meat freshness detection. J Food Meas Charact 13:1411–1422. https://doi.org/10.1007/s11694-019-00057-z

Gouda HS, Pradhan A, Hasanain M, Praharaj S (2020) Nanobiosensors in agriculture. In: Naresh RK (ed) Advances in agriculture sciences, vol 23. AkiNik Publications, New Delhi, pp 11–29. https://doi.org/10.22271/ed.book.751

Gupta BD, Kant R (2018) Recent advances in surface plasmon resonance based fiber optic chemical and biosensors utilizing bulk and nanostructures. Opt Laser Technol 101:144–161. https://doi.org/10.1016/j.optlastec.2017.11.015

Habimana JDD, Ji J, Sun X (2018) Minireview: trends in optical-based biosensors for point-of-care bacterial pathogen detection for food safety and clinical diagnostics. Anal Lett 51(18):2933–2966. https://doi.org/10.1080/00032719.2018.1458104

Hinkley TC, Garing S, Jain P, Williford J, Le Ny AL, Nichols KP, Peters JE, Talbert JN, Nugen SR (2020) A syringe-based biosensor to rapidly detect low levels of *Escherichia coli* (ECOR13)

in drinking water using engineered bacteriophages. Sensors 20:1953. https://doi.org/10.3390/s20071953

Hirakawa Y, Yamasaki T, Harada A, Iwasa S, Narita H, Miyake S (2018) Development of an immunosensor based on surface plasmon resonance for simultaneous residue analysis of three pesticides -boscalid, clothianidin, and nitenpyram- in vegetables. Anal Sci 34:533–539. https://doi.org/10.2116/analsci.17P487

Hosu O, Selvolini G, Marrazza G (2018) Recent advances of immunosensors for detecting food allergens. Curr Opin Electrochem 10:149–156. https://doi.org/10.1016/j.coelec.2018.05.022

Jafarizadeh-Malmiri H, Sayyar Z, Anarjan N, Berenjian A (2019) Nano-sensors in food nanobiotechnology. In: Nanobiotechnology in food: concepts, applications and perspectives. Springer Nature, Cham, pp 81–94. https://doi.org/10.1007/978-3-030-05846-3_6

Jia J, Yan S, Lai X, Xu Y, Liu T, Xiang Y (2018) Colorimetric aptasensor for detection of malachite green in fish sample based on RNA and gold nanoparticles. Food Anal Methods 11:1668–1676. https://doi.org/10.1007/s12161-017-1144-3

Jiang Y, Sun DW, Pu H, Wei Q (2019) Ultrasensitive analysis of kanamycin residue in milk by SERS-based aptasensor. Talanta 197:151–158. https://doi.org/10.1016/j.talanta.2019.01.015

Kim C, Lee H, Devaraj V, Kim WG, Lee Y, Kim Y, Jeong NN, Choi EJ, Baek SH, Han DW, Sun H (2020) Hierarchical cluster analysis of medical chemicals detected by a bacteriophage-based colorimetric sensor array. Nanomaterials 10(1):121. https://doi.org/10.3390/nano10010121

Koh EH, Mun C, Kim C, Park SG, Choi EJ, Kim SH, Dang J, Choo J, Oh JW, Kim DH, Jung HS (2018) M13 bacteriophage/silver nanowire surface-enhanced Raman scattering sensor for sensitive and selective pesticide detection. ACS Appl Mater Interfaces 10:10388–10397. https://doi.org/10.1021/acsami.8b01470

Kumar A, Malinee M, Dhiman A, Sharma TK (2019) Aptamer technology for the detection of foodborne pathogens and toxins. In: Advanced biosensors for health care applications. Elsevier, Amsterdam, pp 45–69. https://doi.org/10.1016/b978-0-12-815743-5.00002-0

Kuralay F (2019) Nanomaterials-based enzyme biosensors for electrochemical applications: recent trends and future prospects. In: New developments in nanosensors for pharmaceutical analysis. Academic Press, London, pp 381–408. https://doi.org/10.1016/b978-0-12-816144-9.00012-2

Ledlod S, Areekit S, Santiwatanakul S, Chansiri K (2020) Colorimetric aptasensor for detecting *Salmonella spp.*, *Listeria monocytogenes*, and *Escherichia coli* in meat samples. Food Sci Technol Int 16:430. https://doi.org/10.1177/1082013219899593

Lee Y, Moon J (2020) Introduction to bio-nanotechnology. Springer. https://doi.org/10.1016/b978-0-323-39080-4.00012-4

Lee JM, Choi EJ, Park J, Devaraj V, Kim C, Han J, Kim WG, Kim K, Kang YC, Kim KH, Oh JW (2019) Improvement of high affinity and selectivity on biosensors using genetically engineered phage by binding isotherm screening. Viruses 11:1–11. https://doi.org/10.3390/v11030248

Li Y, Chen Q, Xu X, Jin Y, Wang Y, Zhang L, Yang W, He L, Feng X, Chen Y (2018) Microarray surface enhanced Raman scattering based immunosensor for multiplexing detection of mycotoxin in foodstuff. Sensors Actuators B Chem 266:115–123. https://doi.org/10.1016/j.snb.2018.03.040

Li C, Hao J, Wu K (2019a) Triethylamine-controlled Cu-BTC frameworks for electrochemical sensing fish freshness. Anal Chim Acta 1085:68–74. https://doi.org/10.1016/j.aca.2019.07.064

Li F, Yu Z, Han X, Lai RY (2019b) Electrochemical aptamer-based sensors for food and water analysis: a review. Anal Chim Acta 1051:1–23. https://doi.org/10.1016/j.aca.2018.10.058

Li Z, Liu C, Sarpong V, Gu Z (2019c) Multisegment nanowire/nanoparticle hybrid arrays as electrochemical biosensors for simultaneous detection of antibiotics. Biosens Bioelectron 126:632–639. https://doi.org/10.1016/j.bios.2018.10.025

Liao Z, Zhang Y, Li Y, Miao Y, Gao S, Lin F, Deng Y, Geng L (2018) Biosensors and bioelectronic microfluidic chip coupled with optical biosensors for simultaneous detection of multiple analytes: a review. Biosens Bioelectron 12:697–706. https://doi.org/10.1016/j.bios.2018.11.032

Liu M, Khan A, Wang Z, Liu Y, Yang G, Deng Y, He N (2019) Aptasensors for pesticide detection. Biosens Bioelectron 130:174–184. https://doi.org/10.1016/j.bios.2019.01.006

López-Cuevas O, Medrano-Félix JA, Castro-Del Campo N, Chaidez C (2019) Bacteriophage applications for fresh produce food safety. Int J Environ Health Res:1–16. https://doi.org/10.1080/09603123.2019.1680819

Lozano MG, García YP, Gonzalez JAS, GBañuelos CV, Escareño MP, Balagurusamy N (2018) Biosensors for food quality and safety monitoring: fundamentals and applications. In: Enzymes in food biotechnology. Academic Press, London, pp 691–709. https://doi.org/10.1016/b978-0-12-813280-7.00040-2

Lu L, Zhu Z, Hu X (2019) Hybrid nanocomposites modified on sensors and biosensors for the analysis of food functionality and safety. Trends Food Sci Technol 90:100–110. https://doi.org/10.1016/j.tifs.2019.06.009

Luna-Moreno D, Sánchez-álvarez A, Islas-Flores I, Canto-Canche B, Carrillo-Pech M, Villarreal-Chiu JF, Rodríguez-Delgado M (2019) Early detection of the fungal banana black Sigatoka pathogen *Pseudocercospora fijiensis* by an SPR immunosensor method. Sensors 19:1–12. https://doi.org/10.3390/s19030465

Luo B, Li X, Yang J, Li X, Xue L, Li X, Gu J, Wang M, Jiang L (2014) Non-enzymatic electrochemical sensors for the detection of hydrogen peroxide based on Cu2O/Cu nanocomposites. Anal Methods 6:1114–1120. https://doi.org/10.1039/c3ay41914b

Lv M, Liu Y, Geng J, Kou X, Xin Z, Yang D (2018) Engineering nanomaterials-based biosensors for food safety detection. Biosens Bioelectron 106:122–128. https://doi.org/10.1016/j.bios.2018.01.049

Ma Q, Wang Y, Jia J, Xiang Y (2018a) Colorimetric aptasensors for determination of tobramycin in milk and chicken eggs based on DNA and gold nanoparticles. Food Chem 249:98–103. https://doi.org/10.1016/j.foodchem.2018.01.022

Ma X, Xu X, Xia Y, Wang Z (2018b) SERS aptasensor for *Salmonella typhimurium* detection based on spiny gold nanoparticles. Food Control 84:232–237. https://doi.org/10.1016/j.foodcont.2017.07.016

Majdinasab M, Hayat A, Marty JL (2018) Aptamer-based assays and aptasensors for detection of pathogenic bacteria in food samples. TrAC - Trends Anal Chem 107:60–77. https://doi.org/10.1016/j.trac.2018.07.016

Malakar S, Paul SK, Jolvis Pou KR (2020) Biotechnological interventions in beverage production. In: Biotechnological Progress and Beverage Consumption, Academic press, Duxford, United Kingdom, pp 1–37. https://doi.org/10.1016/B978-0-12-816678-9.00001-1

Mehrotra P (2016) Biosensors and their applications – a review. J Oral Biol Craniofacial Res 6:153–159. https://doi.org/10.1016/j.jobcr.2015.12.002

Minopoli A, Sakač N, Lenyk B et al (2020) LSPR-based colorimetric immunosensor for rapid and sensitive 17β-estradiol detection in tap water. Sensors Actuators B Chem 308:127699. https://doi.org/10.1016/j.snb.2020.127699

Miyake S, Hirakawa Y, Yamasaki T et al (2020) Simultaneous detection of six different types of pesticides by an immunosensor based on surface plasmon resonance. Anal Sci 36:335–340. https://doi.org/10.2116/analsci.19P333

Mohammad-Razdari A, Ghasemi-Varnamkhasti M, Izadi Z, Rostami S, Ensafi AA, Siadat M, Losson E (2019) Detection of sulfadimethoxine in meat samples using a novel electrochemical biosensor as a rapid analysis method. J Food Compos Anal 82:1–8. https://doi.org/10.1016/j.jfca.2019.103252

Mohan HK, Chee WK, Li Y, Nayak S, Poh CL, Thean AV (2020) A highly sensitive graphene oxide based label-free capacitive aptasensor for vanillin detection. Mater Des 186:108208. https://doi.org/10.1016/j.matdes.2019.108208

Mohana NC, Mithun P, Rao HCY, Mahendra C, Satish S (2020) Nanoparticle applications in sustainable agriculture, poultry, and food: trends and perspective. In: Nanotoxicity. Elsevier, pp 341–354. https://doi.org/10.1016/b978-0-12-819943-5.00016-6

Muniandy S, Teh SJ, Thong KL, Thiha A, Dinshaw IJ, Lai CW, Ibrahim F, Leo BF (2019) Carbon nanomaterial-based electrochemical biosensors for foodborne bacterial detection. Crit Rev Anal Chem 49:510–533. https://doi.org/10.1080/10408347.2018.1561243

Murugaboopathi G, Parthasarathy V, Chellaram C, Anand TP, Vinurajkumar S (2013) Applications of biosensors in food industry. Biosci Biotechnol Res Asia 10:711–714. https://doi.org/10.13005/bbra/1185

Nabok A, Al-Rubaye AG, Al-Jawdah AM, Tsargorodska A, Marty JL, Catanante G, Szekacs A, Takacs E (2019) Novel optical biosensing technologies for detection of mycotoxins. Opt Laser Technol 109:212–221. https://doi.org/10.1016/j.optlastec.2018.07.076

Padilla FM, Thompson RB (2018) Proximal optical sensors for nitrogen management of vegetable crops: a review. Sensors 18(7):2083. 1–23. https://doi.org/10.3390/s18072083

Patel G, Pillai V, Bhatt P, Mohammad S (2020) Application of nanosensors in the food industry. In: Nanosensors for smart cities, part III. Elsevier, Amsterdam, pp 355–368. https://doi.org/10.1016/b978-0-12-819870-4.00020-7

Pawar VS, Verma N, Pawar SD (2020) Overview of different milk and milk products contaminant detections by biosensors. SSRN:1–7. https://doi.org/10.2139/ssrn.3571717

Pechprasarn S, Ittipornnuson K, Jungpanich T (2019) Surface plasmon biosensor platform for food industry. Appl Mech Mater 891:103–108. https://doi.org/10.4028/www.scientific.net/AMM.891.103

Piecková E, Lehotská R, Globanová M (2019) Heat resistant fungi, toxicity and their management by nanotechnologies. In: Nanomycotoxicology treating mycotoxins in the nano way, pp 217–237. https://doi.org/10.1016/B978-0-12-817998-7.00009-4

Połaska M, Sokołowska B (2019) Review bacteriophages—a new hope or a huge problem in the food industry. AIMS Microbiol 5:324–347. https://doi.org/10.3934/microbiol.2019.4.324

Polatoglu I, Ozkan FC (2019) Development of an optical tyrosinase biosensor (TCA) for detection of "Parathion-Methyl". Sens Rev 39:604–611. https://doi.org/10.1108/SR-10-2018-0242

Pourakbari R, Shadjou N, Yousefi H, Isildak I, Yousefi M, Rashidi MR, Khalilzadeh B (2019) Recent progress in nanomaterial-based electrochemical biosensors for pathogenic bacteria. Microchim Acta 186:820. https://doi.org/10.1007/s00604-019-3966-8

Quintela IA, Reyes BGDL, Lin C, Wu VC (2019) Simultaneous colorimetric detection of a variety of *Salmonella spp.* in food and environmental samples by optical biosensing using oligonucleotide-gold nanoparticles. Front Microbiol 10:1–12. https://doi.org/10.3389/fmicb.2019.01138

Ramezani M, Esmaelpourfarkhani M, Taghdisi SM et al (2020) Application of nanosensors for food safety. In: Nanosensors for smart cities. Elsevier, Amsterdam, pp 369–386. https://doi.org/10.1016/b978-0-12-819870-4.00021-9

Rayappan JBB, Nesakumar N, Bhat LR, Gumpu MB, Babu KJ, Jayalatha JBBA (2019) Electrochemical biosensors with nanointerface for food, water quality, and healthcare applications. In: Bioelectrochemical interface engineering, pp 431–468. https://doi.org/10.1002/9781119611103.ch22

Ren Q, Shen X, Sun Y, Fan R, Zhang J (2020) A highly sensitive competitive immunosensor based on branched polyethyleneimine functionalized reduced graphene oxide and gold nanoparticles modified electrode for detection of melamine. Food Chem 304:125397. https://doi.org/10.1016/j.foodchem.2019.125397

Revathi C, Rajendra Kumar RT (2019) Enzymatic and nonenzymatic electrochemical biosensors. In: Fundamentals and sensing applications of 2D materials. Woodhead Publishing, pp 259–300. https://doi.org/10.1016/b978-0-08-102577-2.00007-5

Reynoso EC, Torres E, Bettazzi F, Palchetti I (2019) Trends and perspectives in immunosensors for determination of currently-used pesticides: the case of glyphosate, organophosphates, and neonicotinoids. Biosensors 9(1):20. https://doi.org/10.3390/bios9010020

Riangrungroj P, Bever CS, Hammock BD, Polizzi KM (2019) A label-free optical whole-cell *Escherichia coli* biosensor for the detection of pyrethroid insecticide exposure. Sci Rep 9:1–9. https://doi.org/10.1038/s41598-019-48907-6

Richter Ł, Janczuk-Richter M, Niedziółka-Jönsson J, Paczesny J, Hołyst R (2018) Recent advances in bacteriophage-based methods for bacteria detection. Drug Discov Today 23:448–455. https://doi.org/10.1016/j.drudis.2017.11.007

Riu J, Giussani B (2020) Electrochemical biosensors for the detection of pathogenic bacteria in food. TrAC - Trends Anal Chem 126:115863. https://doi.org/10.1016/j.trac.2020.115863

Rubab M, Shahbaz HM, Olaimat AN, Oh DH (2018) Biosensors for rapid and sensitive detection of *Staphylococcus aureus* in food. Biosens Bioelectron 105:49–57. https://doi.org/10.1016/j.bios.2018.01.023

Saini K, Kaushal A, Gupta S, Kumar D (2019) Rapid detection of *Salmonella enterica* in raw milk samples using Stn gene-based biosensor. 3 Biotech 9:1–9. https://doi.org/10.1007/s13205-019-1957-4

Seol D, Jang D, Oh JW, Cha K, Chung H (2019) Discrimination of phthalate species using a simple phage-based colorimetric sensor in conjunction with hierarchical support vector machine. Environ Res 170:238–242. https://doi.org/10.1016/j.envres.2018.12.030

Sharma R, Raghavarao KSMS (2018) Nanoparticle-based Aptasensors for food contaminant detection. In: Nanomaterials for food applications. Elsevier, Amsterdam, pp 123–145

Sharma A, Khan R, Catanante G, Sherazi TA, Bhand S, Hayat A, Marty JL (2018) Designed strategies for fluorescence-based biosensors for the detection of mycotoxins. Toxins 10:1–19. https://doi.org/10.3390/toxins10050197

Singh V (2018) Bacteriophage-mediated biosensors for detection of foodborne pathogens. In: Singh J., Sharma D., Kumar G., Sharma N. (eds) Microbial Bioprospecting for Sustainable Development. Springer, Singapore, pp 353-384. https://doi.org/10.1007/978-981-13-0053-0_19

Singh K (2020) Nanosensors for food safety and environmental monitoring. In: Thangadurai D, Sangeetha J, Prasad R (eds) Nanotechnology for food, agriculture and environment. Springer, Cham, pp 63–78. https://doi.org/10.1007/978-3-030-31938-0_4

Song SH, Gao ZF, Guo X, Chen GH (2019) Aptamer-based detection methodology studies in food safety. Food Anal Methods 12:966. ; 2019. https://doi.org/10.1007/s12161-019-01437-3

Stevenson HS, Shetty SS, Thomas NJ, Dhamu VN, Bhide A, Prasad S (2019) Ultrasensitive and rapid-response sensor for the electrochemical detection of antibiotic residues within meat samples. ACS Omega 4:6324–6330. https://doi.org/10.1021/acsomega.8b03534

Stone E, Campbell K, Grant I, McAuliffe O (2019) Understanding and exploiting phage–host interactions. Viruses 11:1–26. https://doi.org/10.3390/v11060567

Sultan KS, Ali TA, Fahmy NA, El-Shibiny A (2019) Using millimeter-waves for rapid detection of pathogenic bacteria in food based on bacteriophage. Eng Rep 1:1–15. https://doi.org/10.1002/eng2.12026

Thakur MS, Ragavan KV (2013) Biosensors in food processing. J Food Sci Technol 50:625–641. https://doi.org/10.1007/s13197-012-0783-z

Tilton L, Das G, Yang X, Wisuthiphaet N, Kennedy IM, Nitin N (2019) Nanophotonic device in combination with bacteriophages for enhancing detection sensitivity of *Escherichia coli* in simulated wash water. Anal Lett 52:2203–2213. https://doi.org/10.1080/00032719.2019.1604726

Velasco-Garcia MN, Mottram T (2003) Biosensor technology addressing agricultural problems. Biosyst Eng 84:1–12. https://doi.org/10.1016/S1537-5110(02)00236-2

Vizzini P, Braidot M, Vidic J, Manzano M (2019) Electrochemical and optical biosensors for the detection of *Campylobacter* and *Listeria*: an update look. Micromachines 10:500. https://doi.org/10.3390/mi10080500

Wang Q, Zhao W (2018) Optical methods of antibiotic residues detections: a comprehensive review. Sensors Actuators B Chem 50:238. https://doi.org/10.1016/j.snb.2018.04.097

Wang Z, Ma B, Shen C, Lai OM, Tan CP, Cheong LZ (2019) Electrochemical biosensing of chilled seafood freshness by xanthine oxidase immobilized on copper-based metal–organic framework nanofiber film. Food Anal Methods 12:1715–1724. https://doi.org/10.1007/s12161-019-01513-8

Wei S, Chelliah R, Rubab M, Oh DH, Uddin MJ, Ahn J (2019) Bacteriophages as potential tools for detection and control of *Salmonella spp.* in food systems. Microorganisms 7:1–22. https://doi.org/10.3390/microorganisms7110570

Weng X, Neethirajan S (2018a) Paper-based microfluidic aptasensor for food safety. J Food Saf 38:1–8. https://doi.org/10.1111/jfs.12412

Weng X, Neethirajan S (2018b) Immunosensor based on antibody-functionalized MoS2 for rapid detection of avian coronavirus on cotton thread. IEEE Sensors J 18:4358–4363. https://doi.org/10.1109/JSEN.2018.2829084

Wu Z, He D, Cui B, Jin Z (2018) A bimodal (SERS and colorimetric) aptasensor for the detection of *Pseudomonas aeruginosa*. Microchim Acta 185:1–7. https://doi.org/10.1007/s00604-018-3073-2

Wu K, Ma C, Zhao H, Chen M, Deng Z (2019a) Sensitive aptamer-based fluorescene assay for ochratoxin A based on RNase H signal amplification. Food Chem 277:273–278. https://doi.org/10.1016/j.foodchem.2018.10.130

Wu W, Yu C, Wang Q, Zhao F, He H, Liu C, Yang Q (2019b) Research advances of DNA aptasensors for foodborne pathogen detection. Crit Rev Food Sci Nutr 60:1–16. https://doi.org/10.1080/10408398.2019.1636763

Yan J, Shi Q, You K, Li Y, He Q (2019) Phage displayed mimotope peptide-based immunosensor for green and ultrasensitive detection of mycotoxin deoxynivalenol. J Pharm Biomed Anal 168:94–101. https://doi.org/10.1016/j.jpba.2019.01.051

Yaneva S, Stoykova I, Danalev D, Yotova L (2019) Determination of organophosphorous pesticides in liver samples using an optical biosensor. J Chem Technol Metall 4:831–837. https://doi.org/10.1016/j.bios.2006.05.007

Yazdanparast S, Benvidi A, Abbasi S, Rezaeinasab M (2019) Enzyme-based ultrasensitive electrochemical biosensor using poly(L-aspartic acid)/MWCNT bio-nanocomposite for xanthine detection: a meat freshness marker. Microchem J 149:104000. https://doi.org/10.1016/j.microc.2019.104000

Ye W, Liu T, Zhang W, Zhu M, Liu Z, Kong Y, Liu S (2019) Marine toxins detection by biosensors based on aptamers. Toxins 12:1–22. https://doi.org/10.3390/toxins12010001

Younis MR, Wang C, Younis MA, Xia XH (2020) Use of biosensors for mycotoxins analysis in food stuff. In: Nanobiosensors: from design to applications. Wiley-VCH, Weinheim, pp 171–201

Yu W, Sang Y, Wang T, Liu W, Wang X (2020) Electrochemical immunosensor based on carboxylated single-walled carbon nanotube-chitosan functional layer for the detection of cephalexin. Food Sci Nutr 8:1001–1011. https://doi.org/10.1002/fsn3.1382

Yun Y, Pan M, Wang L, Li S, Wang Y, Gu Y, Yang J, Wang S (2019) Fabrication and evaluation of a label-free piezoelectric immunosensor for sensitive and selective detection of amantadine in foods of animal origin. Anal Bioanal Chem 411:5745–5753. https://doi.org/10.1007/s00216-019-01954-4

Yunus G (2019) Biosensors: an enzyme-based biophysical technique for the detection of foodborne pathogens. In: Enzymes in food biotechnology. Academic Press, pp 723–738. https://doi.org/10.1016/b978-0-12-813280-7.00042-6

Zhang H, Shi Z, Cheng S, Zhang H, Shi Z, Cheng S, Yang Q, Sun X, Guo Y (2019) Ultrasensitive immunosensor for aflatoxin B1 detection based on screen-printed carbon electrode modified by ferrocene @multi-walled carbon nanotubes. Int J Electrochem Sci 14:9170–9180. https://doi.org/10.20964/2019.09.61

Zhou J, Qi Q, Wang C, Qian Y, Liu G, Wang Y, Fu L (2019) Surface plasmon resonance (SPR) biosensors for food allergen detection in food matrices. Biosens Bioelectron 142:111449. https://doi.org/10.1016/j.bios.2019.111449

Chapter 10
Pros and Cons of Nano-Materials as Mineral Supplements in Poultry Feed

Rajendran Mala, Ravichandran Keerthana, and Preetha Mohan

Abstract Poultry is a rapidly growing sector of agriculture that produces meat and egg. Chicken meat and egg are the inexpensive sources of proteins and minerals. In addition to supplying food, poultry industry also offers employment to millions of people. It is a source of rural income and alleviates poverty. Poultry industry strives to produce high-quality meat and egg to meet the food security of the ever-expanding population. The conventional feed is supplemented with antibiotics and inorganic minerals. Antibiotics are used as prophylaxis to prevent birds from avian infectious diseases and contamination by foodborne pathogens. The emergence of multi-drug resistant pathogens and the presence of antibiotics in poultry and meat products restrict their use. Nano-materials has shown its potential to be an alternative of antibiotics and also is being exploited to improve the growth of birds and enrichment of meat and egg. Nano-materials as a feed additive at a very low concentration, aid in the efficient conversion of feed to biomass and products. The positive effect of nano-materials on the growth and performance of broilers and layers are determined by their physico-chemical properties. Further, the use of nano-sensors can also help in detecting avian pathogens at the early stage. Here, we review the potential of nanomaterials in the poultry industry to sustain good level of animal yield, low mortality rate, while preserving the environment and consumer health.

Keywords Absorption · Bioavailability · Feed additive · Nano-material · Selenium nano-material · Nano-sensor · Regulations · Safety · Zinc oxide

R. Mala (✉) · R. Keerthana · P. Mohan
Department of Biotechnology, Mepco Schlenk Engineering College, Sivakasi, Tamil Nadu, India
e-mail: maalsindia@mepcoeng.ac.in

V. K. Maurya et al. (eds.), *Sustainable Agriculture Reviews 55*, Sustainable Agriculture Reviews 55, https://doi.org/10.1007/978-3-030-76813-3_10

10.1 Introduction

The poultry industry is one of the fast-growing sectors of agriculture. The poultry industry substantially contributes to food security and poverty deterioration (Alemayehu et al. 2018; Abu Hatab et al. 2019). It primarily focuses on the production of meat and egg by raising the domesticated birds such as chicken, duck, emu, quails, and turkey. Meat is a good source of protein, iron, selenium, zinc, and vitamin B-complex. Approximately 50% of chicken fat is composed of healthy monounsaturated fats. It is also the rich source of omega 3 fatty acids and polyunsaturated fatty acids. It does not contain trans-fat which causes coronary heart disease. An egg is a nutritious food that supplies calories, protein, minerals, and vitamins. Recently it is considered as a functional food because of the presence of lutein and zeaxanthin. These bioactive compounds are antioxidants and prevent age-related macular disease and cataracts. In addition to the primary product, poultry adds a wide range of by-products such as feathers, shells, oils, skin, and manure.

The world population is projected to reach 8 billion in 2025 and 9.8 billion in 2050 (EL Sabry et al. 2018). To ensure food security to the growing population, agriculture and the poultry sector have to be revolutionized to produce high-quality products in large quantities. Transition in food habits towards chicken meat has increased the production of broiler chickens. Global production of broiler meat in different countries is represented in Fig. 10.1. The United States is the leading producer of broiler chicken meat which accounts for 17% of global production followed by China (14%), Brazil (14%), European Union (13%), and India (5%). High poultry production in East and Southeast Asia and Latin America, especially in China and Brazil is ascribed to the abundant supply of natural sources, grassland

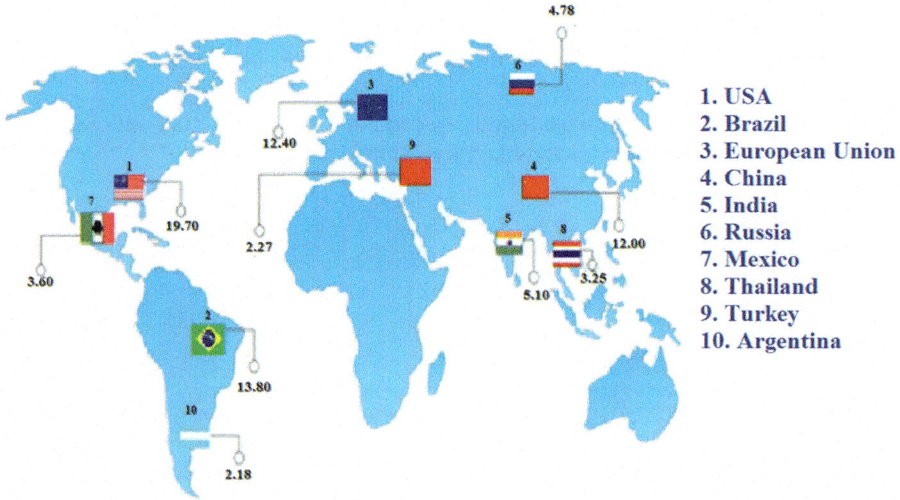

Fig. 10.1 Leading poultry meat producers in the world (*million metric tons*). http://www.fao.org/poultry-production-products/production/en/

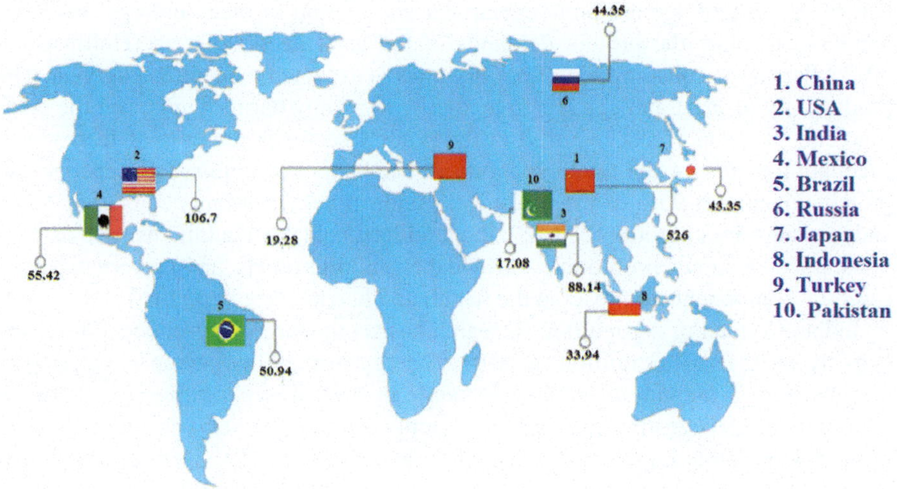

Fig. 10.2 Leading egg producers in the world (*in million metric ton*). http://www.fao.org/poultry-production-products/production/en/

and feed availability, and productivity gains (Wilkinson 2009). Consumption of broiler chicken in Brazil is highest with 45 kg/person/year. The United States ranks second with 43 kg/person/year and China with 10.5 kg/person/year. Consumption rate in India is 3.35 kg/person/year. In India, broiler meat production is increasing at a maximum rate of 8%. Indian poultry is growing impressively due to technological advancement in breeding and feeding (MAFW 2017).

Egg production has also tremendously increased from 15 million tons to 87 million tons between 1960 and 2017. Africa produces eggs at the rate of 250/capita/year. America produces the highest of 880 eggs/capita/year followed by Asia with 675 eggs/capita/year. Australia and New Zealand produce 225 eggs/capita/year (MAFW 2017). Leading egg-producing countries are represented in Fig. 10.2. China is the leading egg producer globally accounting for about 42% followed by the USA (7%) and India (6%). More than 60% of the global output is produced from Asia.

10.2 Growth of Indian Poultry Industry

The poultry sector in India is divided into organized sectors worth Rs. 64,000 crore and unorganized backyard sector worth of Rs.16,000 crore by 2017. As per the 19th livestock census, there was a 729 million poultry population in India with 30% of layers and 40% of broilers Backyard sectors play a major role in preventing poverty and malnutrition. The poultry sector in India is growing at a rate of 10% for meat and 6% for egg (MAFW 2017). India produces approximately 3.97 million tons of eggs and 3.46 million tons of poultry meat/year (Mehta and Nambiar 2007). Indian population is expected to reach 1.65 billion by 2050. Approximately 71% of Indians below 15 years of age are non-vegetarians. Production of meat and egg has to be increased to meet the protein demands of the growing population (Hellin et al. 2015). Per capita consumption of poultry meat is expected to reach 9.2 kg/year. The productivity of meat and egg has to be met without any harmful effect on the environment. The major cost incurred in the poultry sector is the cost of feed which accounts for 70% of the total expenditure. Feed supplies required for energy and protein constitutes 95% of the feed cost. Major mineral nutrients constitute 3–4% and feed additives account for 1–2% the total feed cost. Feed additives such as vitamins, trace elements, probiotics, antioxidants, antimicrobials, and preservatives are essential components to preserve the health and hatchability in poultry.

Indian Council of Agriculture Research has set the target to produce 106 billion eggs by 2020 from 83 million in 2016. The egg availability/person is targeted to achieve 83 eggs /annum from 63 eggs/annum in 2016. There is a huge gap between the demand (180 eggs/person/year) and supply (69 eggs/person/year) which has to be met with technological advancement (Bhatta et al. 2012). Meat production is targeted to be increased from 3.3 million tons in 2016 to 4.20 million tons. Percapita meat availability is expected to reach 3.21 kg/annum by 2020 from 2.22 Kg/annum in 2015 (MAFW 2017).

10.3 Nano-Materials

Nano-materials encompass all materials whose size in any one dimension is less than100 nm (European Commission 2011; ISO 2010; Rauscher et al. 2014). The word “Nano” originates from Greek meaning “dwarf”. European Union broadly defines nano-material as “any intentionally produced material that has one or more dimensions of the order of 100 nm or less or that is composed of discrete functional parts either internally or at the surface, many of which have one or more dimensions of the order of 100 nm or less, including structures, agglomerates, or aggregates, which may have a size above the order of 100 nm but retain properties that are characteristics of the nano scale” (European Parliament and Council 2015). Living systems naturally possess nano-materials such as DNA, proteins, and ribosomes. Size of many viruses are in the nano range (Yokel and Macphail 2011). Ultrafine particles emitted by the combustion of fuels, forest fire, and volcano are also in the nano scale (Oberdorster et al. 2005; USEPA 1994). Engineered nanomaterials are intentionally produced by bottom-up/ top-down methods.

10.3.1 Classification

Nano-materials are classified based on different criteria such as chemical composition, size in different dimensions, and shape. Based on their chemical composition, they are classified into inorganic, organic, and hybrid materials. Based on their size and the dimensions, they are classified as 0 dimensional, 1 dimensional, 2 dimensional, and 3 dimensional nano-materials. Based on their morphology, they are classified as spherical, rods, needle, plate, dendrimers, and whiskers. Silver, copper, zinc, selenium, gold, titanium, and cadmium are primary metal-based nanomaterials are while organic nano-involves wide variety of biomolecules like proteins, carbohydrates, and lipids (Peters et al. 2016). Miniaturization of materials to nanoscale tunes the properties of the material which are entirely different from their bulk counterparts (Hartmann et al. 2012). The high aspect ratio of nano-materials is responsible for their high surface area, reactivity, spectral properties, mechanical strength, and functional properties. Unique Physico-chemical and biological properties of nano-materials make them attractive and promising material for a wide range of applications (Gentile et al. 2016; Jeevanandam et al. 2018).

10.3.2 Synthesis

Two different approaches such as "bottom up" and "top down" are used to synthesize nano-materials. Bottom up approach includes wet chemical synthesis by growth and nucleation of mineral atoms. In contrast to bottom up approach, nano- materials are synthesized by breaking of bulk minerals in top down method (Rajendran et al. 2013). Broadly three different methods like physical, chemical, and biological methods are being used to produce nano-materials. Physical vapor deposition (Mehran et al. 2017), RF plasma (Rashidi and Khosravi-Darani 2011), laser ablation (Kurland et al. 2009; Stötzel et al. 2013) and thermal decomposition (Moloto et al. 2010) are few techniques grouped under physical methods.

Chemical vapor deposition (Fernándezs et al. 2010), ionic gelation (Fernández et al. 2010), sol-gel (Mulens et al. 2013a, b; Sriondee et al. 2018; Yu et al. 2019), co-precipitation (Rahimi et al. 2014; Maleki et al. 2014; Sanchez-Martinez et al. 2018; Zhao et al. 2018) sonochemical synthesis (Okoli et al. 2018; Santibenchakul et al. 2018) and hydrothermal synthesis are few techniques grouped under chemical methods (Obreja et al. 2019; Wongpratat et al. 2015).

In biological synthesis, wide variety of agents like bacteria (Korbekandi et al. 2012; Marshall et al. 2006), fungi (Balaji et al. 2009; Gajbhiye et al. 2009; Fayaz et al. 2010; Binupriya et al. 2010), algae (Chiu et al. 2013; Kannan et al. 2013; Sahoo et al. 2014), plants (Krishnaraj et al. 2010; Mondal et al. 2011; Narayanan and Sakthivel 2008; Jia et al. 2009; Raghunandan et al. 2010) and biomolecules (Akhlaghi et al. 2013; Duan et al. 2015; Boury and Plumejeau 2015; Maruyama et al. 2015) were used to synthesize inorganic nanomaterials.

10.3.3 Application of Nano-Materials in Agriculture, Food and Feed

An excellent review of the application of nanomaterials in agriculture, food, and feed has been compiled by (Peters et al. 2016). Nano-materials have been used to protect plants, improve productivity, bio-farming, food packaging, food processing, preparation of fermented foods, delivery of functional foods, increase the bioavailability of minerals, vitamins, and nutraceuticals.

Approximately, 88% of the application of nano-materials are in the food industry, 9% in agriculture, and only 3% in feed. About half of the nano-materials used in agriculture, food, and feed are inorganic materials while organic nano-carriers such as capsules, emulsion, micelles are prepared using biopolymers. In inorganic materials, metal and metal-based nanomaterials are widely used accounting to 35% and carbon-based are accounts for 6%. Nanocomposites contribute slightly more than carbon-based materials (7%). Approximately 75% of nanoparticles used in agriculture, food, and feed are derived from chitosan, nisin, clay, gold, iron, silver, zinc oxide, titanium dioxide, nanocomposites, silica nanoparticles, and carbon nanotubes (Peters et al. 2014, 2016).

10.3.3.1 Application in Agriculture

In agriculture, the net utilization efficiency of fertilizers and the nutritional quality of agricultural products are increased by nano- fertilizers (Pandey et al. 2010; Mala et al. 2017). Plants are protected from biotic stress by delivering of agro-chemicals through nano-carrier (Sarkar et al. 2015), nano-capsule (Kashyap et al. 2015), nano-emulsion (Campos et al. 2015; Wang et al. 2007b) and hydrogel (Bhagat et al. 2013).

10.3.3.2 Application in Food

In the food industry, nanomaterials are used to deliver the nutraceuticals, antioxidants, and vitamins to increase their stability, solubility, and bioavailability (McClements 2010; Aslani et al. 2014; Chow et al. 2015). Equally, they are used in packaging the food material to improve shelf life. The majority of nanomaterials used in food packaging are based on chitosan, silver, zinc, nanoclays, titanium dioxide (Silvestre et al. 2011; Ramachandraiah et al. 2015; Shatkin and Kim 2015).

10.3.3.3 Application in Poultry

In the poultry industry, unique properties of nano-materials are exploited to improve the health of animals and birds, increase production efficiency and enhance the nutrient quality of meat and egg (Hefferon 2015; Hill and Li 2017; Scott et al. 2016)

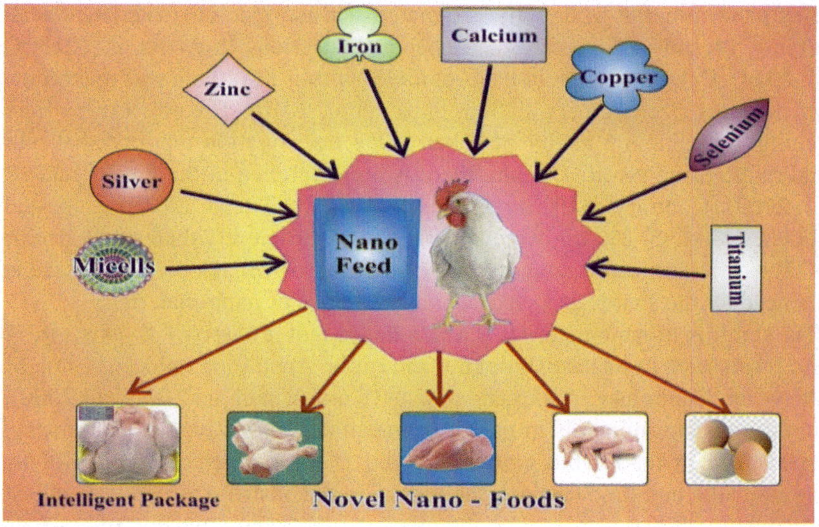

Fig. 10.3 Application of nano-materials in poultry

(Fig. 10.3). Nano-materials are also used as an alternative to antibiotics (Pineda et al. 2012; Gholami-Ahangaran and Zia-Jahromi 2013) where bulk minerals of feed were replaced with nano-minerals derived from silver, copper, iron, zinc, selenium, and chromium. Owing to their nano size, the minerals are taken inside the cells rapidly by endocytosis (Hoet et al. 2004; Gangadoo et al. 2016; Surai et al. 2017; Konkol and Wojnarowski 2018). Their absorption and bioavailability are very high compared to bulk minerals (Mahler et al. 2012; Sarkar et al. 2015). They circulate in the blood for a longer time before getting eliminated by the liver and kidney (Choi et al. 2011; Liao et al. 2010; Zha et al. 2008). Many of the inorganic mineral nutrients are incorporated into the biomolecules and form a part of organic materials.

10.4 Properties of Nano-Materials

Particle dependent properties of nano-materials play a key role in their interaction with cells, diffusion, transport, absorption distribution, bioavailability, and elimination.

10.4.1 Size and Surface Area

Particle size and surface area of nano-materials play a significant role in their interaction cells (Gatoo et al. 2014). The size of nanomaterials used as feed additive varies based on the precursor and method used for synthesis (Cai et al. 2012). The size of nano-minerals is directly associated with surface characteristics, stability, solubility, crystalline structure, and chemical reactions (Luyts et al. 2013; Gatoo et al. 2014). Cellular uptake of nano-particles within 14–20 nm was maximum than other particles size (Luo et al. 2006; Sahay et al. 2010). The effect of particle size on cellular uptake is a matter of debate. One investigation reported that within a broad range of 25 nm to 150 nm, there is no difference in the uptake rate (Roger et al. 2009). Contrary to the report, results by Awaad et al. (2012) suggested that particles within 95–200 nm were absorbed more efficiently than small-sized particles. The different results suggest that in addition to size, the cellular uptake is also influenced by the shape, and surface characteristics of nano-materials.

The stability of nanomaterials is a size-dependent property. TiO_2 exists in 3 polymeric forms such as anatase, brookite, and rutile. Anatase is stable $\leq$11 nm, brookite between 11 nm and 35 nm, and above 35 nm (Zhang and Banfield 2000). The solubility of nano-minerals in the gastrointestinal fluid is higher than micro-sized nutrients. When fat-soluble vitamins A and D are delivered through food-grade nano-emulsion and lipid carriers, the lipases in the gastrointestinal tract digests the lipid constituent and releases the vitamins. As the nano-emulsion offers a greater surface area for the catalytic action of enzymes, the delivery and bioavailability of vitamins are improved (Maurya and Agarwall 2017a, b; Maurya et al. 2020a, b). Greater solubility is associated with greater absorption in the villi of the intestine and its diffusion through the mucosal cells (Nel et al. 2006; Hoet et al. 2004). Uptake of nano minerals by diffusion and endocytosis are 15–250 times more than the conventional minerals (Desai et al. 1996; Mohanraj and Chen 2006) while small-sized nano-materials reside in circulation for a longer time (Sahay et al. 2010). Particles of size less than 500 nm are excreted by liver kidney and colon. Large-sized particles are not absorbed and are excreted in feces (Bertrand and Leroux 2012). The absorption rate of selenium nano-material in the intestine was higher than conventional selenomethionine. Particles above 500 nm are not taken by the cells and cleared from the circulation and are eliminated by mononuclear phagocytosis (Choi et al. 2011; Naahidi et al. 2013). Spherical shapes are endocytosed easily than other shapes.

The proportion of feed converted into useful products like meat and egg (feed conversion ratio) is very high with nano-materials than micro-sized materials. Nano-sized particles and minerals are assimilated readily than bulk-sized particles due to their greater surface area which increases their bioavailability (Gangadoo et al. 2016). The feed conversion ratio of nano selenium was efficient and it improves the health and laying performance of chickens. In the case of micro-sized nutrients, the dose required to supplement is very close to the toxic dose as a high concentration of dose has to be supplemented to make them bioavailable. There is a narrow gap between the required dose and toxic dose in conventional selenium supplementation. With nano-sized selenium, bioavailability is higher leading to widening the gap between the supplemented dose and toxic dose. Similarly, calcium supplemented as nano formulated calcium phosphate and vitamin D3 increased the weight gain and laying performance in chickens (El-Sheikh 2017).

Silver and copper nano-materials are used as an alternative to antibiotics. Nano-materials offer a high surface area for interaction with microbes. Hence their bactericidal activity is high at lowermost concentration than micro-sized metals. Zinc and selenium nano-materials are antioxidants. Nano-materials have a highly reactive surface that binds with oxidants, reactive oxygen species, and free radicals. Nano antioxidants quench oxidative stress more than conventional antioxidants. In contrast to the above mentioned positive effect of nano-materials on chicken's performance, a negative impact on embryo was also documented. Silver nanoparticles of size <35 nm reduced the oxygen uptake by the chicken embryo (Pineda et al. 2012; Sawosz et al. 2012; Hotowy et al. 2012). Nano-materials coated with bile salts pass through the mucus readily (Macierzanka et al. 2011, 2012). Hydrophilic molecules easily pass through the mucus Choi et al. 2011; Naahidi et al. 2013; Maldonado-Valderrama et al. 2011).

10.4.2 Composition

Chemical composition of nano-materials plays a major role in their metabolism. Carbon-based nanoparticles are organic materials. Inorganic nanomaterials are used as mineral supplements and as antimicrobial elements. Biopolymer based organic materials are used as cargo for the delivery of drugs, vaccines, and nutraceuticals. Selenium is the inorganic nano mineral supplemented recently. It is antioxidant and important for the function of the body's antioxidant systems such as glutathione peroxidase. Antioxidant activity was mediated in broiler chickens even at a lowermost concentration of 0.15–1.2 ppm (Bagheri et al. 2015; Fuxiang et al. 2008). Liposomes modified with non-ionic polymers increase mucosal penetration and reached epithelial cells (Chen et al. 2013). Liposomes of small size carrying the bioactive compounds are easily digested and release the contents in the intestine (Salvia-Trujillo et al. 2013). Nano-delivery of Vitamin A and D through protein carriers are not effective due to the defective release from the carrier. Comparatively lipid capsulues, emulsion and micellesrelease effectively increasing their bioavailability (Maurya and Agarwall 2017a, b; Maurya et al. 2020a, b).

10.4.3 Surface Properties

The surface properties of nano-materials include charge, electrochemical reactivity, and hydrophobicity. Thesepropertiesgovern the interaction of nanomaterials with cells and their uptake (Maurya et al. 2016).The digestive system starting from the oral route to the intestine is lined with a mucosal layer. The interaction of nanomaterials with the mucosal layer is essential for their transport and uptake. Irrespective of the size of the material, charge plays a vital role in absorption. Absorption of positively charged 200 nm particle was more than negatively charged 100 nm-sized particles (Wang et al. 2007a; Behzadi et al. 2017). Positively charged minerals interact with the mucosal layer than neutral minerals. Most of the mineral supplements in poultry feed are positively charged. Hence, they are readily absorbed and transported to the systemic (Dawson et al. 2003; Frohlich 2012). Positively charged golden nanoparticles showed greater uptake and enhanced reproduction rate in *D.magna* compared to the same negatively charged golden nanoparticles (Bozich et al. 2014). Neutral or negatively charged particles are not taken nonspecifically and their toxicity is comparatively less than positively charged nanoparticles Hydrophilic nanoparticles are more toxic than lipophilic nanoparticles because of their greater uptake (Amini et al. 2014).

Surface modification alters the stability, solubility, charge, bioavailability, and toxicity of nano-materials (Kirchner et al. 2005; Mahmoudi et al. 2010). The surface properties of nano-materials can be modified using organic compounds like poloxamers, polyethylene, and polyethylene glycol (Pelaz et al. 2015). The surface of nanoparticles modified by polyethylene glycol reduces the toxicity of nanoparticles by lowering the immune response (Amini et al. 2014).

Supplementation of L-cysteine coated iron oxide nano-material in breeder quails improved the bioavailability of iron in the diet and also improved egg production, egg mass, and fertility rate than uncoated iron oxide nano-material (Mohammadi et al. 2017; Bantz et al. 2014). Silver nanomaterial ≤10 nm coupled with threonine and cysteine increased the immunity in chicken (Bhanja et al. 2015). The surface properties of negatively charged SiO_2 nano-materials directly affect the agglomeration and biological activity of nano-materials.

First pass metabolism in the living system is responsible for the detoxification of xenobiotics and drugs. It reduces the bioavailability of drugs in the systemic circulation. To escape from the first-pass metabolism and to increase the bioavailability of minerals, nutraceuticals and vitamins, the surface of the nano-carrier gas to be engineered to be hydrophobic through lipid moieties. Nanoencapsulation of vitamin A and D increase their bioavailability (Maurya et al. 2020a, b).

10.4.4 Agglomeration

Nanoparticles possess a high tendency for agglomeration due to strong attractive forces (Bantz et al. 2014). Physical forces such as Van der Waals, hydrogen bonding, electrostatic, steric, and hydrophobic forces hold the nanoparticles together (Doane and Burda 2013). Agglomeration affect biocompatibility, bioavailability, and stability of nano-materials (Halamoda-Kenzaoui et al. 2017). Agglomerationnanoparticlerely on their size, charge, surrounding pH, and ionic strength (Vippola et al. 2009; Ashraf et al. 2018). Cellular absorption and endocytosis of nano-materials are influenced by their agglomeration. Agglomerated nanoparticles have a larger dimension, which reduces absorption in the gastrointestinal tract (Halamoda-Kenzaoui et al. 2017). Metal nanoparticles such as SiO_2, TiO_2 have been reported to undergo agglomeration whileZnO and Ag are not agglomerated within the gastrointestinal tract. The aggregation of nanoparticles influences their biological function and does not have a beneficial effect similar to unaggregated forms (Miroshnikov et al. 2015).

10.5 Pros of Nano-Materials as Mineral Feed Additives

Nanotechnology is used to increase the absorption, bioavailability, stability of nutrients, nutraceuticals, improve color, taste, aroma, and shelf life of poultry products.

10.5.1 Nano-Material as an Alternative to Antibiotics

The discovery by Jukes (1950) about the growth-promoting effect of aureomycin in pigs laid the foundation for the application of antibiotics in poultry (Jukes et al. 1950; Hui et al. 2017). Many antibiotics are used as growth promoters in poultry (Table 10.1). The Table 10.1 enlists the antibiotics widely used in poultry to increase productivity. Antibiotics increase the growth of chickens by decreasing the infection by avian pathogens (Pan and Yu 2014). Widespread and long-term use of antibiotics has resulted in the emergence of multi-drug-resistant bacteria and the prevalence of antibiotic residues in meat, egg, and environment (Landers et al. 2012). Due to this, the World Health Organization and the European Union banned the use of many antibiotics in poultry feed (Marshall and Levy 2011).

Non-therapeutic alternatives to antibiotics are phytogenic feed additives, enzymes, metals, probiotics, synbiotics, and organic acid (Sethiya 2016). These alternatives target the proliferation of pathogens and increase the beneficial microbiome of the gut (Lillehoj et al. 2018). Such alternatives are less efficient due to the lack of species and target specificity (Salim et al. 2018).

The application of silver nano-material in medicine and health care for its antimicrobial property is well established (Maurya et al. 2016). In poultry also it is used as a substitute to antibiotics. It exerts its lethal effect by interacting with the thiol group of proteins, disrupting the ATP generating electron transport chain complex in mitochondria, and imposing oxidative stress (Sawosz et al. 2012). Other metal oxide nano-materials such as zinc and copper also exerts bactericidal activity by inducing oxidative stress. The free radical generated disrupts the membrane architecture and disrupts the structure of biomolecules. Supplementation of selenium nano-material improved gut health by increasing the presence of *Lactobacillus* and *Faecalibacterium* in broiler chicken while chicken fed with copper silicate also increased *Lactobacillus*and reduced count of *E.coli* (Gangadoo et al. 2018).

Table 10.1 Antibiotics used as feed additive in poultry feed

Antibiotic	Mode of action	Role in poultry	References
Bacitracin Brand-Baci-Rx	Cell wall synthesis inhibitor	Prevents the growth of gasterointestinal bacteria such as *Oscillospira, Peptostreptococcaceae*, and *Erysipelotrichaceae* in the colon	Hofacre et al. (1998) and Proctor and Phillips (2019)
		Prevents necrotic enteritis.	
		Stabilizes cecum microbial population	
ChlortetracyclineBrand-**aureomycin**	Protein synthesis inhibitor	Prevents microbial spoilage of chicken meat by *Pseudomonas, E.coli*	Thatcher and Loit (1961)
Oxytetracycline Brand-Terramycin	Protein synthesis inhibitor	Increases body weight, Prevents respiratory infections.	Feighner and Dashkevicz (1987) and Shaddad et al. (1985)
		Increases the biotransformation of bile acids	
		Increase the nutrient absorption in intestine	
Penicillin Brand-Amoxil	Cell wall synthesis inhibitor	Prevent the growth of pathogenic bacteria	Datta (1969)
Tylosin Brand-Afilosina	Protein synthesis inhibitor	Prevents respiratory diseases caused by *Mycoplasma gallisepticum* and *M. synoviae*	Kowalski et al. (2002)
Bambermycin Brand-Flavo-80	Cell wall synthesis inhibitor	Prevents *Salmonella* infections.	George et al. (1982)
Neomycin Brand- neo-Fradin	Protein synthesis inhibitor	Effective against *Salmonella* infections	Williams (1985)
		Improved feed efficiency, weight gain	
Lincomycin Brand-Lincocin	Protein synthesis inhibitor	Effective against skin or bone infections	Proudfoot et al. (1990)
		Growth promoter	
Streptomycin Brand-Ambistryn S	Protein synthesis inhibitor	Used to treat non-specific infectious enteritis	Bornstein and Samberg (1954)
		Increased growth and egg production	
Erythromycin Brand-Pediazole	Protein synthesis inhibitor	Used for the treatment of chronic mycoplasma causing diseases	Potter et al. (1963)
		Improves egg production	
Oleandomycin Brand-OM-5	Protein synthesis inhibitor	Growth promoting agent	Haritova et al. (2003)
		Antimicrobial agent	
Virginiamycin Brand- Aviax / Stafac [+ Semduramicin]	Protein synthesis inhibitor	Improves the early growth rate,	Dumonceaux et al. (2006), Gadde et al. (2018) and Yates and Schaible (1962)
		Improves feed utilization	
		Increase the lactobacilli population in duodenal loop	

10.5.2 Mechanism of Absorption

Understanding the interaction of nanomaterials with the cells of the gastrointestinal tract will pave the way to apply nano-materials safely to poultry (Lacey 2017). Nano-mineral feed additives are given orally through feed or water. Nano-minerals diffuse through mucus into the cells of the gastrointestinal tract (Bergin and Witzmann 2013). Digestion of food starts from the oral cavity and ends with the intestine.

In the oral cavity, nano-materials primarily contact with the gingival cells (Presland and Dale 2000). The pH of the oral cavity is slightly acidic and facilitates the breakdown of organic materials. When the nano-materials are encapsulated with the organic coatings like chitosan, they are removed in the oral cavity. Moreover, the oral cavity possesses an antimicrobial system that generates hydrogen peroxide. Hydrogen peroxide releases the metal ions from the nano-material through Fentons reaction. Lactoferrin present in the oral cavity stabilizes the nano-emulsion loaded with curcumin (Pinheiro et al. 2016). Salivary flow in the oral cavity prevents the absorption of inorganic nanomaterials. So inorganic nano-materials are rarely or poorly absorbed in the oral cavity (Best et al. 2015). In contrast to inorganic nano-materials, lipid nano-materials are absorbed in the oral cavity (Kotta et al. 2012). Nanomaterials pass through the esophagus within seconds and no absorption occurs there.

The stomach is highly acidic with a pH of 1.5–3.5. At this pH, the structural integrity of nano-material is affected and ions are released from the mineral nano-materials (Yada et al. 2014). Silver, copper, and zinc nanoparticles dissolve at low pH of the stomach (Rajasekaran and Santra 2015). Carbon nano-tubes aggregate in the stomach acidity. Nano-emulsion carrying curcumin or any other nutrient is stable in the stomach. The chemical digestion of nano-emulsion occurs in the duodenum (Wick et al. 2007). Nanoemulsion of zinc oxide is destabilized in the gastric fluid and releases zinc ions increasing its bioavailability (Seok et al. 2013). In the stomach, aggregation of silver nano-materials reduces its bioavailability (Mwilu et al. 2013). From the stomach, the nanomaterials reach the small intestine which is composed of duodenum, jejunum, and ileum. Duodenum is a site of chemical digestion where some of the nanoemulsions are digested. The ileum is 2 m length with a surface area of more than 20 m^2. It is specialized for absorption. Silver nanomaterials that are aggregated in the stomach are dispersed and absorbed in the ileum (Walczak et al. 2013). The bioavailability of nanomaterials in the ileum is high and it reaches systemic circulation (Bergin and Witzmann 2013). The absorption of nano-materials in the colon is very less compared to the intestine. In the gut, the absorbed nano-materials greatly influence the gut microbiome (Taylor et al. 2015).

Uptake of nano-minerals occurs by paracellular, transcellular, carrier-mediated, and receptor-mediated mechanisms (Fig. 10.4). Uptake by endocytosis and transcellular mechanisms are predominant with nano-materials (Liu et al. 2016). Through hepatic circulation, nanomaterials are transported to the liver and spleen (Wang and Luo 2019). As a feed additive, nanoparticles have higher absorption and uptake efficiency than their conventional minerals (Bunglavan et al. 2014; Gunasekaran et al. 2014).

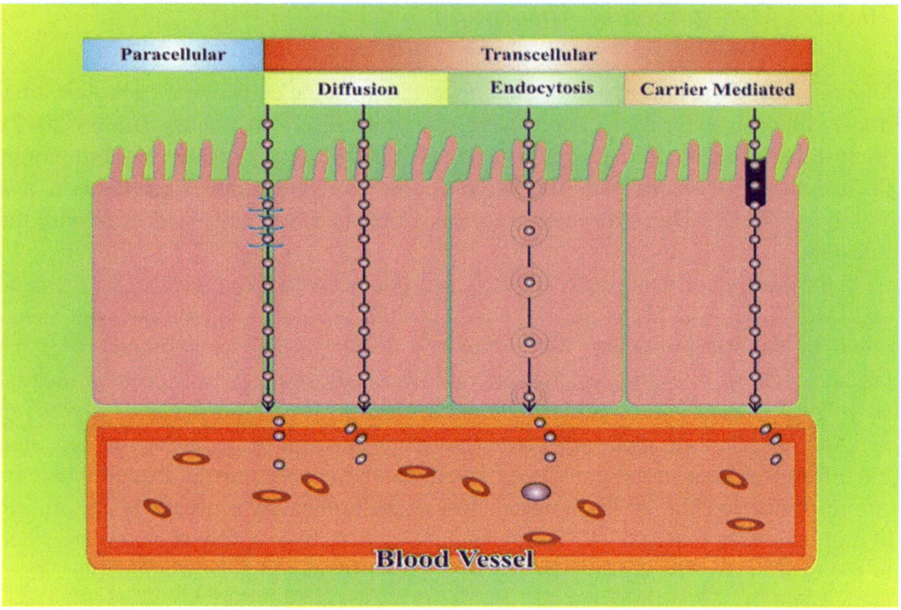

Fig. 10.4 Absorption of nano-materials

10.5.3 Bioavailability

Bioavailability is the proportion of mineral absorbed from the diet and available for biological functions (Maurya and Aggarwal 2017b). FDA defines bioavailability based on the absorption rate and absorption extent. It is defined as "the rate and extent to which the bioactive ingredient or active moiety is absorbed from a product and becomes available at the site of action" (Pathak and Raghuvanshi 2015). The absorption rate is the fastest time in which the absorbed nutrient reaches systemic circulation. The absorption extent defines the extent of a bioactive nutrient is absorbed from the food (Borel et al. 2013; Johnson et al. 2005).

The bioavailability of fat-soluble nutrients is determined by three different factors such as Bioavailability coefficient (F_B .proportion of lipid nutrients released from the nano-carrier into the gastric fluid), Transport coefficient (F_T- ratio of lipid nutrients transported through the intestine) and Mobility coefficient (F_M- route map followed by the lipophilic nutrient to reach systemic circulation). Based on the characteristics of the nutrient, its, absorption, metabolic rate, preferential organ distribution, and the prevailing conditions in the absorbed site, suitable nano-carrier has to be engineered to ensure higher bioavailability (Maurya and Agarwall 2017a). During the process of digestion, the engineered nano-carrier undergoes many transformations throughout the gastrointestinal tract. So the design of the nano-material or the nano-carrier has to be optimized for increased bioavailability (Maurya and Agarwal 2017a). The gastrointestinal tract is 30 ft. long with a surface area of 30 $m^{2.}$

It offers the greatest surface area for the absorption of all nutrients (Helander and Fandriks 2014). The bioavailability of nutrition is dependent on the physiological characteristics of the host and the nutrient. Size, shape, charge, aggregation, composition, functionalization, and solubility of nano-materials determine the bioavailability (Fig. 10.5). Bioavailability is determined by the release of mineral nutrients from the feed matrix, digestion in the stomach and intestine, transport by diffusion through the gastrointestinal tract, systemic distribution, storage, and metabolic rate leading to excretion (Aboalnaja et al. 2016; Aggett 2010; Katouzian and Jafari 2016). The main challenges in mineral bioavailability include chemical instability, poor solubility, and slow absorption in the gastrointestinal tract (Maurya and Aggarwal 2017b). Smaller size, greater surface area, and rapid dissolution of nano-materials encourage greater bioavailability. Based on their particle size, the nanoparticle may be eliminated without uptake or they are absorbed by gastrointestinal tract and reach systemic circulation (Oberdörster et al. 2005). Reduced particle size ensures greater dispensability in biological fluids penetration and absorption of nano-materials (Sessa et al. 2014). Gold nanoparticles with size $\leq$50 nm are absorbed and distributed in different organs. Gold nanoparticles of 10 nm are widely distributed in many organs (De Jong et al. 2008). Water-soluble nano-materials are assimilated faster than insoluble nutrients. The presence of anti-nutritional factors in the feed such as phytate, oxalate, tannin, and polyphenol affect mineral bioavailability (Hailu and Addis 2016). Bioavailability of nano-minerals is concentration-dependent and it differs for each mineral. Bioavailability of copper was high when supplemented at 50 ppm while bioavailability of zinc at 40 mg/kg and 80 mg/kg improved the bioavailability, egg mass, and egg production of layer chicken (Abedini et al. 2018).

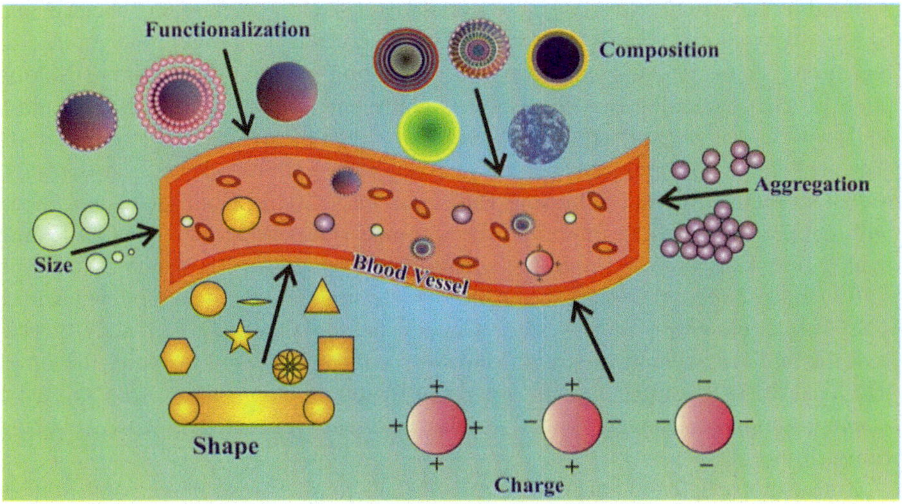

Fig. 10.5 Factors influencing the bioavailability of nano-materials

10.5.4 Health of Poultry

Nano-mineral supplementation in poultry feed improves immunity, antioxidant activity, and gut health. Supplementation of nano selenium in layer chicken improved the intake of selenium, decreased free radicals and increased egg production (Radwan et al. 2015). Selenium is essential for the conversion of thyroxine and triiodotyronine (Surai et al. 2017). Dietary supplementation with selenium nanoparticles (0.9 mg/kg) in chick has displayed improved intestinal health by promoting the abundance of beneficial bacteria, such as *Lactobacillus* and *Faecali bacterium.*

Zinc is an essential component of many metalloenzymes such as carbonic anhydrase and metalloproteinases). It plays a vital role in the metabolism of major biomolecules (Khalid et al. 2014). In animal growth, from embryogenesis to organ formation, skin and feather formation, skeleton muscular development, reproductive performance, the formation of eggshell, and hatchability zinc is essential (Saenmahayak 2007). Zinc supplementation induces molting in chicken at the end of the first laying cycle. During molting, the reproductive tract is rejuvenated and the post molting laying performance will be increased (Brake 1993; Scott and Creger 1976).

The concentration of zinc required to meet the demands of poultry depends upon the age of the animal or bird. Zinc facilitates the efficient conversion of feed to overall weight gain, increase in the organ weights, and laying performance in chickens (Mohammadi et al. 2015). In addition to their role in the growth and performance of poultry, they exhibit antibacterial activity against major infecting pathogens such as *Campylobacter* and *Salmonella* (Khalid et al. 2014).

Avian pathogens pose a major challenge to the revenue generated in poultry farming due to infection and the rapid transmission of infection to healthy birds. The role of nanomaterials as an antibacterial agent to prevent avian disease is summarized in Table 10.2. Silver nano-materials were toxic to pathogenic bacteria and had no toxicity against probiotics such as lactobacilli. By improving the gut microbial flora, it enhances the digestion and absorption of mineral nutrients (Elkloub et al. 2015). Enhancing the immunity of chick embryo by silver chelated amino acids was a positive approach to provide immunity at the earliest stage of bird's life (Bhanja et al. 2015). Supplementation of silver with selenium showed very promising effect on the growth of chickens (Felehgari et al. 2013). Chitosan encapsulated with copper nanoparticle improved the immune status of broiler chicken (Wang et al. 2011). Copper is an important constituent of many enzymes such as ascorbic acid oxidase, superoxide dismutase, and cytochrome oxidase. These enzymes play a key role in the anti-oxidant system. Copper due to its antimicrobial activity, prevent the birds from immune stress. Moreover, copper increase the concentration of RBC, packed cell volume, and the weight of lymphoid organs like spleen and liver. These reasons collectively boost up the immunity of chicken (El-Kazaz and Hafez 2019).

Zinc nanoparticles enhanced the growth and immunity of piglets and poultry (Swain et al. 2016). Antibacterial nano-materials prevent the infection and improve

Table 10.2 Antimicrobial activity of different nano-mineral supplements

Nano-material	Method of synthesis	Mode of action	Benefits	Limitation	References
Zinc oxide	Ball milling	Zn^{2+} ions are released and diffuse into the cell wall	Reduces foodborne bacterial contamination	Supplement dose and method of synthesis, has to be optimized	Basha et al. (2016) and Safaei-Ghomi et al. (2013)
	Thermal evaporation	Direct contact with the pathogen	Improves the beneficial gut microbes, growth and productivity	Burst release of ions during digestion has to be avoided	
	Chemical precipitation	Generation of ROS		Safety of has to assessed before application	
Iron oxide	Ball milling	Fe^{2+} ions are released and diffuse into the cell wall	Reduces food borne bacterial contamination	Easily oxidized	Arakha et al. (2015)
	Thermal evaporation	Direct contact with the pathogen	Improves the beneficial gut microbes, growth and productivity	Stability should be improved	Mohan and Mala (2019)
	Chemical precipitation	Generation of ROS		Supplement dose and method of synthesis, has to be optimized	
	Biological			Burst release of ions during digestion has to be avoided	Saki and Abbasinezhad (2014)
Silver oxide	Ball milling	Direct contact with the pathogen	Improved immune status	Easily oxidized	Gopi et al. (2017)
	Thermal evaporation	Ag^{2+}ions penetrate inside the cell and inactivates enzymes	Improves the beneficial gut microbes, growth and productivity	Stability should be improved	
	Chemical precipitation	Formation of ROS	Reduces food borne contamination	Supplement dose and method of synthesis, has to be optimized	
	Biological	Binding with thiolgroups of proteins		Burst release of ions during digestion has to be avoided	

(continued)

Table 10.2 (continued)

Nano-material	Method of synthesis	Mode of action	Benefits	Limitation	References
Copper oxide	Ball milling	Cu^{2+} ions are released and diffuse into the cell wall	Electrostatic interaction with cell membrane	Easily oxidized	Wang et al. (2011)
	Thermal evaporation	Direct contact with the pathogen	Denaturation of intracellular proteins	Stability should be improved	
	Chemical precipitation	Generation of ROS	Interacts with DNA	Supplement dose and method of synthesis, has to be optimized	
	Biological		Reduces food borne contamination	Burst release of ions during digestion has to be avoided	
Selenium	Ball milling	Induces ROS production	Electrostatic interaction with cell membrane	Supplement dose and method of synthesis, has to be optimized	Huang et al. (2019)
	Thermal evaporation	Disrupts membrane potential	Denaturation of intracellular proteins	Burst release of ions during digestion has to be avoided	
	Ball milling	Depletes ATP	Interacts with DNA	NA	
	Thermal evaporation		Reduces food borne contamination		
	Chemical precipitation		Electrostatic interaction with cell membrane		
	Biological		Denaturation of intracellular proteins		

the health of poultry. The different antibacterial nano-materials and their role in poultry health are summarized in Table 10.2.

All the metal nano-materials displayed concentration-dependent antibacterial efficacy against *Salmonella, Campylobacter, Staphylococcus aureus, Escherichia coli*, and *Listeria monocytogenes* in the order of Au ≥ CuO ≥ ZnO (Duffy et al. 2018; Jones et al. 2008; Xie et al. 2011; Mahmoodi et al. 2018; Zarei et al. 2014). Mycotoxins are the major agents that spoil feed through fungal infections. Zinc oxide nano-materials are effective against potent fungal pathogens such as

Fusariumoxysporum, Aspergillus flavus, Alternariaalternata, Aspergillusniger, Botrytis cinerea, Fusariumoxysporum, F. graminearum, P. citrinum and Penicillium expansum. The membrane structure was disrupted by zinc oxide nanomaterials. The growth of fungi was significantly reduced with very little conidia formation. The reduction in growth is associated with the defective productivity of mycotoxins.

Nutraceuticals refer to ingredients that possess well defined nutritional value, pharmaceutical value, and physiological effect (Andlauer and Fürst 2002). Nutraceuticals such as vitamin E, curcumin, phytosterols, and fatty acids were investigated to deliver through nanocarriers. Nano-materials increase the bioavailability of short-chain fatty acids such as butyric acid (Gangadoo et al. 2018). All investigations related to the supplementation of nano-materials are still in their infancy and it requires an in-depth study related to the biosafety concerns.

Nano-particles are used for targeted delivery and availability of vaccines to elicit optimum immune responses (Cai et al. 2010; Simon et al. 2016). Nano-materials function as an adjuvant to mount a maximum immune response to vaccines and therapeutic agents (Zhao et al. 2014). As an adjuvant they slowly release the active principle and retain them for a longer time in circulation, increasing their immunogenicity (Sekhon 2014). The self-assembled protein-based vaccine was recently developed to offer immunity to birds against the infectious bronchitis virus. The vaccine contains the antigen co displayed with flagellin expressed the highest immunity against (Li et al. 2018). Vaccination for the Avian Influenza Virus used Poly (D, L-lactide-co-glycolide) with a single booster dose (Alkie et al. 2018).

10.5.5 Improved Product Quality

Nano-materials are used to enrich the nutrition of egg and meat, process meat, increase flavor, enhance taste, increase the shelf life, detection of pathogens, and packaging (Gangadoo et al. 2016). Broilers and layers convert feed into food products and excrete the majority of nutrients as waste. Chickens lose 50% of nitrogen and 55% of phosphorus in excretion (Leeson and Summers 2005). Many strategies were evolved to increase the efficiency of feed conversion into meat and egg. Supplementation with nano-materials improves the feed conversion ratio and assimilate the nano-minerals more efficiently than conventional mineral sources.

Selenium in the diet prevents cancer. Selenium content of chicken meat can be designed to have 8.6μg–41μg/100 g by supplementing 0.24 mg of selenium/kg of feed. The concentration of selenium supplied by chicken meat by this method is more than 65% of recommended daily allowances (Yu and Huang 2013). Selenium supplementation through an inorganic form is more efficient than organic form. Selenium concentration of egg can be increased by supplementing feed with selenium nano-material. Similarly, omega 3 and omega 6 fatty acids in meat and egg were increased by supplementation in the diet. The dietary use of selenium nanoparticles in broiler chicken improved the antioxidant status and immunity of the chicken. In meat, it increased taste and the selenium content of the liver and muscles

(Cai et al. 2012). Selenium nano-material supplementation (0.3 mg/Kg) in broiler chicken reduced the serum concentration of malondialdehyde in broiler meat compared to organic and inorganic selenium. Reduced malondialdehyde concentration in meat improves meat quality (Aparna et al. 2018). Broiler chicken supplemented with 0.1875 mg/kg selenium nanoparticles showed a significant increase in superoxide dismutase and glutathione peroxidase activity and decreased malondialdehyde concentration. Supplementation with selenium nano-material decreased the concentration of total cholesterol in the blood of chicken and egg (Radwan et al. 2015). The action of selenium may be mediated through the action on probiotics. Evidence suggests the supplementation of selenium-rich probiotics decreased the blood and egg cholesterol in chicken (Cuiling et al. 2011). Probiotics decrease cholesterol by assimilation (Pereira and Gibson 2002)/ incorporation into cell membrane during growth (Liong and Shah 2005)/convert cholesterol into coprostanol (Lye et al. 2010)/ fermented to produce short-chain fatty acids.

Zinc nano-material at 1/500th of concentration of the conventional zinc increased the layer chicken performance (Mishra et al. 2014). Dietary supplementation of zinc nanoparticle significantly increased the feed conversion efficiency, growth, and weight gain in broiler chicken (Ahmadi et al. 2013; Zhao et al. 2014). Calcium phosphate nano-material at half of the concentration than conventional source increased the growth of broiler chicken (Hassan et al. 2016). Chromium nanoparticles increased the breast and thigh muscle protein content and lowered the cholesterol level at 500μg/kg.

There is hesitation among certain people about the high concentration of cholesterol in eggs. An egg of 60 g supplies 200 mg of cholesterol. Coronary heart disease is directly linked to the hardening of arteries caused by low-density lipoproteins. In egg, cholesterol is present as an emulsion of monounsaturated fats which are beneficial to the human being. Still, efforts are made to produce designer eggs with reduced cholesterol. Supplementation of feed with 125 ppm to 250 ppm of copper nano-material reduced 31% of cholesterol in egg. Supplementation with 8% of garlic in feed reduced 24% of cholesterol in egg (Elkin 2006, 2007).

The stability of color and taste of the meat was improved by the use of micelle encapsulated with antioxidants such as vitamin E, vitamin C, and fatty acids by a German company Aquanova (Alfadul and Elneshwy 2010). Meat and cheese were coated with a 5 nm layer of antioxidants and taste enhancers to increase palatability (Weiss et al. 2006). Sensory quality and marination effect of breast muscle was increased by nano delivery of paprika oleoresin (Yusop et al. 2012). Nanocarriers loaded with vitamin E, C, omega 3 fatty acids, lutein, lycopene, carotenoids, benzoic acid, citric acid, and other organic acids were used to increase the shelf life of foods (Chaudhry and Castle 2011). The role of nanomaterials in improving the quality of meat and egg are listed in Table 10.3.

Table 10.3 Role of nano-materials in improving product quality

Nano-material	Quality improved	Limitations	References
Zinc oxide	Enhanced bioavailability of nutrients Improved egg productivity Increased concentration of zinc in meat and egg Increased shell thickness	Standardize the physic-chemical properties of Nano-material Optimize the dose required	Abdulla et al. (2015), Abedini et al. (2018), Fathi et al. (2016), Feng et al. (2017), Hafez et al. (2017), Mahmoud et.al. (2020) and Ramiah et al. (2019)
Iron oxide	Enhanced the bioavailability of iron improved egg productivity Increased egg mass Increased concentration of iron in meat and egg Increased shell thickness Increased blood hemoglobin content	Standardize the physic-chemical properties of Nano-material Optimize the dose required	Miroshnikov et al. (2017), Nikonov et al. (2011), Rahmatollah et al. (2017) and Saki and Abbasinezhad (2014)
Copper oxide	Improved egg productivity Increased egg mass Increased shell thickness Increased bone weight Free of foodborne contaminants	Standardize the physic-chemical properties of Nano-material Optimize the dose required	Joshua et al. (2016), Ognik et al. (2018), Miroshnikov et al. (2015)
Selenium	Enhanced bioavailability of nutrients Improved egg productivity Increased concentration of selenium in meat and egg Increased shell thickness Reduced cracked shell, reduced cholesterol, reduced MDA content in egg and meat, Higher shelf life Increase in egg weight Breast muscle weight increased with high antioxidant status	Standardize the physic-chemical properties of Nano-material Optimize the dose required	Bakhshalinejad et al. (2018), Cai et al. (2012), Liu et al. (2016), Radwan et al. (2015) and Selim et al. (2015)
Calcium	Improved the calcium absorption and utilization, reduce calcium supplementation and	Standardize the physic-chemical properties of Nano-material Optimize the dose required	Ganjigohari et al. (2018)

10.5.6 Nano-Carriers

Delivery of micronutrients, minerals, and other nutraceuticals through nanocarriers protect the active ingredient from degradation and reduce undesirable effects in the finished product (Heller and Heller 2006; Wen et al. 2006). Silicon nano-material delivers silicic acid in the gut. Delivery in the gut increases the bioavailability and reduces osteoporosis (Canham 2007). Nano-carriers encapsulated with food additives are prepared by the emulsion solvent evaporation method (Song et al. 1997), double emulsion, and evaporation method (Pal et al. 2011), salting out method (Lambert et al. 2001). Nano-encapsulation techniques such as emulsification, lipid carrier, liposomes, cyclodextrin molecular complex, and electrospinning were powerful for the fortification of vitamin D (Maurya et al. 2020a, b). The use of nano-emulsion in the meat industry reduces the fat content of the product without compromising the creaminess, and taste of food (Cushen et al. 2012). Nano-emulsion containing functional foods was used to retain the freshness and reduces the salt required for preservation (Loncina et al. 2013). Nano-emulsion increases the delivery and bioavailability of water-insoluble feed additives (McClements 2013). Nano-nutraceuticals are delivered as amorphous nano-dispersions prepared by co-solvent freeze-drying (Onoue et al. 2010; Yu and Huang 2013). Polymer micelles prepared using starch and amphipathic molecules as core (lipophilic) shell (hydrophilic) nano-particles are used to deliver lipophilic substances (Yu and Huang 2013). Liposomes prepared using e.g., lecithin., cholesterol, or any synthetic phospholipids are used for the delivery of lipophilic substances (Akbarzadeh et al. 2013; Jeetah et al. 2014). Fortification and delivery of fat-soluble vitamins A through lipid nano-carriers and other capsule forms are reviewed extensively (Maurya et al. 2020a, b). Vitamin D is another fat-soluble nutrient whose bioavailability was increased using nano-delivery systems.

10.5.7 Nano-Sensor

Nano-sensors in intelligent packaging is intended to detect microbial pathogens, toxins, and degradation products of food (Duncan 2011; Cushen et al. 2012). Conventional diagnosis of infectious diseases is expensive and consumes a long time. Gaseous and moisture sensors detect the volatile gases and moisture without hampering the package of the food. Estimation of ATP, the degraded product hypoxanthine is one of the food quality indices in seafood. Nano-sensor based on amperometric measurement of hypoxanthine using xanthine oxidase and gold nanoparticle (Cubukcu et al. 2007) was developed as a nanosensor. Other gaseous emissions of amines are also indicators of meat and fish spoilage. Nano-sensor to detect the gases was developed to identify the freshness of food (Duncan 2011; Mills and Hazafy 2009). Nano-sensors are used in the diagnosis of antibiotic residues in meat and animal products to ensure food safety and good quality animal products (Mungroo and Neethirajan 2014; Sekhon 2014).

Detection and elimination of pathogens are essential to ensure food safety and security. Biofunctionalized nanoparticle with a high affinity to adhesins of *Campylobacter jejuni* was used to purge it. Binding of the functionalized nanoparticles to the enteric pathogen prevents its attachment poultry cells (Taylor et al. 2004). The biofunctionalized nano-particle is a core-shell nano-particle. The core was made up of hydrophobic polystyrene and the shell was tethered to polyethylene glycol, sugars, and peptides similar to the poultry cell receptors to which the pathogen binds. Nano-particle with many binding sites at the surface bind with *Campylobacter jejuni* and causes aggregation and elimination of pathogens. Immobilon-polyvinylidene difluoride membrane tagged with gold nanoparticle for the detection of immunoglobulins against avian flu (Emami et al. 2012). Nanosensors employing gold nanoparticles and quantum dots were developed for onsite detection of avian flu H1N1 and H5N1 (Jarocka et al. 2016; Xu et al. 2016). A highly advanced NA-NOSE, an artificial olfactory system was developed to detect the volatile organic compounds profile in cattle infected by *Mycobacterium bovis* (Peled et al. 2012). *Salmonella* and *Campylobacter* are food born enteric pathogens present in the gut of animals. They easily infect people during the handling of animals and through contact with contaminated meat and egg. Nanosensor based on carbon nanotube was used to detect *Salmonella* in chicken meat and egg (Villamizar et al. 2008). Nano-sensors employing magnetic nano-materials was used to detect *E. coli, Salmonella,* and *Listeria monocytogenes* (Chen et al. 2006; Duncan 2011). Microbalance based sensor employing a gold nanoparticle was used to detect pathogenic DNA (Rashidi and Kashravi-Darani 2011; Zhao et al. 2001). Nano-cantilever based detection of pathogenic proteins and DNA and even viruses was developed with high precision and accuracy (Hall 2002).

10.5.8 Food Packaging

The food pack is used as a passive barrier of gases to active and interactive packaging. The packaging provides antimicrobial property and a nano sensor to detect the freshness and spoilage of food. The use of biopolymers based on starch and zein in association with nanoclay as a bio-nanocomposite reduces the use of non-biodegradable plastics in the packaging (Sozer and Kokini 2009). Nanoparticles offer high heat resistance and mechanical property suitable for food packaging Film of clay nanoparticles was used as a barrier to oxygen, carbon dioxide and water to keep the freshness of meat (Brody et al. 2008).

Nano-composite biopolymers embedded with antimicrobial nano metals such as silver, copper, zinc, titanium, and manganese were used to prevent spoilage by food-borne pathogens (Duncan 2011). Silver nanoparticle encapsulates cellulose pad was used to prevent microbial infection of meat (Fernandez et al. 2010). Other silver-containing materials were also used as an antimicrobial packaging (Azeredo 2009;

Loncina et al. 2013; Velebit and Petrovic 2012). Liposomes loaded with nisin the antimicrobial peptide was used to prevent the microbial deterioration of food without affecting the quality of food (Da Silva et al. 2010). Zinc oxide –polypyrrole nano-composites film was developed to resist microbial spoilage of chicken meat. The nanofilm senses the change in storage temperature, microbial contamination, sensory properties, and pH through a change in the electrical resistance of the film (Pirsa and Shamusi 2019). All metal-based nanomaterials are bactericidal by generating reactive oxygen species that nonspecifically kills a broad spectrum of bacteria.

10.5.9 Reduced Feed Cost and Environmental Pollution

The use of imbalanced feed and inappropriate feeding strategy leads to significant economic losses through food wastage, sub-optimal growth, and environmental pollution (Carter and Kim 2013). Nano-mineral supplementation potentially increases mineral absorption and decrease supplement concentration. This reduces feed cost and pollution associated with excess minerals in feed and wastage. The limited supplementation of dicalcium phosphate nano-material in poultry feed would minimize the excretion of calcium and phosphate by about 50% and which in turn reduced the impact of poultry on environmental pollution (Hassan et al. 2016).

10.6 Cons of Nano-Materials as Mineral Feed Additives

Despite advantages, regulatory issues related to safety, toxicity, and environmental pollution due to nano-materials limit their widespread application in food and feed applications.

10.6.1 Safety

The application of nanomaterials in the food industry necessitates stringent measures to be adopted to preserve human health and environmental safety (Cushen et al. 2012). The main routes of entry of nano-materials into the human system are dermal contact, ingestion, and inhalation. The safety of nanomaterials has to be considered based on bio-persistence inside the living system (Chaudhry and Castle 2011). Natural materials prepared as nanostructures are of least concern. Intentionally prepared nano-carriers which are not bio-persistent are of little concern as they pass through the gastrointestinal tract. Metals, metal oxide, and other nano-materials which are bio-persistent and materials whose absorption, distribution, metabolism, and elimination properties remain unknown are of great concern.

10.6.2 Toxicity

The distinctive characteristics of nano-materials not only confer critical benefits but also give toxicity due to their unwanted interactions with different biological compartments (Gupta and Xie 2018). Crohn's disease is caused by the toxicity of nano-materials (Lomer et al. 2002; Molodecky et al. 2012). Nano-materials enter into the cell membrane via receptor-mediated or non-receptor-mediated endocytosis (Binderup et al. 2013). Intracellularly transported nano-materials damage the internal sub-cellular organs and cause genotoxicity by binding to DNA (Soenen et al. 2009; Prasad et al. 2013).

The toxicity of nanomaterials is a size-dependent property. Small-sized particles have more number of particles/volume. The release of ions from the small-sized particles is more than the large-sized nano-materials. Nano-materials induce oxidative stress by generating free radicals. Such free radicals cause hazardous effects in biological systems, by causing DNA damage, lipid oxidation, and subsequent inflammatory reactions (Gatoo et al. 2014). The mortality rate was high in chickens fed with silver nano-material below 12 ppm. It reduced the weight of bursa of Fabricius indicating its toxic effect on hematopoiesis and immunity. The magnitude of toxicity of a nano-material to chickens is dependent on different factors such as the method of synthesis, the presence of residual unreacted precursor, agglomeration, interaction with other minerals, and effect on the gut microbiome. Due to the high reactivity of nanomaterials, it is challenging to determine their toxicity. The toxic effects of different nanomaterials are depicted in Table 10.4. Leucocyte infiltration and change in the mucus composition was recorded in animals to silver nano-material toxicity (Shahare and Yashpal 2013). There is no study on the toxicity of nanomaterials in human beings. Nano-materials used in food packaging may leach into food and enter the system during consumption. There is also data supporting that the nano-material leaching from the food package will be of insufficient concentration to toxicity (EFSA 2016).

When nano-materials enter a living organism through the oral route, throughout their journey from mouth to kidneys, they exert their ill effect. Once nano-materials are released into the systemic circulation, they are distributed to different organs at a different concentration based on their physical-chemical properties (Kreyling et al. 2009). Nano-materials readily accumulate in the liver, spleen, and nervous system. Higher accumulation of gold, silver, iron, silica, carbon nanotubes was observed in spleen and liver (Balasubramanian et al. 2010; De Jong et al. 2013; Hasezaki et al. 2011; Swain et al. 2016). Burst release of metal ions in the stomach or intestine from the nano-formulations causes oxidative stress. Iron oxide nanoparticles release metallic iron which reacts with hydrogen peroxide produced during mitochondrial metabolic activity, generates highly reactive hydroxide free radicals that culminates in cellular damage. This process is termed as Haber –Weiss cycle and Fenton's reaction (Buzea et al. 2007). Nano-materials, exert indirect toxicity by eliciting an immune response against them (Singh et al. 2016; Timbrell 1991; Yoshida et al. 2014). Neonates suffer from asthma on exposure to nanomaterials.

Table 10.4 Toxicity of nano-materials

Name of nano-mineral	Preparation method	Dose supplied	Impact on Health	References
ZnO	Chemical precipitation method	120 mg/kg	Hepatocyte damage Weight loss Reduced hepatic catalase activity	Ahmadi et al. (2013) and Zhao et al. (2014)
CuO	Green synthesis	16 mg/kg	Protein denaturation reduced the Hb Reduced albumin concentration	Maryam and Samaneh (2014) and Faghihi and Samaneh (2014)
Se	Chemical reduction method	1.5 mg/kg	Hyperaemia of submucosal blood vessels and subserosal oedema	Gangadoo et al. (2018)
AgO		5 mg/kg		Ahmadi et al. (2013)

The inhalation route takes less time to cause toxicity (Terzano et al. 2010). Inhaled nanomaterials induce cardiovascular changes through changes in the autonomic nervous system (Kan et al. 2018). The toxicity of nanomaterials to the health of poultry birds is listed in Table 10.4.

10.6.3 Environmental Hazards

Nano-materials are released into the air, water, and soil during preparation, handling, consumption, and excretion by animals and birds (Jeevanandam et al. 2018). The fate of nanomaterials in the environment is determined by its physico-chemical property and interaction with other materials (Maiti et al. 2018). Moreover, the concentration, composition of nanomaterials, and the duration of exposure to nanomaterials, has a profound effect on their toxicity (Rienzie and Adassooriya 2018). Nano-materials cause toxicity by dissolution, direct contact, and co-transport of other contaminants (Mukherjee et al. 2016). Nano-minerals released into the environment from feed waste and poultry litter accumulate in the environment (Bundschuh et al. 2018). The nano-materials are transferred to other organisms in the food chain and lead to biomagnification.

In soil, nano-materials seep through the small pores and cause aggregation of soil particles (Mukhopadhyay 2014). Nano-materials translocated from soil to the plants affect germination and the growth of the plant (Hong et al. 2015; Khodakovskaya et al. 2014). Metal oxide nano-materials reduce the biodiversity of soil microbes. Rain or wind causes the migration of nano-materials from soil to nearby aquatic systems (Aslani et al. 2014). In an aquatic environment, metal nano-materials undergo different transformations such as dissolution, homo-agglomeration, hetero agglomeration, and sedimentation (Ovissipour et al. 2013). The dissolution of ions from metal nanoparticles is dependent on the pH of the interacting medium. Zinc oxide nano-material is highly toxic at 4.5 (Chen et al. 2016). The reactivity of aggregated nano-materials is less than the original nano-materials(Grillo et al. 2015). Nano-materials adhere to the gills, skin, and mucus membrane lining the internal organs, and cause lethal effect (Ovissipour et al. 2013). Zinc oxide nano-materials affect the metabolism of nitrogen-fixing bacteria such as *Azotobacter* (Chai et al. 2015). Organic carbon of soil is an indicator of soil fertility. Rich microbial biomass in soil maintains the soil fertility through a high level of organic carbon (Thakur et al. 2015). Soil contaminated with silver nanoparticles (Antisari et al. 2015), carbon nanotubes (Jin et al. 2013), and copper oxide nano-materials significantly reduced the organic carbon.

Bioaccumulation of nano-materials in aquatic plants and algae depends on size and concentration (Jahan et al. 2017). Bioaccumulation of Ag nano-materials was observed in hornworms fed with tomato plants cultivated in soil contaminated with silver nano-materials (Judy et al. 2011). The dynamics of nitrogen, phosphorus, potassium, magnesium, sulphur, calcium, iron, and other trace minerals were observed in many studies.

The toxicity of nano-materials to unicellular organisms are more than the other higher aquatic organisms. The toxicity of zinc oxide nanomaterials to the microalgae *R. subcapitata* was more than the toxicity of bulk zinc oxide from 0.01 ppm to 0.7 ppm. In addition to size, the shape and hydrodynamic properties of nanomaterials determine the toxicity. The growth stage of algae was most susceptible to toxicity posed by nano-materials (Yue et al. 2017). Carbon nano-tubes are toxic to crabs, larvae of marine organisms, and algae (Kwok et al. 2012). Nano-materials in the aquatic system damage the DNA of organisms and cause genotoxicity (Rodriguez-Garraus et al. 2020).

Nano-materials not only exert toxicity in soil and soil microbes but also to vegetables (Ghosh et al. 2010; Hong et al. 2015; Pittol et al. 2017; Lopez-Moreno et al. 2018). The dynamics of nitrogen, phosphorus, potassium, magnesium, sulphur, calcium, iron, and other trace minerals were altered by the nanomaterials. Smaller sized nano-materials are more toxic due to their larger surface area available for interaction with the target.

Silver nano-materials particles of size $\leq$20 nm were highly toxic to L929 fibroblasts and mouse peritoneal macrophage cell lines (RAW264.7) than larger size nano-materials (Park et al. 2011). Spherical nano-materials are more toxic to Smulow–Glickman gingival epithelial cells, oral mucosa fibroblasts, normal human bronchial epithelial cells and lung fibroblasts (WI-38) than rod-shaped nanomaterials (Chen et al. 2016). Needle shaped nanomaterials fierce through the cells disrupting the cell membrane and their toxicity is more than spherical structures (Doshi and Mitragotri 2010). Uptake of positively charged particles is more than negatively charged materials and their toxicity was increased with increased bioavailability (Lin et al. 2010). Coating of metal oxide nanomaterials with chitosan or any other biocompatible polymers reduce their toxicity by reduced immunogenicity (Agnihotri et al. 2004).

Nano-materials are used in all these applications based on the hypothesis that the toxic dose for the human being is far away from the lower organisms. Non-toxicity

Table 10.5 Environmental hazards of nano-materials

Nano-material	Environmental impact	References
Zinc oxide	Reduce soil microbial biomass, Induce imbalance in biogeochemical cycles Bioaccumulation and biomagnification of nanoparticles. Reduce germination at higher dose Reduce the growth and development of embryos Hematological abnormalities in terrestrial animals	Boonyanitipong et al. (2011), Dimkpa et al. (2012), Feizi et al. (2013), Rajput (2017) and Zhu et al. (2009)
Copper oxide	Reduce soil microbial biomass Induce imbalance in biogeochemical cycles Bioaccumulation and biomagnification of nanoparticles Reduce germination at higher dose Decrease root growth Affects the absorbance of minerals from the soil Affects the redox balance of the soil and other organisms inhabiting soil and water	Dimkpa et al. (2012), Keller et al. (2017) and Rajput et al. (2020)
Iron	In soil, shows less or no toxicity, affects In plants, bioaccumulation affects photosynthesis and reduction in metabolic rate, inhibition of plantlet growth In water, bioaccumulation controls the productivity and algal growth	Zhu et al. (2008)
Silver oxide	In soil, affects the reproduction of earthworms, reduction in microbial biomassdue to antimicrobial activity In plants, exhibits adverse effect on root and shoot growth, seed germination, Inhibits the growth of aquatic plant	Justin and Armstrong (1991), Pokhrel and Dubey (2013), Schlich and Hund-Rinke (2015) and Vannini et al. (2014)
Titanium dioxide	Reduce soil microbial biomass Bioaccumulation and biomagnification of nanoparticles Reduce germination at higher dose Decrease root growth Decrease the concentration of cholorophyll Reduce ythe photosynthetic rate	Rafique et al. (2018)

of TiO_2 (Yemmireddy and Hung 2015) and ZnO (Gunalan et al. 2012) to humans supported the hypothesis. Nano-materials enter a human system through the skin (Buzea et al. 2007), respiratory tract (Buzea et al. 2007), gastrointestinal tract (Szentkuti 1997; Hoet et al. 2004. The summary of environmental hazards imposed by nano-materials is represented in Table 10.5.

10.7 Regulatory Aspects of Nano-Materials

With the advent of nano-based products in the consumer market, serious concerns were raised related to the regulatory framework for nanomaterials (Cushen et al. 2012). Regulations related to the application of nanomaterials in food, feed, medicine, and cosmetics was discussed elaborately in the literature (Claudia et al. 2016).

The definition of nanomaterial is based on size, number of surface area. Scientific Committee on Emerging and Newly IdentifiedHealth Risks defines nano-materials as whose size in any one dimension is 1 nm–100 nm (SCENIHR 2015). Based on the size distribution, an unambiguous criterion for defining nano-material is that more than 50% of the material size should be distributed in nanoscale within 100 nm. Volume specific surface area of the nanomaterial must be 60 m^2/cm^3 for a perfect sphere (Kreyling et al. 2010). Regulatory approaches is linked to safety, risk sanalysis, transparency, the welfare of animals, and environmental protection (Coles and Frewer 2013). Some international regulations for nano-materials include Registration, Evaluation, Authorization, and Restriction of Chemicals (REACH), Environmental protection Agency (EPA), Australian Pesticides and Veterinary Medicines Authority (AVMPA), Organisation for Economic Co-operation and Development (OECD), Food and Agricultural Organization (FAO) and World Health Organization (WHO).

Framing regulatory policy for nanomaterials is challenging because of the diverse range of nano-materials, varieties of protocols used for biosynthesis. According to the European Union, all nano-materials fall under REACH (Registration, Evaluation, Authorisation and Restriction of Chemical substances) regulation (EC) No. 1907/2006. Nanomaterials have to ensure the lack of adverse effects on human health and the environment (EC 2011). Many EU regulations are used to regulate nanomaterials use in food and feed (EU 2002, 2004, 2006, 2008, 2010, 2011).

In the USA, nano-materials are regulated by Environmental Protection Agency which considers nano-materials as chemical substances regulated by Toxic Substances Control Act (USEPA 2015). As per The General Food Law Regulation (EC) No. 178/2002 (EU 2002), nano-materials are not directly included under food. But it applies that food containing nano-material should be safe for human consumption. Nano-materials added as an additive in the food as one of the ingredient falls under the scope of Regulation (EC) No. 1333/2008 (EU 2008). According to this legislation, the nanoscale feed additive must be assessed for its safety and must be included in the Union list before marketing. Nano-materials which are permitted before the approval as per Regulation (EC) No. 1333/2008 will be reassessed by European Food Safety Authority (EFSA 2016) according to Regulation (EU) 257/2010 (EU 2010). EFSA recommends the particle size for approval. If the particle size of the nanomaterial used in food differs from the approved one, then it will be considered as a different additive. It must get new approval (EU 2008).

According to the novel food regulation, foods containing engineered nanomaterials will be considered as a novel food. As per the regulation (EU) No. 1169/2011 (EU 2011), novel food containing engineered nanomaterials should be listed in the ingredients. The name should be suffixed with the word "nano" within brackets. The word "nano" is not necessary if the nano-material changes into non-nano form after addition to the food.

Nonfood contact nano-materials which are used in packaging are governed by Regulation (EC) No. 1935/2004 (EU 2004). Accordingly, the nano-material shall be prepared as per good manufacturing practices. They should not be transferred to the food inside the package and cause any change in the food composition, taste, aroma, and should not cause any adverse effect. Titanium nitride is one of the nano-material approved and listed in Annex I of Regulation (EU) No. 10/2011. Nano-materials used in active and intelligent packing are governed by Regulation (EC) No. 450/2009 (EU 2009) should be assessed case by case. Along with the Regulation (EU) No. 10/2011, certain conditions are laid to be used in intelligent and active packaging. The nano-material must be located behind the functional barrier and its migration must be below the given value. A feed or feed additive in nano form should not be fed to live animals if it lacks safety According to Regulation (EC) No. 178/2002 (EU 2002). The safety of the feed or feed additive should be assessed and has been authorized in accordance with Regulation (EC) No. 1831/2003 (EU 2003).

In India, the regulations for the use of nano-material in food are controlled by The Food Safety and Standards Act 2006 (FSSAI 2006). It establishes Food Safety and Standards Authority (FSSA) and sets standards for regulating the production, distribution, storage, and import of food. It regulates the application of nano-materials in food processing, production, and use of new functional materials, new product development, and storage (Institute of Food Technologists 2006). Regulations for food additives added for nutritional or nonnutritional value, packaging, processing, storage, transport, are followed under Section 3(k). Section 3(r) deals with nano-materials used for packing. According to the section, "food safety audit" is defined as "Systematic and functionally independent examination of food safety measures adopted by manufacturing units to determine whether such measures and related results meet with objectives of food safety and the claims made in that behalf". FSSA is empowered under Section 16(3), to take all measures to undertake action for any unforeseen effect of nanomaterials used in food. As per Section 8(1.f), it is mandatory to provide public information disclosure about the health risks that might emerge from the use of risk causing substances in food.

Environmental disposal of nano-materials is under the control of Environment Protection Act, 1986, Water Act, 1974, and Air Act, 1981. Ministry of Health regulates the application of nano-materials through Central Drugs Standard Control Organisation (CDSCO) which is governed by Directorate General of Health Services, India. Various regulatory measures applicable to the utility of nano-materials in food and medicine were discussed in the literature (Chowdhury 2006). The Government had launched Nano Science and Technology Initiative (NSTI) and "Nano Mission" to undertake research activities and to address risk issues of nanotechnology. The nation also lacks effective nano hazards regulations and an appeal for resources and expertise to cope with the hazards of nanotechnology (Rajput 2017).

10.8 Consumer Acceptance

Public acceptance has a direct implication on the commercialization and policy-making for nano-based food products. In spite of the availability of many nano-based products in the market, public knowledge, and awareness about their functions, benefits, cost-effectiveness and toxicities are still in infancy (Gehrke 2017). Lack of knowledge and unfamiliarity with the Nanotechnology limits consumer acceptance (Yue et al. 2017). Only 11% of nano-enabled products in the market are food and beverages. Three nano food products in the market are canola oil, a chocolate slim shake drink, and 'Nanotea'. Chocolate slim shake drink contains nanoclusters of silica-coated with antioxidants cocoa coating (Kroese et al. 2009; WWICS 2007). Many nanoceuticals products containing vitamins, antioxidants, antimicrobials (Nanoceuticals™ from RBC Life Sciences® Inc. USA), nano calcium, magnesium (Nano Calcium/Magnesium from Mag-I-Cal.com USA) and selenium (Nanotea from Shenzhen Become Industry & Trade Co., Ltd. China) are available (Chaudhry et al. 2008). A survey in Australia revealed that only 7% of people accepted the nano-food, 33% rejected and 63% wanted to have more information about nano-foods (MARS 2008). Till now, no poultry product containing engineered nanomaterials are available in the market. Poultry feed supplement containing a multivitamin solution is marketed by ZDHF Pharma, Hubei, China. It is a nano-emulsion containing vitamin D3, A, B1, B2, B3, E, and other constituents. The product claims high stability, availability, and solubility of vitamins. Safety and future risk of using nano-foods are the major concern among people (Joubert et al. 2020). Consumer preference for environmentally safe products (Kriwy and Mecking 2011). Perception towards animal welfare standards plays a complex role in public and societal approval and acceptance (Lagerkvist and Hess 2010). Knowledge and awareness about the toxicity of nanomaterials to a living being and environmental hazards may have a negative impact the consumer acceptance (Sodano et al. 2016).

The population is heterogeneous and the perception of people differs significantly with the product. Awareness should be created among targeted people to change their attitude about nano-food products (Kim et al. 2014). Consumer acceptance can be improved by imparting awareness and benefits of nano-foods. Gaining social trust will increase the market value of nano-foods (Giles et al. 2015). Communication systems such as TV, YouTube, tick-tock, newspapers, magazines, blogs, and web sites, peer to peer communication can be exploited to create awareness among people about the benefits of nano-foods (Bostrom and Lofstedt 2010; Ho et al. 2010). Socio-economic and socio-psychological factors determine the acceptance of nano-foods. The Health benefits of nano-materials have to be portrayed well along with the standard values set by the regulatory authorities.

10.9 Future Prospects

The cost of feed that accounts for the majority of the input can be reduced by using nano-materials. By appropriately manipulating the feed composition with desired nano-materials, designer meat and eggs can be produced. Nutritional quality of eggs can be tailored to suit babies, adults, pregnant women, lactating mothers, diabetic patients, cardiac patients, and geriatric people. To make the nano-foods acceptable to consumers, regulatory policies have to be framed based on the safety of nano-formulations used in the poultry. To generate revenue, and contribute to national productivity, the technology has to reach the unorganized poultry sector. The methodology of preparation of nanomaterials has to be optimized and it has to be standardized as per the regulatory policies. With technological support, meat and eg should be processed to value-added products. To investigate the impact of nanomaterials on chicken health and laying performance, a large number of trials have to be undertaken starting from the first day till the functionally mature chicken in broiler and till the end of laying stage in layers. The investigation must be replicated to be statistically significantt in all environmental conditions.

10.10 Conclusion

The main role of nano-materials as a source of minerals/feed additives/carriers/ sensors in the poultry industry is to improve the livelihood of birds which culminates in the production of good quality meat and egg. The main bottleneck in translating the promising bench results into the plate is the lack of standard operating procedures about the production of nano-materials and guidelines regarding the physicochemical properties of nanomaterials to be used in food and feed. The stability of nanomaterials, their transformation within the food/feed matrix, their interaction with other bulk and nano-materials were not addressed in many studies. Severals studies have used different concentrations of nanomaterials for different duration of the experiment ranging from few days to weeks. Moreover, the effects were studied in different breeds of layer, and broiler chicken.No study has completely investigated the differential distribution of nanomaterials in different organs at regular intervals. No report is available related to the impact of nano-supplements on laying performance, the health of poultry, and the quality of egg for the entire duration of laying. The effect of nano-materials on different types of cells has to be investigated at *invitro* and *in vivo* level with the same type and characteristics of nano-material.

It is imperative to investigate the safety of these novel nano-foods by feeding these foods to other models like mice/rats /rabbits. If the nano-food claims enrichment of certain nutrients, then their bioavailability in different animal models like mice/rats /rabbits has to be studied. For example, if the nano-egg is claimed to be rich in iron, then it has to be tested in an iron deficiency animal model to alleviate anemia.

To translate the results reported in the literature to the industrial scale, standard operating procedures must be devised for the synthesis and characteristics of nanomaterials. A complete study has to be conducted with nano-materials of uniform characteristics as a feed additive with each genetic variety of breeds for the entire productivity period. To obtain a consistent outcome in the quality of meat and egg using nano-materials, the physico-chemical characteristics, the required dose, and the duration of supplementation should be standardized and optimized. The safety and cytotoxicity of the nano-materials used in the study have to be investigated in minute details to ensure approval for nano-food. To minimize the cost of feed with protein and energy sources, investigations can be initiated for their slow and sustained delivery. The nano-feed must be available in all areas at an economic price.

Acknowledgments The authors would like to thank The Principal and Head of the department, Department of Biotechnology for the constant support and encouragement.

References

Abdulla NR, Mohd Zamri AN, Sabow AB, Kareem KY, Nurhazirah S, Ling FH, Loh TC (2015) Physico- chemical properties of breast muscle in broiler chickens fed probiotics, antibiotics or antibiotic–probiotic mix. J Appl Anim Res 45:67–70. https://doi.org/10.1080/09712119.2015.1124330

Abedini M, Shariatmadari F, Karimi Torshizi MA, Ahmadi H (2018) Effects of zinc oxide nanoparticles on the egg quality, immune response, zinc retention, and blood parameters of laying hens in the late phase of production. J Anim Physiol Anim Nutr (Berl) 102:736–745. https://doi.org/10.1111/jpn.12871

Aboalnaja KO, Yaghmoor S, Kumosani TA, McClements DJ (2016) Utilization of nanoemulsions to enhance bioactivity of pharmaceuticals, supplements, and nutraceuticals: Nanoemulsion delivery systems and nanoemulsion excipient systems. Expert Opin Drug Deliv 13:1327–1336. https://doi.org/10.1517/17425247.2016.1162154

Abu Hatab A, Cavinato MER, Lagerkvist CJ (2019) Urbanization, livestock systems and food security in developing countries: a systematic review of the literature. Food Sec 11:279–299. https://doi.org/10.1007/s12571-019-00906-1

Aggett PJ (2010) Population reference intakes and micronutrient bioavailability: a European perspective. Am J Clin Nutr 91:1433S–1437S. https://doi.org/10.3945/ajcn.2010.28674c

Agnihotri SA, Mallikarjuna NN, Aminabhavi TM (2004) Recent advances on chitosan-based micro-and nanoparticles in drug delivery. J Control Release 100:5–28. https://doi.org/10.1016/j.jconrel.2004.08.010

Ahmadi F, Khah MM, Saman J, Zarneshan A, Loghman A, Salehifar P (2013) The effect of dietary silver nanoparticles on performance, immune organs, and lipid serum of broiler chickens during starter period. Int J Biosci 3:95–100. https://doi.org/10.12692/ijb/3.5.95-100

Akbarzadeh A, Rezaei-Sadabady R, Davaran S, Joo SW, Zarghami N, Hanifehpour Y, Samiei M, Kouhi M, Nejati-Koshki N (2013) Liposome: classification, preparation, and applications. Nanoscale Res Lett 8:102. https://doi.org/10.1186/1556-276x-8-102

Akhlaghi SP, Peng B, Yao Z, Tam KC (2013) Sustainable nanomaterials derived from polysaccharides and amphiphilic compounds. Soft Matter 9:7905–7918. https://doi.org/10.1039/c3sm50358e

Alemayehu, Beuving J, Ruben R (2018) Risk preferences and farmers' livelihood strategies: a case study from eastern Ethiopia. J Int Dev 30:1369–1391. https://doi.org/10.1002/jid.3341

Alfadul S, Elneshwy A (2010) Use of nanotechnology in food processing, packaging and safety – review. Afr J Food Agric Nutr Dev 10(6):2719–2739. https://doi.org/10.4314/ajfand.v10i6.58068

Alkie TN, Yitbarek A, Taha-Abdelaziz K, Astill J, Sharif S (2018) Characterization of immunogenicity of avian influenza antigens encapsulated in PLGA nanoparticles following mucosal and subcutaneous delivery in chickens. PLoS One 13:e0206324. https://doi.org/10.1371/journal.pone.0206324

Amini SM, Gilaki M, Karchani M (2014) Safety of nanotechnology in food industries. Electron Physician 6:962–968. https://doi.org/10.14661/2014.962-968

Andlauer W, Fürst P (2002) Nutraceuticals: a piece of history, present status and outlook. Food Res Int 35:171–176. https://doi.org/10.1016/s0963-9969(01)00179-x

Antisari LV, Carbone S, Gatti A, Vianello G, Nannipieri P (2015) Uptake and translocation of metals and nutrients in tomato grown in soil polluted with metal oxide (CeO(2), Fe(3)O(4), SnO(2), TiO(2)) or metallic (Ag, Co, Ni) engineered nanoparticles. Environ Sci Pollut Res Int 22:1841–1853. https://doi.org/10.1007/s11356-014-3509-0

Aparna V, Melge AR, Rajan VK, Biswas R, Jayakumar R, Gopi Mohan C (2018) Carboxymethylated i-carrageenan conjugated amphotericin B loaded gelatin nanoparticles for treating intracellular Candida glabrata infections. Int J Biol Macromol 110:140–149. https://doi.org/10.1016/j.ijbiomac.2017.11.126

Arakha M, Pal S, Samantarrai D, Panigrahi TK, Mallick BC, Pramanik K, Jha S (2015) Antimicrobial activity of iron oxide nanoparticle upon modulation of nanoparticle-bacteria interface. Sci Rep 5:14813. https://doi.org/10.1038/srep14813

Ashraf MA, Peng W, Zare Y, Rhee KY (2018) Effects of size and aggregation/agglomeration of nanoparticles on the interfacial/interphase properties and tensile strength of polymer nanocomposites. Nanoscale Res Lett 13:214. https://doi.org/10.1186/s11671-018-2624-0

Aslani F, Bagheri S, Muhd Julkapli N, Juraimi AS, Hashemi FS, Baghdadi A (2014) Effects of engineered nanomaterials on plants growth: an overview. Sci World J 2014:641759. https://doi.org/10.1155/2014/641759

Awaad A, Nakamura M, Ishimura K (2012) Imaging of size-dependent uptake and identification of novel pathways in mouse Peyer's patches using fluorescent organosilica particles. Nanomedicine 8:627–636. https://doi.org/10.1016/j.nano.2011.08.009

Azeredo HMC (2009) Nanocomposites for food packaging applications. Food Res Int 42:1240–1253. https://doi.org/10.1016/j.foodres.2009.03.019

Bagheri M, Golchin-Gelehdooni S, Mohamadi M, Tabidian A (2015) Comparative effects of nano, mineral and organic selenium on growth performance, immunity responses and total antioxidant activity in broiler chickens. IJBPAS 4:583–595

Bakhshalinejad R, Akbari Moghaddam Kakhki R, Zoidis E (2018) Effects of different dietary sources and levels of selenium supplements on growth performance, antioxidant status and immune parameters in Ross 308 broiler chickens. Br Poult Sci 59:81–91. https://doi.org/10.1080/00071668.2017.1380296

Balaji DS, Basavaraja S, Deshpande R, Mahesh DB, Prabhakar BK, Venkataraman A (2009) Extracellular biosynthesis of functionalized silver nanoparticles by strains of *Cladosporium cladosporioides* fungus. Colloids Surf B: Biointerfaces 68:88–92. https://doi.org/10.1016/j.colsurfb.2008.09.022

Balasubramanian SK, Jittiwat J, Manikandan J, Ong CN, Yu LE, Ong WY (2010) Biodistribution of gold nanoparticles and gene expression changes in the liver and spleen after intravenous administration in rats. Biomaterials 31:2034–2042. https://doi.org/10.1016/j.biomaterials.2009.11.079

Bantz C, Koshkina O, Lang T, Galla HJ, Kirkpatrick CJ, Stauber RH, Maskos M (2014) The surface properties of nanoparticles determine the agglomeration state and the size of the particles under physiological conditions. Beilstein J Nanotechnol 5:1774–1786. https://doi.org/10.3762/bjnano.5.188

Basha K, Lakshmi K, Sugantha (2016) Ammonia sensor and antibacterial activities of green zinc oxide nanoparticles. Sens Bio-Sens Res 10:34–40. https://doi.org/10.1016/j.sbsr.2016.08.007

Behzadi S, Serpooshan V, Tao W, Hamaly MA, Alkawareek MY, Dreaden EC, Brown D, Alkilany AM, Farokhzad OC, Mahmoudi M (2017) Cellular uptake of nanoparticles: journey inside the cell. Chem Soc Rev 46:4218–4244. https://doi.org/10.1039/c6cs00636a

Bergin IL, Witzmann FA (2013) Nanoparticle toxicity by the gastrointestinal route: evidence and knowledge gaps. Int J Biomed Nanosci Nanotechnol 3:163–210. https://doi.org/10.1504/ijbnn.2013.054515

Bertrand N, Leroux JC (2012) The journey of a drug-carrier in the body: an anatomo-physiological perspective. J Control Release 161:152–163. https://doi.org/10.1016/j.jconrel.2011.09.098

Best M, Phillips G, Fowler C, Rowland J, Elsom J (2015) Characterisation and cytotoxic screening of metal oxide nanoparticles putative of interest to oral healthcare formulations in non-keratinised human oral mucosa cells in vitro. Toxicol In Vitro 30:402–411. https://doi.org/10.1016/j.tiv.2015.09.022

Bhagat D, Samanta SK, Bhattacharya S (2013) Efficient management of fruit pests by pheromone nanogels. Sci Rep 3:1294. https://doi.org/10.1038/srep01294

Bhanja S, Hotowy A, Mehra M, Sawosz E, Pineda L, Vadalasetty K, Chwalibog A (2015) In ovo administration of silver nanoparticles and/or amino acids influence metabolism and immune gene expression in chicken embryos. Int J Mol Sci 16:9484–9503. https://doi.org/10.3390/ijms16059484

Bhatta R, Jash S, Corbon G (2012) NIANP-Annual Report 2011-2012, National Institute of Animal Nutrition and Physiology, Bengaluru, Karnataka

Binderup ML, Bredsdorff L, Beltoft VM, Mortensen A, Löschner K, Löschner K, Larsen EH, Eriksen FD (2013) Systemic absorption of nanomaterials by oral exposure. Part of the "Better control of nano" initiative 2012–2015. Danish Environmental Protection Agency. http://www2.mst.dk/Udgiv/publications/2013/09/978-87-93026-51-3.pdf

Binupriya AR, Sathishkumar M, Yun SI (2010) Biocrystallization of silver and gold ions by inactive cell filtrate of *Rhizopus stolonifer*. Colloids Surf B: Biointerfaces 79:531–534. https://doi.org/10.1016/j.colsurfb.2010.05.021

Boonyanitipong, Kositsup B, Kumar P, Sunandan B, Joydeep D (2011) Toxicity of zno and tio2 nanoparticles on germinating rice seed Oryza sativa l. Int J Biosci Biochem Bioinf 1(4):282. https://doi.org/10.7763/ijbbb.2011.v1.53

Borel P, Preveraud D, Desmarchelier C (2013) Bioavailability of vitamin E in humans: an update. Nutr Rev 71:319–331. https://doi.org/10.1111/nure.12026

Bornstein S, Samberg Y (1954) The therapeutic effect of streptomycin on infectious coryza of chickens caused by *Hemophilus gallinarum*. II. Isolation and culture of *Hemophilus gallinarum*, and some of its biochemical reaction. Am J Vet Res 15:612–616. https://doi.org/10.3382/ps.0340896

Bostrom A, Löfstedt RE (2010) Nanotechnology risk communication past and prologue. Risk Anal 30:1645–1662. https://doi.org/10.1111/j.1539-6924.2010.01521.x

Boury B, Plumejeau S (2015) Metal oxides and polysaccharides: an efficient hybrid association for materials chemistry. Green Chem 17:72–88. https://doi.org/10.1039/c4gc00957f

Bozich JS, Lohse SE, Torelli MD, Murphy CJ, Hamers RJ, Klaper RD (2014) Surface chemistry, charge and ligand type impact the toxicity of gold nanoparticles to Daphnia magna. Environ Sci Nano 1:260–270. https://doi.org/10.1039/c4en00006d

Brake J (1993) Recent advances in induced molting. Poult Sci 72:929–931. https://doi.org/10.3382/ps.0720929

Brody AL, Bugusu B, Han JH, Sand CK, McHugh TH (2008) Scientific status summary. Innovative food packaging solutions. J Food Sci 73:R107–R116. https://doi.org/10.1111/j.1750-3841.2008.00933.x

Bundschuh M, Juliane F, Simon L, Moira SM, George M, Gabriele ES, Ralf S, Stephan W (2018) Nanoparticles in the environment: where do we come from, where do we go to? Environ Sci Eur 30(1):1–7. https://doi.org/10.1186/s12302-018-0132-6

Bunglavan SJ, Garg AK, Dass RS, Shrivastava S (2014) Use of nanoparticles as feed additives to improve digestion and absorption in livestock. Livest Res Int 2:36–47

Buzea C, Pacheco II, Robbie K (2007) Nanomaterials and nanoparticles: sources and toxicity. Biointerphases 2:MR17–MR71. https://doi.org/10.1116/1.2815690

Cai Z, Wang Y, Zhu LJ, Liu ZQ (2010) Nanocarriers: a general strategy for enhancement of oral bioavailability of poorly absorbed or pre-systemically metabolized drugs. Curr Drug Metab 11:197–207. https://doi.org/10.2174/138920010791110836

Cai SJ, Wu CX, Gong LM, Song T, Wu H, Zhang LY (2012) Effects of nano-selenium on performance, meat quality, immune function, oxidation resistance, and tissue selenium content in broilers. Poult Sci 91:2532–2539. https://doi.org/10.3382/ps.2012-02160

Campos EV, de Oliveira JL, da Silva CM, Pascoli M, Pasquoto T, Lima R, Abhilash PC, Fraceto LF (2015) Polymeric and solid lipid nanoparticles for sustained release of carbendazim and tebuconazole in agricultural applications. Sci Rep 5:13809. https://doi.org/10.1038/srep13809

Canham LT (2007) Nanoscale semiconducting silicon as a nutritional food additive. Nanotechnology 18:185704. https://doi.org/10.1088/0957-4484/18/18/185704
Carter SD, Kim H (2013) Technologies to reduce environmental impact of animal wastes associated with feeding for maximum productivity. Anim Front 3:42–47. https://doi.org/10.2527/af.2013-0023
Chai H, Yao J, Sun J, Zhang LW, Zhu M, Ceccanti B (2015) The effect of metal oxide nanoparticles on functional bacteria and metabolic profiles in agricultural soil. Bull Environ Contam Toxicol 94:490–495. https://doi.org/10.1007/s00128-015-1485-9
Chaudhry Q, Castle L (2011) Food applications of nanotechnologies: an overview of opportunities and challenges for developing countries. Trends Food Sci Technol 22:595–603. https://doi.org/10.1016/j.tifs.2011.01.001
Chaudhry Q, Scotter M, Blackburn J, Ross B, Boxall A, Castle L, Aitken R, Watkins R (2008) Applications and implications of nanotechnologies for the food sector. Food Addit Contam 25(3):241–258. https://doi.org/10.1080/02652030701744538
Chen H, Weiss J, Shahidi F (2006) Nanotechnology in nutraceuticals and functional foods. J Food Technol 60:30–36
Chen D, Xia D, Li X, Zhu Q, Yu H, Zhu C, Gan Y (2013) Comparative study of Pluronic® F127-modified liposomes and chitosan-modified liposomes for mucus penetration and oral absorption of cyclosporine A in rats. Int J Pharm 449:1–9. https://doi.org/10.1016/j.ijpharm.2013.04.002
Chen CW, Huang JH, Lai TC, Jan YH, Hsiao M, Chen CH, Hwu YK, Liu RS (2016) Evaluation of the intracellular uptake and cytotoxicity effect of TiO2 nanostructures for various human oral and lung cells under dark conditions. Toxicol Res 5:303–311. https://doi.org/10.1039/c5tx00312a
Chiu CY, Ruan L, Huang Y (2013) Biomolecular specificity controlled nanomaterial synthesis. Chem Soc Rev 42:2512–2527. https://doi.org/10.1039/c2cs35347d
Choi CH, Zuckerman JE, Webster P, Davis ME (2011) Targeting kidney mesangium by nanoparticles of defined size. Proc Natl Acad Sci U S A 108:6656–6661. https://doi.org/10.1073/pnas.1103573108
Chow PY, Gue SZ, Leow SK, Goh LB (2015) Solid self-microemulsifying system (S-SMECS) for enhanced bioavailability and pigmentation of highly lipophilic bioactive carotenoid. Powder Technol 274:199–204. https://doi.org/10.1016/j.powtec.2015.01.020
Chowdhury N (2006) Nanotechnology regulation in India: a framework for exploring the risks and opportunities. Econ Polit Wkly 18:4730–4733
Claudia B, Tabea P, Kerstin S, Evamaria K, Dirk WL (2016) An update of definitions and regulations regarding nanomaterials in foods and other consumer products. In: Grumezescu AM (ed) Novel approaches of nanotechnology in food. Academic, Amsterdam, pp 1–19. https://doi.org/10.1016/b978-0-12-804308-0.00001-7
Coles D, Frewer LJ (2013) Nanotechnology applied to European food production – a review of ethical and regulatory issues. Trends Food Sci Technol 34:32–43. https://doi.org/10.1016/j.tifs.2013.08.006
Cubukcu M, Timur S, Anik U (2007) Examination of performance of glassy carbon paste electrode modified with gold nanoparticle and xanthine oxidase for xanthine and hypoxanthine detection. Talanta 74:434–439. https://doi.org/10.1016/j.talanta.2007.07.039
Cuiling P, Yuxin Z, Shengfa FL, Fu C, Shunyi Q, Xianshi W, Hong Z, Kehe H (2011) Effect of selenium-enriched probiotics on laying performance, egg quality, egg selenium content, and egg glutathione peroxidase activity. J Agric Food Chem 59:11424–11431. https://doi.org/10.1021/jf202014k
Cushen M, Kerry J, Morris M, Cruz-Romero M, Cummins E (2012) Nanotechnologies in the food industry – recent developments, risks and regulation. Trends Food Sci Technol 24:30–46. https://doi.org/10.1016/j.tifs.2011.10.006
Da Silva MP, Daroit DJ, Brandelli A (2010) Food applications of liposome-encapsulated antimicrobial peptides. Trends Food Sci Technol 21:284–292. https://doi.org/10.1016/j.tifs.2010.03.003

Datta N (1969) Penicillin in poultry feed. Br Med J 4(5685):741. https://doi.org/10.1136/bmj.4.5685.741-a

Dawson M, Wirtz D, Hanes J (2003) Enhanced viscoelasticity of human cystic fibrotic sputum correlates with increasing microheterogeneity in particle transport. J Biol Chem 278:50393–50401. https://doi.org/10.1074/jbc.m309026200

De Jong WH, Hagens WI, Krystek P, Burger MC, Sips AJ, Geertsma RE (2008) Particle size-dependent organ distribution of gold nanoparticles after intravenous administration. Biomaterials 29:1912–1919. https://doi.org/10.1016/j.biomaterials.2007.12.037

De Jong WH, Van Der Ven LT, Sleijffers A, Park MV, Jansen EH, Van Loveren H, Vandebriel RJ (2013) Systemic and immunotoxicity of silver nanoparticles in an intravenous 28 days repeated dose toxicity study in rats. Biomaterials 34:8333–8343. https://doi.org/10.1016/j.biomaterials.2013.06.048

Desai MP, Labhasetwar V, Amidon GL, Levy RJ (1996) Gastrointestinal uptake of biodegradable microparticles: effect of particle size. Pharm Res 13:1838–1845. https://doi.org/10.1023/a:1016085108889

Dimkpa C, Mclean J, Latta D, Manangón E, Britt D, William J, Maxim B, Anne A (2012) CuO and ZnO nanoparticles: phytotoxicity, metal speciation, and induction of oxidative stress in sand-grown wheat. J Nanopart Res 14:1–15. https://doi.org/10.1007/s11051-012-1125-9

Doane T, Burda C (2013) Nanoparticle mediated non-covalent drug delivery. Adv Drug Deliv Rev 65:607–621. https://doi.org/10.1016/j.addr.2012.05.012

Doshi N, Mitragotri S (2010) Needle-shaped polymeric particles induce transient disruption of cell membranes. J R Soc Interface 7:S403. https://doi.org/10.1098/rsif.2010.0134.focus

Duan H, Wang D, Li Y (2015) Green chemistry for nanoparticle synthesis. Chem Soc Rev 44:5778–5792. https://doi.org/10.1039/c4cs00363b

Duffy LL, Osmond-McLeod MJ, Judy J, King T (2018) Investigation into the antibacterial activity of silver, zinc oxide and copper oxide nanoparticles against poultry-relevant isolates of Salmonella and Campylobacter. Food Control 92:293–300. https://doi.org/10.1016/j.foodcont.2018.05.008

Dumonceaux TJ, Hill JE, Briggs SA, Amoako KK, Hemmingsen SM, Van Kessel AG (2006) Enumeration of specific bacterial populations in complex intestinal communities using quantitative PCR based on the chaperonin-60 target. J Microbiol Methods 64:46–62. https://doi.org/10.1016/j.mimet.2005.04.006

Duncan TV (2011) Applications of nanotechnology in food packaging and food safety: barrier materials, antimicrobials and sensors. J Colloid Interface Sci 363:1–24. https://doi.org/10.1016/j.jcis.2011.07.017

EC (2011) REACH implementation project. Substance identification of nanomaterials. European Commission, Joint Research Centre, Brussels

EFSA (2016) Safety assessment of the substance zinc oxide nanoparticles, for use in food contact materials. EFSDA J14:4401–4408

El Sabry MI, McMillin KW, Sabliov CM (2018) Nanotechnology considerations for poultry and livestock production systems – a review. Ann Anim Sci 18:319–334. https://doi.org/10.1515/aoas-2017-0047

El-kazaz SE, Hafez MH (2019) Evaluation of copper nanoparticles and copper sulfate effect on immune status, behavior, and productive performance of broilers. J Adv Vet Anim Res 7(1):16–25. https://doi.org/10.5455/javar.2020.g388

Elkin RG (2006) Reducing shell egg cholesterol content. I. Overview, genetic approaches, and nutritional strategies. Worlds Poult Sci J 62:665–687. https://doi.org/10.1017/s0043933906001206

Elkin RG (2007) Reducing shell egg cholesterol content. II. Review of approaches utilizing non-nutritive dietary factors or pharmacological agents and an examination of emerging strategies. Worlds Poult Sci J 63:5–32. https://doi.org/10.1017/s0043933907001249

Elkloub K, Moustafa ME, Ghazalah AA, Rehan AAA (2015) Effect of dietary nanosilver on broiler performance. Int J Poult Sci 14:177–182. https://doi.org/10.3923/ijps.2015.177.182

El-Sheikh M (2017) Application of nanotechnologies in poultry production. Nutr Food Sci 3(2):555610. https://doi.org/10.19080/nfsij.2017.03.555610

Emami T, Madani R, Rezayat SM, Golchinfar F, Sarkar S (2012) Applying of gold nanoparticle to avoid diffusion of the conserved peptide of avian influenza nonstructural protein from membrane in Western blot. J Appl Poult Res 21:563–566. https://doi.org/10.3382/japr.2011-00456

EU European Commission (2011) Regulation (Eu) No 1169/2011 of the European parliament and of the Council of 25 october 2011 on the provision of food information to consumers, amending Regulations (EC) No 1924/2006 and (EC) No 1925/2006 of the European parliament and of the Council, and repealing commission directive 87/250/EEC, Council directive 90/496/EEC, commission directive 1999/10/EC, directive 2000/13/EC of the European parliament and of the Council, commission directives 2002/67/EC and 2008/5/EC and commission regulation (EC) No 608/2004. Off J Eur Comm L 304:18

EU European Parliament and Council (2015) Regulation (EC) 2015/2283 of the European parliament and of the Council of 25 november 2015 on novel foods. In E. Union (Ed.). Off J Eur Comm L 327:1

EU European Union (2002) Regulation (EC) No. 178/2002 of the European Parliament and of the council of 28 January 2002 laying down the general principles and requirements of food law, establishing the European Food Safety Authority and laying down procedures in matters of food safety. Off J Eur Comm L 31:1–24

EU European Union (2003) Regulation (EC) No. 1831/2003 of the European Parliament and of the council of 22 September 2003 on additives for use in animal nutrition. Off J Eur Comm L 268:29–43

EU European Union (2004) Regulation (EC) No. 1935/2004 of the European Parliament and the Council of 27 October 2004 on materials and articles intended to come into contact with food and repealing Directives 80/590/EEC and 89/109/EEC. Off J Eur Comm L 338:4–17

EU European Union (2006) Regulation (EC) No. 1907/2006 of the European Parliament and of the Council of 18 December 2006 concerning the Registration, Evaluation, Authorisation and Restriction of Chemicals (REACH), establishing a European Chemicals Agency, amending Directive 1999/45/EC and repealing Council Regulation (EEC) No. 793/93 and Commission Regulation (EC) No. 1488/94 as well as Council Directive 76/769/EEC and Commission Directives 91/155/ EEC, 93/67/EEC, 93/105/EC and 2000/21/EC. Off J Eur Comm L 136:3–280

EU European Union (2008) Regulation (EC) No. 1333/2008 of the European Parliament and of the council of 16 December 2008 on food additives. Off J Eur Comm L 354:16–33

EU European Union (2009) Commission Regulation (EC) No. 450/2009 of 29 May 2009 on active and intelligent materials and articles intended to come into contact with food. Off J Eur Comm L 135:3–11

EU European Union (2010) Commission Regulation (EU) No. 257/2010 of 25 March 2010 setting up a programme for the re-evaluation of approved food additives in accordance with Regulation (EC) No. 1333/2008 of the European Parliament and of the Council on food additives. Off J Eur Comm L 80:19–27

EU European Union (2011) Regulation (EU) No. 1169/2011 of the European Parliament and of the Council of 25 October 2011 on the provision of food information to consumers, amending Regulations (EC) No. 1924/2006 and (EC) No.1925/2006 of the European Parliament and of the Council, and repealing Commission Directive 87/250/EEC, Council Directive 90/496/EEC, Commission Directive 1999/10/EC, Directive 2000/13/EC of the European Parliament and of the Council, Commission Directives 2002/67/EC and 2008/5/EC and Commission Regulation (EC) No. 608/2004. Off J Eur Comm L 304:18–63

Faghihi F, Samaneh Z (2014) Effect of copper oxide nanoparticles on liver enzymes activity in broilers. Mol Biol Res Commun 3:131–131

Fathi M, Haydari M, Tanha T (2016) Effects of zinc oxide nanoparticles on antioxidant status, serum enzymes activities, biochemical parameters and performance in broiler chickens. J Livestock Sci Technol 4:7–13

Fayaz AM, Balaji K, Girilal M, Yadav R, Kalaichelvan PT, Venketesan R (2010) Biogenic synthesis of silver nanoparticles and their synergistic effect with antibiotics: a study against gram-positive and gram-negative bacteria. Nanomedicine 6:103–109. https://doi.org/10.1016/j.nano.2009.04.006

Feighner SD, Dashkevicz MP (1987) Subtherapeutic levels of antibiotics in poultry feeds and their effects on weight gain, feed efficiency, and bacterial cholyltaurine hydrolase activity. Appl Environ Microbiol 53:331–336. https://doi.org/10.1128/aem.53.2.331-336.1987

Feizi H, Kamali M, Jafari L, Rezvani Moghaddam P (2013) Phytotoxicity and stimulatory impacts of nanosized and bulk titanium dioxide on fennel (Foeniculum vulgare mill). Chemosphere 91:506–511. https://doi.org/10.1016/j.chemosphere.2012.12.012

Felehgari KF, Ahmadi, Ardashir AR, Kurdestany H, Khah MM (2013) The effect of dietary silver nanoparticles on performance, immune organs, and lipid serum of broiler chickens during starter period. Int J Biosci (IJB) 3:95–100. https://doi.org/10.12692/ijb/3.5.95-100

Feng Y, Min L, Zhang W, Liu J, Hou Z, Chu M, Li L, Shen W, Zhao Y, Zhang H (2017) Zinc oxide nanoparticles influence microflora in ileal digesta and correlate well with blood metabolites. Front Microbiol 8:992. https://doi.org/10.3389/fmicb.2017.00992

Fernandez A, Picouet P, Lloret E (2010) Reduction of the spoilage-related microflora in absorbent pads by silver nanotechnology during modified atmosphere packaging of beef meat. J Food Prot 73:2263–2269. https://doi.org/10.4315/0362-028x-73.12.2263

Frohlich E (2012) The role of surface charge in cellular uptake and cytotoxicity of medical nanoparticles. Int J Nanomedicine 7:5577–5591. https://doi.org/10.2147/ijn.s36111

FSSAI, Government of India 2006. The Food Safety and Standards Act, 2006. Gazette ofIndia (extraordinary) Part-II, Section 1, Issue No. 40, Act No. 34 of 2006, dated 24 August 2006

Fuxiang W, Huiying R, Fenghua Z, Jinquan S, Jianyang J, Wenli L (2008) Effects of nano- selenium on the immune functions and antioxidant abilities of broiler chickens. Chin Agri Sci Bull 2:831–835

Gadde UD, Oh S, Lillehoj HS, Lillehoj EP (2018) Antibiotic growth promoters virginiamycin and bacitracin methylene disalicylate alter the chicken intestinal metabolome. Sci Rep 8:3592. https://doi.org/10.1038/s41598-018-22004-6

Gajbhiye M, Kesharwani J, Ingle A, Gade A, Rai M (2009) Fungus-mediated synthesis of silver nanoparticles and their activity against pathogenic fungi in combination with fluconazole. Nanomedicine 5:382–386. https://doi.org/10.1016/j.nano.2009.06.005

Gangadoo S, Stanley D, Hughes RJ, Moore RJ, Chapman J (2016) Nanoparticles in feed: progress and prospects in poultry research. Trends Food Sci Technol 58:115–126. https://doi.org/10.1016/j.tifs.2016.10.013

Gangadoo S, Dinev I, Chapman J, Hughes RJ, Van TTH, Moore RJ, Stanley D (2018) Selenium nanoparticles in poultry feed modify gut microbiota and increase abundance of *Faecalibacterium prausnitzii*. Appl Microbiol Biotechnol 102:1455–1466. https://doi.org/10.1007/s00253-017-8688-4

Ganjigohari S, Ziaei N, Ramzani Ghara A, Tasharrofi S (2018) Effects of nanocalcium carbonate on egg production performance and plasma calcium of laying hens. J Anim Physiol Anim Nutr (Berl) 102:e225–ee32. https://doi.org/10.1111/jpn.12731

Gatoo MA, Naseem S, Arfat MY, Dar AM, Qasim K, Zubair S (2014) Physicochemical properties of nanomaterials: implication in associated toxic manifestations. Biomed Res Int 2014:498420. https://doi.org/10.1155/2014/498420

Gehrke PJ (2017) Public understanding of nanotechnology: how publics know. In: Nano-publics. Springer, Cham. https://doi.org/10.1007/978-3-319-69611-9_2

Gentile A, Ruffino F, Grimaldi MG (2016) Complex-morphology metal-based nanostructures: fabrication, characterization, and applications. Nanomaterials (Basel) 6(6):110. https://doi.org/10.3390/nano6060110

George BA, Fagerberg DJ, Quarles CL, Fenton JM, McKinley GA (1982) Effect of bambermycins on quantity, prevalence, duration, and antimicrobial resistance of Salmonella typhimurium in experimentally infected broiler chickens. Am J Vet Res 43:299–303

Gholami-Ahangaran M, Zia-Jahromi N (2013) Nanosilver effects on growth parameters in experimental aflatoxicosis in broiler chickens. Toxicol Ind Health 29:121–125. https://doi.org/10.1177/0748233711425078

Ghosh M, Bandyopadhyay M, Mukherjee A (2010) Genotoxicity of titanium dioxide (TiO2) nanoparticles at two trophic levels: plant and human lymphocytes. Chemosphere 81:1253–1262. https://doi.org/10.1016/j.chemosphere.2010.09.022

Giles EL, Kuznesof S, Clark B, Hubbard C, Frewer LJ (2015) Consumer acceptance of and willingness to pay for food nanotechnology: a systematic review. J Nanopart Res 17(12):467. https://doi.org/10.1007/s11051-015-3270-4

Gopi M, Pearlin B, Kumar RD, Shanmathy M, Prabakar G (2017) Role of nanoparticles in animal and poultry nutrition: modes of action and applications in formulating feed additives and food processing. Int J Pharmacol 13:724–731. https://doi.org/10.3923/ijp.2017.724.731

Grillo R, Rosa AH, Fraceto LF (2015) Engineered nanoparticles and organic matter: a review of the state-of-the-art. Chemosphere 119:608–619. https://doi.org/10.1016/j.chemosphere.2014.07.049

Gunalan S, Sivaraj R, Rajendran V (2012) Green synthesized ZnO nanoparticles against bacterial and fungal pathogens. Prog Nat Sci Mater Int 22:693–700. https://doi.org/10.1016/j.pnsc.2012.11.015

Gunasekaran T, Haile T, Nigusse T, Dhanaraju MD (2014) Nanotechnology: an effective tool for enhancing bioavailability and bioactivity of phytomedicine. Asian Pac J Trop Biomed 4:S1–S7. https://doi.org/10.12980/apjtb.4.2014c980

Gupta R, Xie H (2018) Nanoparticles in daily life: applications, toxicity and regulations. J Environ Pathol Toxicol Oncol 37:209–230. https://doi.org/10.1615/jenvironpatholtoxicoloncol.2018026009

Hafez A, Hegazi SM, Bakr AA, Shishtawy HE (2017) Effect of zinc oxide nanoparticles on growth performance and absorptive capacity of the intestinal villi in broiler chickens. Life Sci J 14:67–72

Hailu AA, Addis G (2016) The content and bioavailability of mineral nutrients of selected wild and traditional edible plants as affected by household preparation methods practiced by local community in Benishangul Gumuz regional state, Ethiopia. Int J Food Sci 2016:7615853. https://doi.org/10.1155/2016/7615853

Halamoda-Kenzaoui B, Ceridono M, Urban P, Bogni A, Ponti J, Gioria S, Kinsner-Ovaskainen A (2017) The agglomeration state of nanoparticles can influence the mechanism of their cellular internalisation. J Nanobiotechnol 15:48. https://doi.org/10.1186/s12951-017-0281-6

Hall RH (2002) Biosensor technologies for detecting microbiological foodborne hazards. Microbes Infect 4:425–432. https://doi.org/10.1016/s1286-4579(02)01556-3

Haritova A, Lashev L, Pashov D (2003) Pharmacokinetics of enrofloxacin in lactating sheep. Res Vet Sci 74:241–245. https://doi.org/10.1016/s0034-5288(03)00003-1

Hartmann NB, Legros S, Von der Kammer F, Hofmann T, Baun A (2012) The potential of TiO2 nanoparticles as carriers for cadmium uptake in Lumbriculus variegatus and Daphnia magna. Aquat Toxicol 118:1–8. https://doi.org/10.1016/j.aquatox.2012.03.008

Hasezaki T, Isoda K, Kondoh M, Tsutsumi Y, Yagi K (2011) Hepatotoxicity of silica nanoparticles with a diameter of 100 nm. Die Pharm Int J Pharm Sci 66:698–703

Hassan HMA, Samy A, El-Sherbin AE, Mohamed MA, Abd-Elsame MO (2016) Application of nano-dicalcium phosphate in broiler nutrition: performance and excreted calcium and phosphorus. Asian J Anim Vet Adv 11:477–483. https://doi.org/10.3923/ajava.2016.477.483

Hefferon KL (2015) Nutritionally enhanced food crops; progress and perspectives. Int J Mol Sci 16:3895–3914. https://doi.org/10.3390/ijms16023895

Helander HF, Fandriks L (2014) Surface area of the digestive tract – revisited. Scand J Gastroenterol 49:681–689. https://doi.org/10.3109/00365521.2014.898326

Heller M, Heller MJ (2006) Nanotechnology for cancer diagnostics and therapeutics. Nanomed Nanotechnol Biol Med 4(2):301. https://doi.org/10.1016/j.nano.2006.10.104

Hellin, Krishna VV, Erenstein O, Boeber C (2015) India's poultry revolution: implications for its sustenance and the global poultry trade. Int Food Agribusiness Manag Rev 18:151–164

Hill EK, Li J (2017) Current and future prospects for nanotechnology in animal production. J Anim Sci Biotechnol 8(1):26. https://doi.org/10.1186/s40104-017-0157-5

Ho SS, Scheufele DA, Corley EA (2010) Making sense of policy choices: understanding the roles of value predispositions, mass media, and cognitive processing in public attitudes toward nanotechnology. J Nanopart Res 12:2703–2715. https://doi.org/10.1007/s11051-010-0038-8

Hoet PH, Bruske-Hohlfeld I, Salata OV (2004) Nanoparticles – known and unknown health risks. J Nanobiotechnol 2:12. https://doi.org/10.1186/1477-3155-2-12

Hofacre CL, Froyman R, Gautrias B, George B, Goodwin MA, Brown J (1998) Use of aviguard and other intestinal bioproducts in experimental *Clostridium perfringens*-associated necrotizing enteritis in broiler chickens. Avian Dis 1:579–584. https://doi.org/10.2307/1592685

Hong J, Rico CM, Zhao L, Adeleye AS, Keller AA, Peralta-Videa JR, Gardea-Torresdey JL (2015) Toxic effects of copper-based nanoparticles or compounds to lettuce (*Lactuca sativa*) and alfalfa (*Medicago sativa*). Environ Sci Process Impacts 17:177–185. https://doi.org/10.1039/c4em00551a

Hotowy A, Sawosz E, Pineda L, Sawosz F, Grodzik M, Chwalibog A (2012) Silver nanoparticles administered to chicken affect VEGFA and FGF2 gene expression in breast muscle and heart. Nanoscale Res Lett 7:418. https://doi.org/10.1186/1556-276x-7-418

Huang T, Holden JA, Heath DE, O'Brien-Simpson NM, O'Connor AJ (2019) Engineering highly effective antimicrobial selenium nanoparticles through control of particle size. Nanoscale 11:14937–14951. https://doi.org/10.1039/c9nr04424h

Hui S, Mahfuz SU, Nahar MJ, Mo C, Ganfu Z, Zhongjun L (2017) Inclusion of probiotic on chicken performance and immunity: a review. Int J Poult Sci 16:328–335. https://doi.org/10.3923/ijps.2017.328.335

Institute of Food Technologists (2006) Food nanotechnology. Scientific status summary on potential applications of nanotechnology in the food industry. http://members.ift.org/NR/rdonlyres/FA6CF1C9–5E70–4A0C-9300–6A8D450A7D06/0/ednanotech.pdf

ISO (2010) ISO nanotechnologies eVocabulary part 1: core terms. International Organization for Standardization. DD ISO/TS 80004-1:2010

Jahan S, Yusoff IB, Alias YB, Afba B (2017) Reviews of the toxicity behavior of five potential engineered nanomaterials (ENMs) into the aquatic ecosystem. Toxicol Rep 4:211–220. https://doi.org/10.1016/j.toxrep.2017.04.001

Jarocka U, Sawicka R, Gora-Sochacka A, Sirko A, Dehaen W, Radecki J, Radecka H (2016) An electrochemical immunosensor based on a 4, 4′-thiobisbenzenethiol self-assembled monolayer for the detection of hemagglutinin from avian influenza virus H5N1. Sensors Actuators B Chem 228:25–30. https://doi.org/10.1016/j.snb.2016.01.001

Jeetah R, Bhaw-Luximon A, Jhurry D (2014) Nanopharmaceutics: phytochemical-based controlled or sustained drug-delivery systems for cancer treatment. J Biomed Nanotechnol 10:1810–1840. https://doi.org/10.1166/jbn.2014.1884

Jeevanandam J, Barhoum A, Chan YS, Dufresne A, Danquah MK (2018) Review on nanoparticles and nanostructured materials: history, sources, toxicity and regulations. Beilstein J Nanotechnol 9:1050–1074. https://doi.org/10.3762/bjnano.9.98

Jia L, Zhang Q, Li Q, Song H (2009) The biosynthesis of palladium nanoparticles by antioxidants in Gardenia jasminoides Ellis: long lifetime nanocatalysts for p-nitrotoluene hydrogenation. Nanotechnology 20:385601. https://doi.org/10.1088/0957-4484/20/38/385601

Jin L, Son Y, Yoon TK, Kang YJ, Kim W, Chung H (2013) High concentrations of single-walled carbon nanotubes lower soil enzyme activity and microbial biomass. Ecotoxicol Environ Saf 88:9–15. https://doi.org/10.1016/j.ecoenv.2012.10.031

Johnson JL, Mistry VV, Vukovich MD, Hogie-Lorenzen T, Hollis BW, Specker BL (2005) Bioavailability of vitamin D from fortified process cheese and effects on vitamin D status in the elderly. J Dairy Sci 88:2295–2301. https://doi.org/10.3168/jds.s0022-0302(05)72907-6

Jones N, Ray B, Ranjit KT, Manna AC (2008) Antibacterial activity of ZnO nanoparticle suspensions on a broad spectrum of microorganisms. FEMS Microbiol Lett 279:71–76. https://doi.org/10.1111/j.1574-6968.2007.01012.x

Joshua PP, Valli C, Balakrishnan V (2016) Effect of in ovo supplementation of nano forms of zinc, copper, and selenium on post-hatch performance of broiler chicken. Vet World 9:287–294. https://doi.org/10.14202/vetworld.2016.287-294

Joubert IA, Geppert M, Ess S, Nestelbacher R, Gadermaier G, Duschl A, Himly M (2020) Public perception and knowledge on nanotechnology: a study based on a citizen science approach. NanoImpact 17:100201. https://doi.org/10.1016/j.impact.2019.100201

Judy JD, Unrine JM, Bertsch M (2011) Evidence for biomagnification of gold nanoparticles within a terrestrial food chain. Environ Sci Technol 45:776–781. https://doi.org/10.1021/es103031a

Jukes TH, Stokstad ELR, Tayloe RR, Cunha TJ, Edwards HM, Meadows GB (1950) Growth-promoting effect of aureomycin on pigs. Arch Biochem 26:324–325. https://doi.org/10.3382/ps.0290611

Justin SHFW, Armstrong W (1991) Evidence for the involvement of ethene in aerenchyma formation in adventitious roots of rice (*Oryza sativa L.*). New Phytol 118:49–62. https://doi.org/10.1111/j.1469-8137.1991.tb00564.x

Kan H, Pan D, Castranova V (2018) Engineered nanoparticle exposure and cardiovascular effects: the role of a neuronal-regulated pathway. Inhal Toxicol 30:335–342. https://doi.org/10.1080/08958378.2018.1535634

Kannan RR, Arumugam R, Ramya D, Manivannan K, Anantharaman P (2013) Green synthesis of silver nanoparticles using marine macroalga Chaetomorpha linum. Appl Nanosci 3:229–233. https://doi.org/10.1007/s13204-012-0125-5

Kashyap PL, Xiang X, Heiden (2015) Chitosan nanoparticle based delivery systems for sustainable agriculture. Int J Biol Macromol 77:36–51. https://doi.org/10.1016/j.ijbiomac.2015.02.039

Katouzian I, Jafari SM (2016) Nano-encapsulation as a promising approach for targeted delivery and controlled release of vitamins. Trends Food Sci Technol 53:34–48. https://doi.org/10.1016/j.tifs.2016.05.002

Keller AA, Adeleye AS, Conway JR, Garner KL, Zhao L, Cherr GN, Zuverza-Mena N (2017) Comparative environmental fate and toxicity of copper nanomaterials. NanoImpact 7:28–40. https://doi.org/10.1016/j.impact.2017.05.003

Khalid N, Ahmed A, Bhatti MS, Randhawa MA, Ahmad A, Rafaqat R (2014) A question mark on zinc deficiency in 185 million people in Pakistan--possible way out. Crit Rev Food Sci Nutr 54:1222–1240. https://doi.org/10.1080/10408398.2011.630541

Khodakovskaya M, Bong-Soo K, Jong K, Alimohammadi M, Enkeleda D, Thikra M, Carl C (2014) Carbon nanotubes as plant growth regulators: effects on tomato growth, reproductive system, and soil microbial community. Small 9(1):115–123. https://doi.org/10.1002/smll.201201225

Kim YR, Lee EJ, Park SH, Kwon HJ, An SS, Son SW, Seo YR, Pie JE, Yoon M, Kim JH, Kim MK (2014) Comparative analysis of nanotechnology awareness in consumers and experts in South Korea. Int J Nanomedicine 9(Suppl 2):21–27. https://doi.org/10.2147/ijn.s57921

Kirchner C, Javier AM, Susha AS, Rogach AL, Kreft O, Sukhorukov GB, Parak WJ (2005) Cytotoxicity of nanoparticle-loaded polymer capsules. Talanta 67:486–491. https://doi.org/10.1016/j.talanta.2005.06.042

Konkol D, Wojnarowski K (2018) The use of nanominerals in animal nutrition as a way to improve the composition and quality of animal products. J Chem 2018:1–7. https://doi.org/10.1155/2018/5927058

Korbekandi H, Iravani S, Abbasi S (2012) Optimization of biological synthesis of silver nanoparticles using *Lactobacillus casei* subsp. Casei. J Chem Technol Biotechnol 87:932–937. https://doi.org/10.1002/jctb.3702

Kotta S, Khan AW, Pramod K, Ansari SH, Sharma RK, Ali J (2012) Exploring oral nanoemulsions for bioavailability enhancement of poorly water-soluble drugs. Expert Opin Drug Deliv 9:585–598. https://doi.org/10.1517/17425247.2012.668523

Kowalski C, Rolinski Z, Zan R, Wawron W (2002) Pharmacokinetics of tylosin in broiler chickens. Pol J Vet Sci 5:127–130

Kreyling WG, Semmler-Behnke M, Seitz J, Scymczak W, Wenk A, Mayer P, Takenaka S, Oberdorster G (2009) Size dependence of the translocation of inhaled iridium and carbon nanoparticle aggregates from the lung of rats to the blood and secondary target organs. Inhal Toxicol 21(1):55–60. https://doi.org/10.1080/08958370902942517

Kreyling WG, Semmler-Behnke M, Chaudhry Q (2010) A complementary definition of nanomaterial. Nano Today 5:165–168. https://doi.org/10.1016/j.nantod.2010.03.004

Krishnaraj C, Jagan EG, Rajasekar S, Selvakumar P, Kalaichelvan PT, Mohan N (2010) Synthesis of silver nanoparticles using Acalypha indica leaf extracts and its antibacterial activity against water borne pathogens. Colloids Surf B: Biointerfaces 76:50–56. https://doi.org/10.1016/j.colsurfb.2009.10.008

Kriwy P, Mecking RA (2011) Health and environmental consciousness, costs of behaviour and the purchase of organic food. Int J Consum Stud 36:30–37. https://doi.org/10.1111/j.1470-6431.2011.01004.x

Kroese FM, Evers C, De Ridder DTD (2009) How chocolate keeps you slim. The effect of food temptations on weight watchinggoal importance, intentions, and eating behavior. Appetite 53:430–433. https://doi.org/10.1016/j.appet.2009.08.002

Kurland HD, Grabow J, Staupendahl G, Müller FA, Müller E, Dutz S, Bellemann ME (2009) Magnetic iron oxide nanopowders produced by CO2 laser evaporation—"in situ" coating and particle embedding in a ceramic matrix. J Magn Magn Mater 321:1381–1385. https://doi.org/10.1016/j.jmmm.2009.02.042

Kwok KW, Auffan M, Badireddy AR, Nelson CM, Wiesner MR, Chilkoti A, Liu J, Marinakos SM, Hinton DE (2012) Uptake of silver nanoparticles and toxicity to early life stages of Japanese medaka (Oryzias latipes): effect of coating materials. Aquat Toxicol 120–121:59–66. https://doi.org/10.1016/j.aquatox.2012.04.012

Lacey J (2017) Bioavailability of nanomaterials and interaction with cells. Innov Food Sci Emerg Technol:81–96. https://doi.org/10.1016/b978-0-323-42980-1.00005-4

Lagerkvist CJ, Hess S (2010) A meta-analysis of consumer willingness to pay for farm animal welfare. Eur Rev Agric Econ 38:55–78. https://doi.org/10.1093/erae/jbq043

Lambert G, Fattal E, Couvreur P (2001) Nanoparticulate systems for the delivery of antisense oligonucleotides. Adv Drug Deliv Rev 47:99–112. https://doi.org/10.1016/s0169-409x(00)00116-2

Landers TF, Cohen B, Wittum TE, Larson EL (2012) A review of antibiotic use in food animals: perspective, policy, and potential. Public Health Rep 127:4–22. https://doi.org/10.1177/003335491212700103

Leeson S, Summers JD (2005) Commercial poultry nutrition. University Press, Nottingham. https://doi.org/10.7313/upo9781904761099

Li J, Helal ZH, Karch CP, Mishra N, Girshick T, Garmendia A, Burkhard P, Khan MI (2018) A self-adjuvanted nanoparticle based vaccine against infectious bronchitis virus. PLoS One 13:e0203771. https://doi.org/10.1371/journal.pone.0203771

Liao CD, Hung WL, Jan KC, Yeh AI, Ho CT, Hwang LS (2010) Nano/sub-microsized lignan glycosides from sesame meal exhibit higher transport and absorption efficiency in Caco-2 cell monolayer. Food Chem 119:896–902. https://doi.org/10.1016/j.foodchem.2009.07.056

Lillehoj H, Liu Y, Calsamiglia S, Fernandez-Miyakawa ME, Chi F, Cravens RL, Oh S, Gay CG (2018) Phytochemicals as antibiotic alternatives to promote growth and enhance host health. Vet Res 49:76. https://doi.org/10.1186/s13567-018-0562-6

Lin J, Zhang H, Chen Z, Zheng Y (2010) Penetration of lipid membranes by gold nanoparticles: insights into cellular uptake, cytotoxicity, and their relationship. ACS Nano 4:5421–5429. https://doi.org/10.1021/nn1010792

Liong MT, Shah NP (2005) Acid and bile tolerance and cholesterol removal ability of lactobacilli strains. J Dairy Sci 88(1):55–66. https://doi.org/10.3168/jds.S0022-0302(05)72662-X

Liu GX, Jiang GZ, Lu KL, Li XF, Zhou M, Zhang DD, Liu WB (2016) Effects of dietary selenium on the growth, selenium status, antioxidant activities, muscle composition and meat quality of blunt snout bream, Megalobrama amblycephala. Aquac Nutr 23:777–787. https://doi.org/10.1111/anu.12444

Lomer MC, Thompson RP, Powell JJ (2002) Fine and ultrafine particles of the diet: influence on the mucosal immune response and association with Crohn's disease. Proc Nutr Soc 61:123–130. https://doi.org/10.1079/pns2001134

Loncina J, Ivanovic J, Baltic T, Dokmanovic M, Duric J, Boskovic M, Baltic ZM (2013) Active system packaging of meat and meat products. Vet J Republic Srpska 13:5–16

Lopez-Moreno ML, Cedeno-Mattei Y, Bailon-Ruizf SJ, Vazquez-Nunez E, Hernandez-Viezcas JA, De La Rosa G, Perales-Perez OJ, Peralta-Videa JR, Gardea-Torresdey JL (2018) Environmental behavior of coated NMs: physicochemical aspects and plant interactions. J Hazard Mater 347:196–217. https://doi.org/10.1016/j.jhazmat.2017.12.058

Luo Y, Chen D, Ren L, Zhao X, Qin J (2006) Solid lipid nanoparticles for enhancing vinpocetine's oral bioavailability. J Control Release 114:53–59. https://doi.org/10.1016/j.jconrel.2006.05.010

Luyts K, Napierska D, Nemery B, Hoet PH (2013) How physico-chemical characteristics of nanoparticles cause their toxicity: complex and unresolved interrelations. Environ Sci Process Impacts 15:23–38. https://doi.org/10.1039/c2em30237c

Lye HS, Rusu G, Liong MT (2010) Removal of cholesterol by lactobacilli via incorporation and conversion to coprostanol. J Dairy Sci 93(4):1383–1392. https://doi.org/10.3168/jds.2009-2574

Macierzanka A, Rigby NM, Corfield AP, Wellner N, Böttger F, Mills ENC, Mackie AR (2011) Adsorption of bile salts to particles allows penetration of intestinal mucus. Soft Matter 7(18):8077–8084. https://doi.org/10.1039/c1sm05888f

Macierzanka A, Bottger F, Rigby NM, Lille M, Poutanen K, Mills EN, Mackie AR (2012) Enzymatically structured emulsions in simulated gastrointestinal environment: impact on interfacial proteolysis and diffusion in intestinal mucus. Langmuir 28:17349–17362. https://doi.org/10.1021/la302194q

MAFW Ministry of Agriculture & Farmers Welfare (2017) National action plan for egg & poultry-2022, for doubling farmers' income by 2022. Department of Animal Husbandry, Dairying & Fisheries, Government of India, New Delhi

Mahler GJ, Esch MB, Tako E, Southard TL, Archer SD, Glahn RP, Shuler ML (2012) Oral exposure to polystyrene nanoparticles affects iron absorption. Nat Nanotechnol 7:264–271. https://doi.org/10.1038/nnano.2012.3

Mahmoodi S, Elmi A, Hallaj Nezhadi S (2018) Copper nanoparticles as antibacterial agents. J Mol Pharm Org Process Res 6(1):1–7. https://doi.org/10.4172/2329-9053.1000140

Mahmoud UT, Abdel-Mohsein HS, Mahmoud MAM, Amen OA, Hassan RIM, Abd-El-Malek AM, Rageb SMM, Waly HSA, Othman AA, Osman MA (2020) Effect of zinc oxide nanoparticles on broilers' performance and health status. Trop Anim Health Prod 3:1–2

Mahmoudi M, Simchi A, Imani M, Shokrgozar MA, Milani AS, Hafeli UO, Stroeve P (2010) A new approach for the in vitro identification of the cytotoxicity of superparamagnetic iron oxide nanoparticles. Colloids Surf B: Biointerfaces 75:300–309. https://doi.org/10.1016/j.colsurfb.2009.08.044

Maiti D, Tong X, Mou X, Yang K (2018) Carbon-based nanomaterials for biomedical applications: a recent study. Front Pharmacol 9:1401. https://doi.org/10.3389/fphar.2018.01401

Mala R, Selvaraj RCA, Sundaram VB, Rajan R, Gurusamy UM (2017) Evaluation of nano structured slow release fertilizer on the soil fertility, yield and nutritional profile of *Vigna radiata*. Recent Pat Nanotechnol 11:50–62. https://doi.org/10.2174/1872210510666160727093554

Maldonado-Valderrama J, Wilde P, Macierzanka A, Mackie A (2011) The role of bile salts in digestion. Adv Colloid Interf Sci 165:36–46. https://doi.org/10.1016/j.cis.2010.12.002

Maleki A, Rahimi R, Maleki S, Hamidi N (2014) Synthesis and characterization of magnetic bromochromate hybrid nanomaterials with triphenylphosphine surface-modified iron oxide nanoparticles and their catalytic application in multicomponent reactions. RSC Adv 4(56):29765–29771. https://doi.org/10.1039/c4ra04654d

MARS (2008) Australian community attitudes HEld about nanotechnology – trends 2005–2008, (Commissioned by Department of Innovation, Industry, Science and Research (DIISR) – Nanotechnology Strategy). Market Attitude Research Services Pty Ltd., Sydney

Marshall BM, Levy SB (2011) Food animals and antimicrobials: impacts on human health. Clin Microbiol Rev 24:718–733. https://doi.org/10.1128/cmr.00002-11

Marshall MJ, Beliaev AS, Dohnalkova AC, Kennedy DW, Shi L, Wang Z, Boyanov MI, Lai B, Kemner KM, McLean JS, Reed SB, Culley DE, Bailey VL, Simonson CJ, Saffarini DA, Romine MF, Zachara JM, Fredrickson JK (2006) c-Type cytochrome-dependent formation of U(IV) nanoparticles by Shewanella oneidensis. PLoS Biol 4:e268. https://doi.org/10.1371/journal.pbio.0040268

Maruyama T, Fujimoto Y, Maekawa T (2015) Synthesis of gold nanoparticles using various amino acids. J Colloid Interface Sci 447:254–257. https://doi.org/10.1016/j.jcis.2014.12.046

Maryam G, Samaneh Z (2014) The effect of copper oxide nanoparticles as feed additive on some the blood proteins of broiler chickens. Biochem Biophys Res Commun 3:144–144

Maurya VK, Aggarwal M (2017a) Enhancing bio-availability of vitamin D by Nano-engineered based delivery systems-An overview. Int J Curr Microbiol App Sci 6:340–353. https://doi.org/10.20546/ijcmas.2017.607.040

Maurya VK, Aggarwal M (2017b) Factors influencing the absorption of vitamin D in GIT: an overview. J Food Sci Technol 54(12):3753–3765. https://doi.org/10.1007/s13197-017-2840-0

Maurya S, Bhardwaj AK, Gupta KK, Agarwal S, Kushwaha A, Vk C, Pathak RK, Gopal R, Uttam KN, Singh AK, Verma V, Singh MP (2016) Green synthesis of silver nanoparticles using Pleurotus and its bactericidal activity. Cell Mol Biol 62(3):1000131

Maurya VK, Aggarwal M, Ranjan V, Gothandam KM (2020a) Improving bioavailability of vitamin A in food by encapsulation: an update. In: Nanoscience in medicine. Springer, Cham, pp 117–145. https://doi.org/10.1007/978-3-030-29207-2_4

Maurya VK, Bashir K, Aggarwal M (2020b) Vitamin D microencapsulation and fortification: trends and technologies. J Steroid Biochem Mol Biol 196:105489. https://doi.org/10.1016/j.jsbmb.2019.105489

McClements DJ (2010) Design of nano-laminated coatings to control bioavailability of lipophilic food components. J Food Sci 75:R30–R42. https://doi.org/10.1111/j.1750-3841.2009.01452.x

McClements DJ (2013) Utilizing food effects to overcome challenges in delivery of lipophilic bioactives: structural design of medical and functional foods. Expert Opin Drug Deliv 10:1621–1632. https://doi.org/10.1517/17425247.2013.837448

Mehran QM, Fazal MA, Bushroa AR, Rubaiee S (2017) A critical review on physical vapor deposition coatings applied on different engine components. Crit Rev Solid State Mater Sci 43(2):158–175. https://doi.org/10.1080/10408436.2017.1320648

Mehta R, Nambiar RG (2007) The poultry industry in India. In: FAO conference on poultry in the 21st century. Bangkok. http://www.fao.org/ag/againfo/home/events/bangkok2007/docs/part1/1_5.pdf

Mills A, Hazafy D (2009) Nanocrystalline SnO2-based, UVB-activated, colourimetric oxygen indicator. Sensors Actuators B Chem 136:344–349. https://doi.org/10.1016/j.snb.2008.12.048

Miroshnikov S, Yausheva E, Sizova E, Miroshnikova E (2015) Comparative assessment of effect of copper nano- and microparticles in chicken. Orient J Chem 31:2327–2336. https://doi.org/10.13005/ojc/310461

Miroshnikov SA, Yausheva EV, Sizova EA, Kosyan DB, Donnik IM (2017) Research of opportunities for using iron nanoparticles and amino acids in poultry nutrition. Int J Geomate 13:124–131. https://doi.org/10.21660/2017.40.99216

Mishra A, Swain RK, Mishra SK, Panda N, Sethy K (2014) Growth performance and serum biochemical parameters as affected by nano zinc supplementation in layer chicks. Indian J Anim Nutr 31:384–388

Mohammadi F, Ahmadi F, Andi MA (2015) Effect of zinc oxide nanoparticles on carcass parameters, relative weight of digestive and lymphoid organs of broiler fed wet diet during the starter period. Int J Biosci 6:389–394. https://doi.org/10.12692/ijb/6.2.389-394

Mohammadi H, Farzinpour A, Vaziry A (2017) Reproductive performance of breeder quails fed diets supplemented with L-cysteine-coated iron oxide nanoparticles. Reprod Domest Anim 52:298–304. https://doi.org/10.1111/rda.12902

Mohan P, Mala R (2019) A review on the effect of ZnO nanomaterial as supplement in poultry farming. In: AIP conference proceedings. AIP Publishing LLC, p 020030. https://doi.org/10.1063/1.5100715

Mohanraj VJ, Chen Y (2006) Nanoparticles – a review. Trop J Pharm Res 5(1):561–573. https://doi.org/10.4314/tjpr.v5i1.14634

Molodecky NA, Soon IS, Rabi DM, Ghali WA, Ferris M, Chernoff G, Benchimol EI, Panaccione R, Ghosh S, Barkema HW, Kaplan GG (2012) Increasing incidence and prevalence of the inflammatory bowel diseases with time, based on systematic review. Gastroenterology 142:46–54. https://doi.org/10.1053/j.gastro.2011.10.001

Moloto N, Revaprasadu N, Moloto MJ, O'Brien P, Raftery J (2010) N,N′-diisopropylthiourea and N,N′-dicyclohexyl-thiourea zinc(II) complexes as precursors for the synthesis of ZnS nanoparticles. S Afr J Sci 105(7–8):258–263. https://doi.org/10.4102/sajs.v105i7/8.43

Mondal S, Roy N, Laskar RA, Sk I, Basu S, Mandal D, Begum NA (2011) Biogenic synthesis of Ag, Au and bimetallic Au/Ag alloy nanoparticles using aqueous extract of mahogany (Swietenia mahogani JACQ.) leaves. Colloids Surf B: Biointerfaces 82:497–504. https://doi.org/10.1016/j.colsurfb.2010.10.007

Mukherjee A, Majumdar S, Servin AD, Pagano L, Dhankher OP, White JC (2016) Carbon nanomaterials in agriculture: a critical review. Front Plant Sci 7:172. https://doi.org/10.3389/fpls.2016.00172

Mukhopadhyay SS (2014) Nanotechnology in agriculture: prospects and constraints. Nanotechnol Sci Appl 7:63–71. https://doi.org/10.2147/nsa.s39409

Mulens, Morales M, Del P, Barber DF (2013a) Development of magnetic nanoparticles for cancer gene therapy: a comprehensive review. ISRN Nanomater 1:14. https://doi.org/10.1155/2013/646284

Mulens V, Morales MD, Barber DF (2013b) Development of magnetic nanoparticles for cancer gene therapy: a comprehensive review. Int Sch Res Notices 1:14

Mungroo NA, Neethirajan S (2014) Biosensors for the detection of antibiotics in poultry industry-a review. Biosensors (Basel) 4:472–493. https://doi.org/10.3390/bios4040472

Mwilu SK, El Badawy AM, Bradham K, Nelson C, Thomas D, Scheckel KG, Tolaymat T, Ma L, Rogers KR (2013) Changes in silver nanoparticles exposed to human synthetic stomach fluid: effects of particle size and surface chemistry. Sci Total Environ 447:90–98. https://doi.org/10.1016/j.scitotenv.2012.12.036

Naahidi S, Jafari M, Edalat F, Raymond K, Khademhosseini A, Chen P (2013) Biocompatibility of engineered nanoparticles for drug delivery. J Control Release 166:182–194. https://doi.org/10.1016/j.jconrel.2012.12.013

Narayanan KB, Sakthivel N (2008) Coriander leaf mediated biosynthesis of gold nanoparticles. Mater Lett 62:4588–4590. https://doi.org/10.1016/j.matlet.2008.08.044

Nel A, Xia T, Madler L, Li N (2006) Toxic potential of materials at the nanolevel. Science 311:622–627. https://doi.org/10.1126/science.1114397

Nikonov IN, Folmanis YG, Folmanis GE, Kovalenko LV, Laptev GY, Egorov IA, Fisinin VI, Tananaev IG (2011) Iron nanoparticles as a food additive for poultry. Dokl Biol Sci 440:328–331. https://doi.org/10.1134/s0012496611050188

Oberdorster G, Oberdorster E, Oberdorster J (2005) Nanotoxicology: an emerging discipline evolving from studies of ultrafine particles. Environ Health Perspect 113:823–839. https://doi.org/10.1289/ehp.7339

Obreja P, Cristea D, Dinescu A, Romaniţan C (2019) Influence of surface substrates on the properties of ZnO nanowires synthesized by hydrothermal method. Appl Surf Sci 463:1117–1123. https://doi.org/10.1016/j.apsusc.2018.08.191

Ognik K, Sembratowicz I, Cholewinska E, Jankowski J, Kozlowski K, Juskiewicz J, Zdunczyk Z (2018) The effect of administration of copper nanoparticles to chickens in their drinking water on the immune and antioxidant status of the blood. Anim Sci J 89:579–588. https://doi.org/10.1111/asj.12956

Okoli CU, Kuttiyiel KA, Cole J, McCutchen J, Tawfik H, Adzic RR, Mahajan D (2018) Solvent effect in sonochemical synthesis of metal-alloy nanoparticles for use as electrocatalysts. Ultrason Sonochem 41:427–434. https://doi.org/10.1016/j.ultsonch.2017.09.049

Onoue S, Takahashi H, Kawabata Y, Seto Y, Hatanaka J, Timmermann B, Yamada S (2010) Formulation design and photochemical studies on nanocrystal solid dispersion of curcumin with improved oral bioavailability. J Pharm Sci 99:1871–1881. https://doi.org/10.1002/jps.21964

Ovissipour M, Rasco B, Sablani SS (2013) Impact of engineered nanoparticles on aquatic organisms. J Fish Livest Prod 1:106. https://doi.org/10.4172/2332-2608.1000e106

Pal SL, Jana U, Manna PK, Mohanta GP, Manavalan R (2011) Nanoparticle: an overview of preparation and characterization. J Appl Pharm Sci 1:228–234

Pan D, Yu Z (2014) Intestinal microbiome of poultry and its interaction with host and diet. Gut Microbes 5:108–119. https://doi.org/10.4161/gmic.26945

Pandey AC, Sanjay S, Yadav S (2010) Application of ZnO nanoparticles in influencing the growth rate of *Cicer arietinum*. J Exp Nanosci 5:488–497. https://doi.org/10.1080/17458081003649648

Park MV, Neigh AM, Vermeulen JP, de la Fonteyne LJ, Verharen HW, Briedé JJ, Van Loveren H, de Jong WH (2011) The effect of particle size on the cytotoxicity, inflammation, developmental toxicity and genotoxicity of silver nanoparticles. Biomaterials 32:9810–9817. https://doi.org/10.1016/j.biomaterials.2011.08.085

Pathak K, Raghuvanshi S (2015) Oral bioavailability: issues and solutions via nanoformulations. Clin Pharmacokinet 54:325–357. https://doi.org/10.1007/s40262-015-0242-x

Pelaz B, Del Pino P, Maffre P, Hartmann R, Gallego M, Rivera-Fernandez S, de la Fuente JM, Nienhaus GU, Parak WJ (2015) Surface functionalization of nanoparticles with polyethylene glycol: effects on protein adsorption and cellular uptake. ACS Nano 9:6996–7008. https://doi.org/10.1021/acsnano.5b01326

Peled N, Ionescu R, Nol P, Barash O, McCollum M, VerCauteren K, Haick H (2012) Detection of volatile organic compounds in cattle naturally infected with Mycobacterium bovis. Sensors Actuators B Chem 171:588–594. https://doi.org/10.1016/j.snb.2012.05.038

Pereira DI, Gibson GR (2002) Cholesterol assimilation by lactic acid bacteria and bifidobacteria isolated from the human gut. Appl Environ Microbiol 68(9):4689–4693. https://doi.org/10.1128/AEM.68.9.4689-4693.2002

Peters R, Brandhoff P, Weigel S, Marvin H, Bouwmeester H, Aschberger K, Mech A (2014) Inventory of nanotechnology applications in the agricultural, feed and food sector. EFSA Support Publ 11(7):621E. https://doi.org/10.2903/sp.efsa.2014.en-621

Peters RJ, Bouwmeester H, Gottardo S, Amenta V, Arena M, Brandhoff P, Marvin HJ, Mech A, Moniz FB, Pesudo LQ, Rauscher H (2016) Nanomaterials for products and application in agriculture, feed and food. Trends Food Sci Technol 54:155–164. https://doi.org/10.1016/j.tifs.2016.06.008

Pineda L, Chwalibog A, Sawosz E, Lauridsen C, Engberg R, Elnif J, Hotowy A, Sawosz F, Gao Y, Ali A, Moghaddam HS (2012) Effect of silver nanoparticles on growth performance, metabolism and microbial profile of broiler chickens. Arch Anim Nutr 66:416–429. https://doi.org/10.1080/1745039x.2012.710081

Pinheiro AC, Coimbra MA, Vicente AA (2016) In vitro behaviour of curcumin nanoemulsions stabilized by biopolymer emulsifiers – effect of interfacial composition. Food Hydrocoll 52:460–467. https://doi.org/10.1016/j.foodhyd.2015.07.025

Pirsa S, Shamusi T (2019) Intelligent and active packaging of chicken thigh meat by conducting nano structure cellulose-polypyrrole-ZnO film. Mater Sci Eng C Mater Biol Appl 102:798–809. https://doi.org/10.1016/j.msec.2019.02.021

Pittol M, Tomacheski D, Simoes DN, Ribeiro VF, Santana RMC (2017) Macroscopic effects of silver nanoparticles and titanium dioxide on edible plant growth. Environ Nanotechnol Monitor Manage 8:127–133. https://doi.org/10.1016/j.enmm.2017.07.003

Pokhrel LR, Dubey B (2013) Evaluation of developmental responses of two crop plants exposed to silver and zinc oxide nanoparticles. Sci Total Environ 452–453:321–332. https://doi.org/10.1016/j.scitotenv.2013.02.059

Potter LM, Ryan FA, Matterson LD, Singsen EP, Tlustohowicz J (1963) Effects of erythromycin on performance of laying hens. Poult Sci J 42:1400–1406. https://doi.org/10.3382/ps.0421400

Prasad RY, Wallace K, Daniel KM, Tennant AH, Zucker RM, Strickland J, Dreher K, Kligerman AD, Blackman CF, Demarini DM (2013) Effect of treatment media on the agglomeration of titanium dioxide nanoparticles: impact on genotoxicity, cellular interaction, and cell cycle. ACS Nano 7:1929–1942. https://doi.org/10.1021/nn302280n

Presland RB, Dale BA (2000) Epithelial structural proteins of the skin and oral cavity: function in health and disease. Crit Rev Oral Biol Med 11:383–408. https://doi.org/10.1177/10454411000110040101

Proctor A, Phillips GJ (2019) Differential effects of bacitracin methylene disalicylate (bmd) on the distal colon and cecal microbiota of young broiler chickens. Front Vet Sci 6:114. https://doi.org/10.3389/fvets.2019.00114

Proudfoot FG, Hulan HW, Jackson ED, Salisbury CD (1990) Effect of lincomycin as a growth promoter for broiler chicks. Br Poult Sci 31:181–187. https://doi.org/10.1080/00071669008417244

Radwan NL, Eldin TAS, Zaiat AAE, Mostafa MASA (2015) Effect of dietary nano-selenium supplementation on selenium content and oxidative stability in table eggs and productive performance of laying hens. Int Poult Sci J 14:161–176. https://doi.org/10.3923/ijps.2015.161.176

Rafique R, Zahra Z , Virk N , Shahid M, Pinelli E, Park TJ, Kallerhoff J, Arshad M (2018) Dose-dependent physiological responses of Triticum aestivum L. to soil applied TiO2 nanoparticles: alterations in chlorophyll content, H2O2 production, and genotoxicity. Agric Ecosyst Environ 255:95–101. https://doi.org/10.1016/j.agee.2017.12.010

Raghunandan D, Bedre MD, Basavaraja S, Sawle B, Manjunath SY, Venkataraman A (2010) Rapid biosynthesis of irregular shaped gold nanoparticles from macerated aqueous extracellular dried clove buds (*Syzygium aromaticum*) solution. Colloids Surf B: Biointerfaces 79:235–240. https://doi.org/10.1016/j.colsurfb.2010.04.003

Rahimi R, Maleki A, Maleki S, Morsali A, Rahimi MJ (2014) Synthesis and characterization of magnetic dichromate hybrid nanomaterials with triphenylphosphine surface modified iron oxide nanoparticles (Fe3O4@SiO2@PPh3@Cr2O72−). Solid State Sci 28:9–13. https://doi.org/10.1016/j.solidstatesciences.2013.11.013

Rahmatollah D, Farzinpour A, Vaziry A, Sadeghi G (2017) Effect of replacing dietary FeSO4with cysteine-coated Fe3O4nanoparticles on quails. Ital J Anim Sci 17:121–127. https://doi.org/10.1080/1828051x.2017.1345662

Rajasekaran P, Santra S (2015) Hydrothermally treated chitosan hydrogel loaded with copper and zinc particles as a potential micronutrient-based antimicrobial feed additive. Front Vet Sci 2:62. https://doi.org/10.3389/fvets.2015.00062

Rajendran D, Thulasi A, Jash S, Selvaraju S, Rao SBN (2013) Synthesis and application of nano minerals in livestock industry. In: Animal nutrition and reproductive physiology (recent concepts). Satish Serial Publishing House, Delhi, pp 517–530

Rajput N (2017) Development of anotechnology in India: a review. IOSR J Appl Phys (IOSR-JAP) 9:45–50. https://doi.org/10.9790/4861-0903034550

Rajput V, Minkina T, Ahmed B, Sushkova S, Singh R, Soldatov M, Laratte B, Fedorenko A, Mandzhieva S, Blicharska E, Musarrat J, Saquib Q, Flieger J, Gorovtsov A (2020) Interaction of copper-based nanoparticles to soil, terrestrial, and aquatic systems: critical review of the state of the science and future perspectives. Rev Environ Contam Toxicol 252:51–96. https://doi.org/10.1007/398_2019_34

Ramachandraiah K, Han SG, Chin KB (2015) Nanotechnology in meat processing and packaging: potential applications – a review. Asian Australas J Anim Sci 28:290–302. https://doi.org/10.5713/ajas.14.0607

Ramiah SK, Awad EA, Mookiah S, Idrus Z (2019) Effects of zinc oxide nanoparticles on growth performance and concentrations of malondialdehyde, zinc in tissues, and corticosterone in broiler chickens under heat stress conditions. Poult Sci 98:3828–3838. https://doi.org/10.3382/ps/pez093

Rashidi L, Khosravi-Darani K (2011) The applications of nanotechnology in food industry. Crit Rev Food Sci Nutr 51:723–730. https://doi.org/10.1080/10408391003785417

Rauscher H, Roebben G, Sanfeliu AB, Emons H, Gibson N, Koeber R, Linsinger T, Rasmussen K, Sintes JR, Sokull-Klüttgen B, Stamm H (2014) Towards a review of the EC recommendation for a definition of the term "nanomaterial". Eur Union 10:36237

Rienzie R, Adassooriya NM (2018) Toxicity of nanomaterials in agriculture and food. In: Nanomaterials: ecotoxicity, safety, and public perception. Springer, Cham, pp 207–234. https://doi.org/10.1007/978-3-030-05144-0_11

Rodriguez-Garraus A, Azqueta A, Vettorazzi A, Lopez de Cerain A (2020) Genotoxicity of silver nanoparticles. Nanomaterials (Basel) 85(7):743–750. https://doi.org/10.3390/nano10020251

Roger E, Lagarce F, Garcion E, Benoit J (2009) Lipid nanocarriers improve paclitaxel transport throughout human intestinal epithelial cells by using vesicle-mediated transcytosis. J Control Release 140:174–181. https://doi.org/10.1016/j.jconrel.2009.08.010

Saenmahayak B (2007) Complexed trace mineral supplementation of broiler diets. Auburn University, Auburn

Safaei-Ghomi J, Ghasemzadeh MA, Zahedi S (2013) ZnO nanoparticles: a highly effective and readily recyclable catalyst for the one-pot synthesis of 1, 8-dioxo-decahydroacridine and 1, 8-dioxooctahydro-xanthene derivatives. J Mex Chem Soc 57:01–07. https://doi.org/10.29356/jmcs.v57i1.228

Sahay GD, Alakhova Y, Kabanov AV (2010) Endocytosis of nanomedicines. J Control Release 145:182–195. https://doi.org/10.1016/j.jconrel.2010.01.036

Sahoo PC, Kausar F, Lee JH, Han JI (2014) Facile fabrication of silver nanoparticle embedded CaCO3 microspheres via microalgae-templated CO2 biomineralization: application in antimicrobial paint development. RSC Adv 7:32562–32569. https://doi.org/10.1039/c4ra03623a

Saki AA, Abbasinezhad RAA (2014) Iron nanoparticles and methionine hydroxy analogue chelate in ovo feeding of broiler chickens. Int J Nanosci Nanotechnol 10(3):187–196

Salim HM, Huque KS, Kamaruddin KM, Beg M (2018) Global restriction of using antibiotic growth promoters and alternative strategies in poultry production. Sci Prog 101:52–75. https://doi.org/10.3184/003685018x15173975498947

Salvia-Trujillo L, Qian C, Martin-Belloso O, McClements DJ (2013) Influence of particle size on lipid digestion and beta-carotene bioaccessibility in emulsions and nanoemulsions. Food Chem 141:1472–1480. https://doi.org/10.1016/j.foodchem.2013.03.050

Sanchez-Martinez A, Ceballos-Sanchez O, Koop-Santa C, López-Mena ER, Orozco-Guareño E, García-Guaderrama M (2018) N-doped TiO2 nanoparticles obtained by a facile coprecipitation method at low temperature. Ceram Int 44:5273–5283. https://doi.org/10.1016/j.ceramint.2017.12.140

Santibenchakul S, Sirijaturaporn P, Mekprasart W, Pechrapa W (2018) Ga-doped ZnO nanoparticles synthesized by sonochemical-assisted process. Mater Today: Proc 5:13865–13869. https://doi.org/10.1016/j.matpr.2018.02.030

Sarkar B, Bhattacharjee S, Daware A, Tribedi P, Krishnani KK, Minhas PS (2015) Selenium nanoparticles for stress-resilient fish and livestock. Nanoscale Res Lett 10(1):371. https://doi.org/10.1186/s11671-015-1073-2

Sawosz F, Pineda L, Hotowy A, Jaworski S, Prasek M (2012) Influence of Ag nanoparticles, ATP and biocomplex of Ag nanoparticles with ATP on morphology of chicken embryo pectoral muscle. Anim Sci 51:127–132

SCENIHR Scientific Committee on Emerging and Newly IdentifiedHealth Risks (2015) Opinion on potential health effects of exposure to electromagnetic fields. Bioelectromagnetics 36(6):480–484. https://doi.org/10.1002/bem.21930

Schlich K, Hund-Rinke K (2015) Influence of soil properties on the effect of silver nanomaterials on microbial activity in five soils. Environ Pollut 196:321–330. https://doi.org/10.1016/j.envpol.2014.10.021
Scott JT, Creger CR (1976) The use of dietary zinc as an effective molting agent in laying hens. Poult Sci 55:2089
Scott A, Vadalasetty KP, Sawosz E, Łukasiewicz M, Vadalasetty RKP, Jaworski S, Chwalibog A (2016) Effect of copper nanoparticles and copper sulphate on metabolic rate and development of broiler embryos. Anim Feed Sci Technol 220:151–158. https://doi.org/10.1016/j.anifeedsci.2016.08.009
Sekhon BS (2014) Nanotechnology in agri-food production: an overview. Nanotechnol Sci Appl 7:31–53. https://doi.org/10.2147/nsa.s39406
Selim NA, Radwan NL, Youssef SF, Eldin TAS, Elwafa SA (2015) Effect of inclusion inorganic, organic or nano selenium forms in broiler diets on: 1-growth performance, carcass and meat characteristics. Int J Poult Sci 14:135–143. https://doi.org/10.3923/ijps.2015.135.143
Seok SH, Cho WS, Park JS, Na Y, Jang A, Kim H, Cho Y, Kim T, You JR, Ko S, Kang B, Lee JK, Jeong J, Che JH (2013) Rat pancreatitis produced by 13-week administration of zinc oxide nanoparticles: biopersistence of nanoparticles and possible solutions. J Appl Toxicol 33:1089–1096. https://doi.org/10.1002/jat.2862
Sessa M, Balestrieri ML, Ferrari G, Servillo L, Castaldo D, D'Onofrio N, Donsi F, Tsao R (2014) Bioavailability of encapsulated resveratrol into nanoemulsion-based delivery systems. Food Chem 147:42–50. https://doi.org/10.1016/j.foodchem.2013.09.088
Sethiya NK (2016) Review on natural growth promoters available for improving gut health of poultry: an alternative to antibiotic growth promoters. Asian J Poult Sci 10:1–29. https://doi.org/10.3923/ajpsaj.2016.1.29
Shaddad SAI, Wasfi IA, Maglad MA, Adam SEI (1985) The effect of oxytetracycline on growth and lipid metabolism in poultry. Comp Biochem Physiol C Comp Pharmacol 80:375–380. https://doi.org/10.1016/0742-8413(85)90071-4
Shahare B, Yashpal M (2013) Toxic effects of repeated oral exposure of silver nanoparticles on small intestine mucosa of mice. Toxicol Mech Methods 23:161–167. https://doi.org/10.3109/15376516.2013.764950
Shatkin JA, Kim B (2015) Cellulose nanomaterials: life cycle risk assessment, and environmental health and safety roadmap. Environ Sci Nano 2:477–499. https://doi.org/10.1039/c5en00059a
Silvestre C, Duraccio D, Cimmino S (2011) Food packaging based on polymer nanomaterials. Prog Polym Sci 36:1766–1782. https://doi.org/10.1016/j.progpolymsci.2011.02.003
Simon LC, Stout RW, Sabliov C (2016) Bioavailability of orally delivered alpha-tocopherol by poly(lactic-co-glycolic) acid (PLGA) nanoparticles and chitosan covered PLGA nanoparticles in F344 rats. Nanobiomedicine (Rij) 3:8. https://doi.org/10.5772/63305
Singh PK, Jairath G, Ahlawat SS (2016) Nanotechnology: a future tool to improve quality and safety in meat industry. J Food Sci Technol 53:1739–1749. https://doi.org/10.1007/s13197-015-2090-y
Sodano V, Gorgitano MT, Verneau F, Vitale CD (2016) Consumer acceptance of food nanotechnology in Italy. Br Food J 118:714–733. https://doi.org/10.1108/BFJ-06-2015-0226
Soenen SJ, Illyes E, Vercauteren D, Braeckmans K, Majer Z, De Smedt SC, De Cuyper M (2009) The role of nanoparticle concentration-dependent induction of cellular stress in the internalization of non-toxic cationic magnetoliposomes. Biomaterials 30:6803–6813. https://doi.org/10.1016/j.biomaterials.2009.08.050
Song C, Labhasetwar V, Murphy H, Qu X, Humphrey W, Shebuski R, Levy R (1997) Formulation and characterization of biodegradable nanoparticles for intravascular local drug delivery. J Control Release 43:197–212. https://doi.org/10.1016/s0168-3659(96)01484-8
Sozer N, Kokini JL (2009) Nanotechnology and its applications in the food sector. Trends Biotechnol 27:82–89. https://doi.org/10.1016/j.tibtech.2008.10.010

Sriondee M, Dungsuwan W, Thountom S (2018) Synthesis and characterization of Bi0.5(Na1-xKx)0.5TiO3 powders by sol–gel combustion method with glycine fuel. Ceram Int 44:S168–SS71. https://doi.org/10.1016/j.ceramint.2018.08.122

Stötzel C, Kurland HD, Grabow J, Dutz S, Müller E, Sierka M, Müller FA (2013) Control of the crystal phase composition of FexOy nanopowders prepared by CO2 laser vaporization. Cryst Growth Des 13:4868–4876. https://doi.org/10.1021/cg4010533

Surai PF, Kochish II, Velichko OA (2017) Nano-Se assimilation and action in poultry and other monogastric animals: is gut microbiota an answer? Nanoscale Res Lett 12:612. https://doi.org/10.1186/s11671-017-2383-3

Swain PS, Rao SBN, Rajendran D, Dominic G, Selvaraju S (2016) Nano zinc, an alternative to conventional zinc as animal feed supplement: a review. Anim Nutr 2:134–141. https://doi.org/10.1016/j.aninu.2016.06.003

Szentkuti L (1997) Light microscopical observations on luminally administered dyes, dextrans, nanospheres and microspheres in the pre-epithelial mucus gel layer of the rat distal colon. J Control Release 46:233–242. https://doi.org/10.1016/s0168-3659(96)01600-8

Taylor S, Qu L, Kitaygorodskiy A, Teske J, Latour RA, Sun YP (2004) Synthesis and characterization of peptide-functionalized polymeric nanoparticles. Biomacromolecules 5:245–248. https://doi.org/10.1021/bm034326m

Taylor AA, Marcus IM, Guysi RL, Walker SL (2015) Metal oxide nanoparticles induce minimal phenotypic changes in a model colon gut microbiota. Environ Eng Sci 32:602–612. https://doi.org/10.1089/ees.2014.0518

Terzano C, Di Stefano F, Conti V, Graziani E, Petroianni A (2010) Air pollution ultrafine particles: toxicity beyond the lung. Eur Rev Med Pharmacol Sci 14:809–821

Thakur MP, Milcu A, Manning P, Niklaus PA, Roscher C, Power S, Reich PB, Scheu S, Tilman D, Ai, Guo HF, Ji R, Pierce S, Ramirez NG, Richter AN, Steinauer K, Strecker T, Vogel A, Eisenhauer (2015) Plant diversity drives soil microbial biomass carbon in grasslands irrespective of global environmental change factors. Glob Chang Biol 21:4076–4085. https://doi.org/10.1111/gcb.13011

Thatcher FS, Loit A (1961) Comparative microflora of chlortetracycline-treated and nontreated poultry with special reference to public health aspects. Appl Microbiol 9:39–45. https://doi.org/10.1128/aem.9.1.39-45.1961

Timbrell J (1991) Principles of biochemical toxicology. Taylor & Francis Ltd, Abingdon

USEPA Environmental Protection Agency (1994) Office of Research and Development: air quality criteria for particulate matter. Washington, DC, 3 600/P-95-001cF

Vannini C, Domingo G, Onelli E, De Mattia F, Bruni I, Marsoni M, Bracale M (2014) Phytotoxic and genotoxic effects of silver nanoparticles exposure on germinating wheat seedlings. J Plant Physiol 171:1142–1148. https://doi.org/10.1016/j.jplph.2014.05.002

Velebit B, Petrovic Z (2012) Antimicrobial packaging in food industry. Tehnologija Mesa 53:71–79. https://doi.org/10.5937/tehmesa1201071v

Villamizar RA, Maroto A, Rius FX, Inza I, Figueras MJ (2008) Fast detection of Salmonella Infantis with carbon nanotube field effect transistors. Biosens Bioelectron 24:279–283. https://doi.org/10.1016/j.bios.2008.03.046

Vippola M, Falck GC, Lindberg HK, Suhonen S, Vanhala E, Norppa H, Savolainen K, Tossavainen A, Tuomi T (2009) Preparation of nanoparticle dispersions for in-vitro toxicity testing. Hum Exp Toxicol 28:377–385. https://doi.org/10.1177/0960327109105158

Walczak AP, Fokkink R, Peters R, Tromp P, Herrera Rivera ZE, Rietjens IM, Hendriksen PJ, Bouwmeester H (2013) Behaviour of silver nanoparticles and silver ions in an in vitro human gastrointestinal digestion model. Nanotoxicology 7:1198–1210. https://doi.org/10.3109/17435390.2012.726382

Wang T, Luo Y (2019) Biological fate of ingested lipid-based nanoparticles: current understanding and future directions. Nanoscale 11:11048–11063. https://doi.org/10.1039/c9nr03025e

Wang JJ, Sanderson BJ, Wang H (2007a) Cyto- and genotoxicity of ultrafine TiO2 particles in cultured human lymphoblastoid cells. Mutat Res 628:99–106. https://doi.org/10.1016/j.mrgentox.2006.12.003

Wang L, Li X, Zhang G, Dong J, Eastoe J (2007b) Oil-in-water nanoemulsions for pesticide formulations. J Colloid Interface Sci 314:230–235. https://doi.org/10.1016/j.jcis.2007.04.079

Wang C, Wang MQ, Ye SS, Tao WJ, Du YJ (2011) Effects of copper-loaded chitosan nanoparticles on growth and immunity in broilers. Poult Sci 90:2223–2228. https://doi.org/10.3382/ps.2011-01511

Weiss J, Takhistov P, McClements DJ (2006) Functional materials in food nanotechnology. J Food Sci 71:R107–RR16. https://doi.org/10.1111/j.1750-3841.2006.00195.x

Wen HW, Decory TR, Borejsza-Wysocki W, Durst RA (2006) Investigation of NeutrAvidin-tagged liposomal nanovesicles as universal detection reagents for bioanalytical assays. Talanta 68:1264–1272. https://doi.org/10.1016/j.talanta.2005.07.032

Wick P, Manser P, Limbach LK, Dettlaff-Weglikowska, Krumeich F, Roth S, Stark WJ, Bruinink A (2007) The degree and kind of agglomeration affect carbon nanotube cytotoxicity. Toxicol Lett 168:121–131. https://doi.org/10.1016/j.toxlet.2006.08.019

Wilkinson J (2009) The globalization of agribusiness and developing world food systems. Mon Rev 61:29. https://doi.org/10.14452/mr-061-04-2009-08_4

Williams BJ (1985) The effects of neomycin and oxytetracycline alone or combined upon the incidence of salmonellosis in broiler chickens. Poult Sci 64:1455–1457. https://doi.org/10.3382/ps.0641455

Wongpratat U, Maensiri S, Swatsitang E (2015) EXAFS study of cations distribution dependence of magnetic properties in Co1−xZnxFe2O4 nanoparticles prepared by hydrothermal method. Microelectron Eng 146:68–75. https://doi.org/10.1016/j.mee.2015.03.059

WWICS (2007) A nanotechnology consumer products inventory. Woodrow Wilson International Center for Scholars (WWICS), Project on Emerging Technologies (data set as at September 2007), Washington

Xie Y, He Y, Irwin PL, Jin T, Shi X (2011) Antibacterial activity and mechanism of action of zinc oxide nanoparticles against campylobacter jejuni. Appl Environ Microbiol 77:2325–2331. https://doi.org/10.1128/aem.02149-10

Xu L, Wang R, Kelso LC, Ying Y, Li Y (2016) A target-responsive and size-dependent hydrogel aptasensor embedded with QD fluorescent reporters for rapid detection of avian influenza virus H5N1. Sensors Actuators B Chem 234:98–108. https://doi.org/10.1016/j.snb.2016.04.156

Yada RY, Buck N, Canady R, DeMerlis C, Duncan T, Janer G, Thurmond S (2014) Engineered nanoscale food ingredients: evaluation of current knowledge on material characteristics relevant to uptake from the gastrointestinal tract. Compr Rev Food Sci Food Saf 13:730–744. https://doi.org/10.1111/1541-4337.12076

Yates JD, Schaible PJ (1962) Virginiamycin as an antibiotic for poultry feeds. Nature 194:183–184. https://doi.org/10.1038/194183b0

Yemmireddy VK, Hung YC (2015) Effect of binder on the physical stability and bactericidal property of titanium dioxide (TiO2) nanocoatings on food contact surfaces. Food Control 57:82–88. https://doi.org/10.1016/j.foodcont.2015.04.009

Yokel RA, Macphail RC (2011) Engineered nanomaterials: exposures, hazards, and risk prevention. J Occup Med Toxicol 6:7. https://doi.org/10.1186/1745-6673-6-7

Yoshida T, Yoshioka Y, Takahashi H, Misato K, Mori T, Hirai T, Nagano K, Abe Y, Mukai Y, Kamada H, Tsunoda S, Nabeshi H, Yoshikawa T, Higashisaka K, Tsutsumi Y (2014) Intestinal absorption and biological effects of orally administered amorphous silica particles. Nanoscale Res Lett 9:532. https://doi.org/10.1186/1556-276x-9-532

Yu H, Huang Q (2013) Bioavailability and delivery of nutraceuticals and functional foods using nanotechnology. Bio-Nanotechnol 1:593–604. https://doi.org/10.1002/9781118451915.ch35

Yu S, Jing W, Tang M, Xu T, Yin W, Kang B (2019) Fabrication of Nd:YAG transparent ceramics using powders synthesized by citrate sol-gel method. J Alloys Compd 772:751–759. https://doi.org/10.1016/j.jallcom.2018.09.184

Yue Y, Li X, Sigg L, Suter MJ, Pillai S, Behra R, Schirmer K (2017) Interaction of silver nanoparticles with algae and fish cells: a side by side comparison. J Nanobiotechnol 15:16. https://doi.org/10.1186/s12951-017-0254-9

Yusop SM, O'Sullivan MG, Preuß M, Weber H, Kerry JF, Kerry JP (2012) Assessment of nanoparticle paprika oleoresin on marinating performance and sensory acceptance of poultry meat. LWT Food Sci Technol 46:349–355. https://doi.org/10.1016/j.lwt.2011.08.014

Zarei M, Jamnejad A, Khajehali E (2014) Antibacterial effect of silver nanoparticles against four foodborne pathogens. Jundishapur J Microbiol 7:e8720. https://doi.org/10.5812/jjm.8720

Zha LY, Xu ZR, Wang MQ, Gu LY (2008) Chromium nanoparticle exhibits higher absorption efficiency than chromium picolinate and chromium chloride in Caco-2 cell monolayers. J Anim Physiol Anim Nutr (Berl) 92:131–140. https://doi.org/10.1111/j.1439-0396.2007.00718.x

Zhang HZ, Banfield JF (2000) Understanding polymorphic phase transformation behavior during growth of nanocrystalline aggregates: insights from TiO2. J Phys Chem 104:3481–3487. https://doi.org/10.1021/jp000499j

Zhao HQ, Lin L, Li JR, Tang JA, Duan MX, Jiang L (2001) DNA biosensor with high sensitivity amplified by gold nanoparticles. J Nanopart Res 3:321–323. https://doi.org/10.1023/a:1017502630894

Zhao CY, Tan SX, Xiao XY, Qiu XS, Pan JQ, Tang ZX (2014) Effects of dietary zinc oxide nanoparticles on growth performance and antioxidative status in broilers. Biol Trace Elem Res 160:361–367. https://doi.org/10.1007/s12011-014-0052-2

Zhao S, Guo J, Li W, Guo H, You B (2018) Fabrication of cobalt aluminate nanopigments by coprecipitation method in threonine waterborne solution. Dyes Pigments 151:130–139. https://doi.org/10.1016/j.dyepig.2017.12.062

Zhu H, Han J, Xiao JQ, Jin Y (2008) Uptake, translocation, and accumulation of manufactured iron oxide nanoparticles by pumpkin plants. J Environ Monit 10:713–717. https://doi.org/10.1039/b805998e

Zhu X, Wang J, Zhang X, Chang Y, Chen Y (2009) The impact of ZnO nanoparticle aggregates on the embryonic development of zebrafish (Danio rerio). Nanotechnology 20:195103. https://doi.org/10.1088/0957-4484/20/19/195103

Index

V. K. Maurya et al. (eds.), *Sustainable Agriculture Reviews 55*, Sustainable Agriculture Reviews 55, https://doi.org/10.1007/978-3-030-76813-3

The manufacturer's authorised representative in the EU is Springer
Nature Customer Service Centre GmbH, Europaplatz 3, 69115 Heidelberg,
Germany. If you have any concerns regarding our products, please
contact ProductSafety@springernature.com

Printed and bound by CPI Group (UK) Ltd, Croydon, CR0 4YY

30/09/2026

02225491-0010